Overview

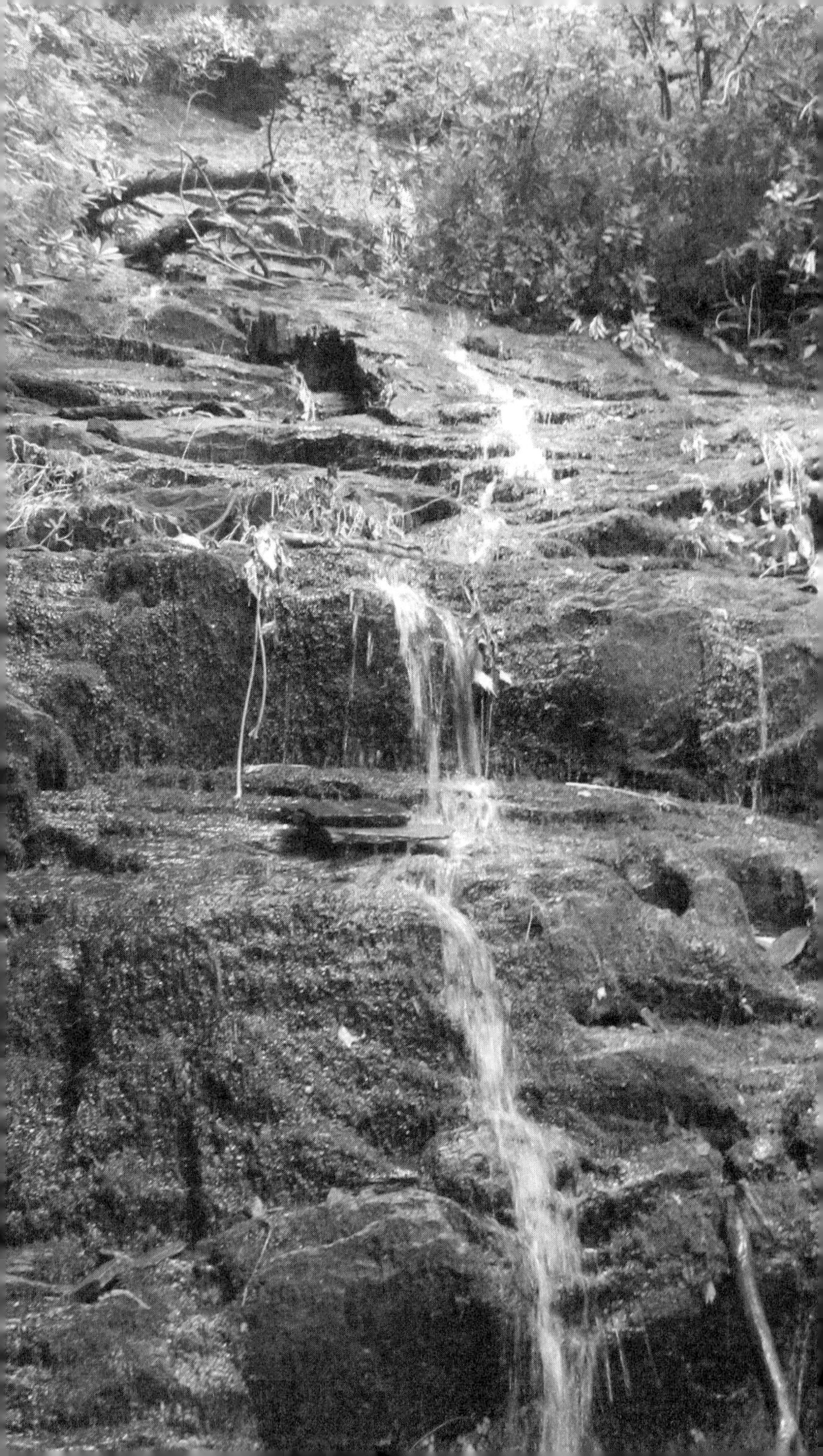

Five-Star Trails

Roanoke and the New River Valley

40 Spectacular Hikes in Virginia's Southern Appalachians

Johnny Molloy

MENASHA RIDGE PRESS
menasharidge.com

Five-Star Trails: Roanoke and the New River Valley

Published by Menasha Ridge Press
Printed in the United States of America
Distributed by Publishers Group West
First edition, first printing

Project editor: Ritchey Halphen
Cover design and cartography: Scott McGrew
Text design: Annie Long
Cover and interior photos: Johnny Molloy, except where noted
Copyeditor: Kate McWhorter Johnson
Proofreaders: Emily C. Beaumont, Julie Hall Bosché, Vanessa Lynn Rusch
Indexer: Ann Weik Cassar / Cassar Technical Services

Frontispiece: Rock Castle Cascades spills steeply toward the trail. *(See Hike 40, page 240.)*

Cataloging-in-Publication Data is on file with the Library of Congress.

ISBN: 978-1-63404-056-3; eISBN: 978-1-63404-057-0

MENASHA RIDGE PRESS
An imprint of AdventureKEEN
2204 First Ave. S., Suite 102
Birmingham, AL 35233
800-443-7227, fax 205-326-1012

FSC
MIX
Paper
FSC® C011935

RAINFOREST ALLIANCE CERTIFIED

Visit menasharidge.com for a complete listing of our books and for ordering information. Contact us at our website, at facebook.com/menasharidge, or at twitter.com/menasharidge with questions or comments. To find out more about who we are and what we're doing, visit blog.menasharidge.com.

Table of Contents

Dedication

This book is for Keri Anne Molloy.

Acknowledgments

THANKS TO ALL THE PEOPLE who have constructed, maintained, and advocated for trails in the greater Roanoke and New River Valley region. Keep on hikin'!

—Johnny Molloy

Preface

ROANOKE AND THE NEW RIVER VALLEY—Western Virginia, if you will—is an outdoorsy place. The area is strategically located within easy reach of a wide array of paddling, camping, and especially hiking destinations. Jefferson National Forest offers huge swaths of public lands and waters to explore. Add in the Blue Ridge Parkway's recreational opportunities, plus a wealth of state and local parks and preserves, and you end up with an outdoor lover's paradise.

Geographically speaking, Roanoke, Blacksburg, and the surrounding communities couldn't be better situated for hikers who wish to traverse a variety of terrain and trails. Centered on the Roanoke River and New River Valleys and their tributaries as they course through the high and mighty Appalachians, the land offers waterfalls, overlooks, and geologically fascinating locales. To the east, the rolling Piedmont presents yet another physical province to explore.

Pathways aplenty wind through the region. The Appalachian Trail (AT) is the centerpiece of the trail network. The world's most famous footpath enters the area near Pearisburg and Angels Rest, a stellar hike included in this guide. From here, the AT works through Mountain Lake Wilderness, then passes north of Roanoke near Daleville before continuing onward. In this section are some of the region's most famous hikes, including the Roanoke hiker's triple crown: Dragons Tooth, McAfee Knob, and the Tinker Cliffs, all of which are included in this guide.

But there's much more to hiking here than just the AT. Have you been to Sentinel Point and the Falls of Mill Creek? How about the Potts Valley Rail Trail? That's where this book comes into play—to help you discover a variety of trails in Roanoke and the New River Valley that together create the region's mosaic of hiking experiences.

This book details 40 of the area's best hikes. They head to overlooks, waterfalls, and wildernesses as well as scenic, cultural, and historical sites, along with lakes and rivers. The Southern Appalachians are an incredibly scenic land—a place where mountains tower thousands of feet above fertile valleys, where crashing cataracts plunge into deep forests, where brawling rivers cut deep gorges through majestic highlands.

It's where Cascade Falls makes its grand plunge into a natural swimming pool and along the way to the falls you traverse a rugged canyon. It's where hikers walk the Allegheny Trail to a historic fire tower to gain magnificent views and witness one of America's best raptor migrations. Other trails take you through biological wonderlands, such as Poor Mountain Natural Area Preserve, where the world's largest concentration of piratebush accentuates views and cascades. The strange but wonderful waterfalls of Falls Ridge Preserve, flowing over some of the largest calcium carbonate displays on the planet, are made better by trailside bluffs and caves.

Speaking of waterfalls, vertical variation and ample rain create an abundance of waterfalls in these parts. In addition to the cataracts already mentioned, there are waterfalls in The Nature Conservancy's Bottom Creek Gorge—Virginia's second-highest at 200 feet—along Lick Branch, and astride the Lower Hoop Hole Loop. Add to that waterfalls along the Blue Ridge Parkway—Fallingwater Cascades drops 100 or so feet, and the family-friendly hike to the falls is enhanced by mountain views. You can make a longer loop at Apple Orchard Falls, where water disperses into multiple spills then filters through a rock jumble as it passes underneath a trail bridge. At the falls of Rock Castle Gorge, the mountain chasm creates lesser but continual cascades as well as waterfalls along tributaries of Rock Castle Creek.

And there are still more falls, including Roaring Run Falls, a long white spiller that is the highest of several cascades tumbling through the canyon of Roaring Run. That recreation area also presents Old Dominion history, where you can see the preserved Roaring Run Furnace, a silent stone edifice of the past.

Other vestiges of days gone by can be found at the Johnson Farm in the Peaks of Otter, where you can visit a restored 1930s

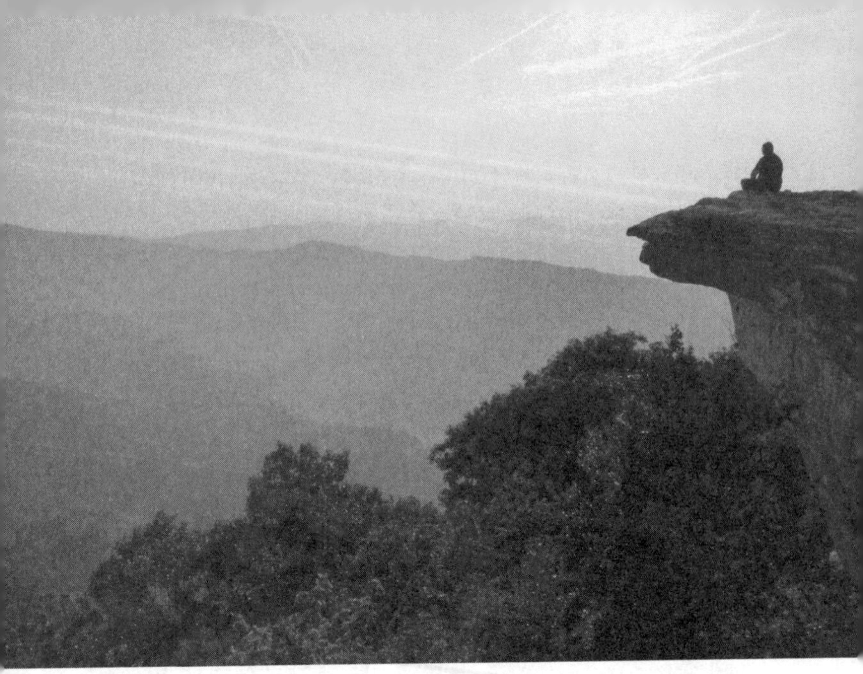

SUPERLATIVE VIEWS AND SCENERY, LIKE THIS VISTA FROM McAFEE KNOB, CHARACTERIZE HIKING AROUND ROANOKE AND THE NEW RIVER VALLEY.
(See Hike 20, page 128.)

mountain farm via a route leading past visually exciting rock formations. Explore Park boasts a trail-accessible display of old and re-created structures, from a one-room schoolhouse to a frontier fort. Smart View on the Blue Ridge Parkway has the restored W. J. Trail cabin. The Fenwick Mines Walk visits a former mining community of yesteryear, a place where you can find the past and rediscover a forgotten waterfall.

What about hikes with solitude? Take the Sulphur Ridge Circuit climbing Patterson Mountain, and loop through lesser-trod terrain to finally join a historic wagon road to close the circuit. The Upper Hoop Hole Trail stretches more than 10 miles in length and presents miles and miles of hiking where you can commune with nature one-on-one. The Flat Peter Loop rambles remote reaches of the Jefferson National Forest, crossing streams and mountain passes and through bottomland meadows where peaks rise in majestic mantles.

And that's not all: This guide includes still more hiking possibilities. Walk the shores of Smith Mountain Lake at Smith Mountain

Lake Community Park, or take a longer waterside trek—including a visit to an island—at Smith Mountain Lake State Park. These two hikes lie within the Piedmont east of Roanoke. Other Piedmont hikes include Franklin County's Waid Park, where an extensive network of paths will excite skeptical first-time visitors, and Grassy Hill Natural Area Preserve, where you can gain views of Rocky Mount and appreciate the plants of the Virginia state natural area.

Who can forget the views to be had on Western Virginia hikes? Bald Knob and Bear Cliffs in the Mountain Lake Conservancy deliver a visual feast, as do panoramas from Kelly Knob, along Tinker Mountain near Hay Rock, just below the Audie Murphy Monument, and in multiples from Flat Top. And how can we leave out the vista from aptly named Smart View?

Then there are family hikes and other classics that are used by locals for regular exercise. Both Mill Mountain Park and Chestnut Ridge are within easy striking distance of Roanoke. The trails of Pandapas Pond near Blacksburg make for fun family strolls, as does the Craig Creek Loop over by New Castle. The trails of Read Mountain Preserve are close to Roanoke, too, for a quick getaway.

Hikes in this book range from just under 2 miles to more than 10 miles, creating opportunities for hikers of all ages and accommodating your desires for hikes of multiple lengths, depending on mood, time, and company. Therefore, the best hikes of Roanoke and the New River Valley can mean a ramble through the remote highland backcountry, a trek to a crashing cascade, or a quick escape to an eye-popping vista. It all depends on your disposition, company and desires. So not only is the "where to hike" component covered, but so is "what type of hike." As far as when: You can hike year-round here in Western Virginia, but most of us will be hiking spring through fall. However, the varied elevations of hikes within make winter hiking a viable and desirable option. The important thing is getting out there and enjoying the wonderful trails and terrain of this scenic slice of the Old Dominion.

The variety of hikes contained within these pages reflects the variety of opportunities in Roanoke and the New River Valley. I've sought to include hikes covering routes of multiple lengths, ranging from easy to difficult. Trail configurations are diverse as well—including out-and-back hikes, loops, and balloons. Hike settings vary from developed county parks to the back of beyond.

The routes befit a range of athletic prowess and hiking experience. Simply scan through the table of contents, randomly flip through the book, or check the Recommended Hikes list (see next section). Find your hike, then get out there and enjoy it. Bring a friend, too. Enjoying nature in the company of another is a great way to enhance your relationship as well as escape from television, the Internet, and other electronic chains that bind us to the daily grind.

One last thing—there is a reason I live in the shadow of the Southern Appalachians. Having written outdoor guidebooks covering 26 states, I truly believe that these highlands comprise the best part of the best country on God's green earth. May this book help you enjoy the wonderful, rewarding trails of Roanoke and the New River Valley.

Recommended Hikes

Best for Scenery

Best for Wildlife

Best for Seclusion

Best for Kids

Best for Dogs

Best for Water Lovers

Best for Waterfalls

Best for History

Best for Geology

Best for Wildflowers

Best for Views

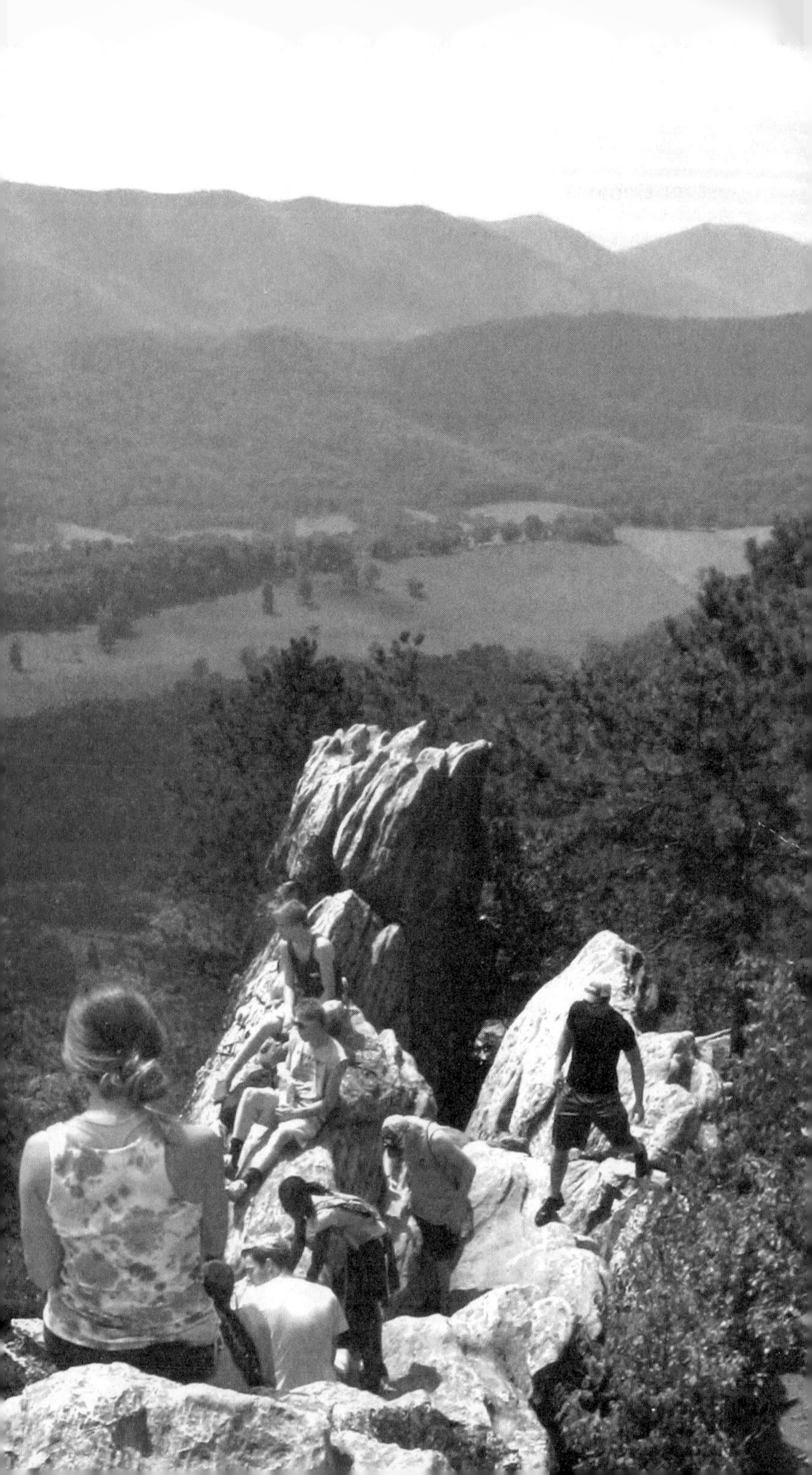

Introduction

About This Book

Five Star Hikes: Roanoke and the New River Valley details 40 fantastic hikes in Western Virginia. It presents an array of treks that reflect the magnificence of the area, ranging from the ridges and valleys of the New River north to Roaring Run and the James River, then east to the Peaks of Otter area along the Blue Ridge Parkway, then down to the Piedmont and Smith Mountain Lake and the lands between. The greater Roanoke and New River Valley area is an ideal jumping-off point for hikers, where trails course through the superlative beauty of the Blue Ridge Mountains, the Alleghany Highlands, and hills that give way to lowlands. These destinations include local, state, and national parks as well as national forests. All this adds up to a hiker's nirvana.

I believe this area to be one of the best outdoor hubs in the United States. Proximity to seemingly endless outdoor opportunities—hiking, paddling, bicycling, camping, hunting, fishing, nature study, and more—vastly enhances the quality of life here. To our west and north, we have large tracts of federal forestland: Virginia's Jefferson National Forest and West Virginia's Monongahela National Forest. Hundreds of miles of trails lace these mountain lands. The geologically fascinating mountains of Western Virginia lead into deep canyons, wild waterfalls, and unique rock features.

The hikes in this book cover destinations in all four cardinal directions, from the untamed grandeur of Mountain Lake Wilderness to the west to trail-laced Waid Park to the east to the lofty Peaks of Otter area to the north to one of the state's best hiking destinations—Rock Castle Gorge—to the south.

The climate is ideal for hiking; we have four distinct and beautiful seasons. If you like winter, the mountains rising more than 4,000

***OPPOSITE:* DRAGONS TOOTH IS CROWNED WITH A NARROW PRECIPICE THAT AFFORDS AN EXCITING VIEW.** *(See Hike 22, page 138.)*

feet deliver all the snow the average hiker wants. Yet there are many mild days perfect for trail trekkers, especially in the lower Piedmont and the Roanoke Valley. The elevation and terrain variations make spring exciting, too, as the season of rebirth grows its way from the New River and Roanoke River to the high country. Wildflowers follow. Summer finds many of us escaping to cool waters and to refreshing mountaintops where heat-relieving breezes blow. During fall, Western Virginia's incredible variety of trees explodes in annual color displays brought on by warm, dry days and cool nights.

How do you get started? Peruse this book, pick out a hike, and strike out on the trail. The wide assortment of paths, distances, difficulties, and destinations will suit any hiker's mood and company. And try them all—the varied hikes will leave you appreciating the nature of this region more than you ever imagined. Enjoy!

Roanoke and the New River Valley's Geographic Divisions

The hikes in this book are divided into six geographic regions. The first covers hikes down the **New River Valley** and the highlands immediately northeast, even a pair of hikes within the boundaries of West Virginia. The hikes here include Pandapas Pond, very near Blacksburg. Down the New River Valley, you can visit Cascade Falls, Angels Rest, and the Falls of Mill Creek. Hike to wild mountaintops, stony ridges, or remote wildernesses.

The **Lower Craig Creek Valley** section includes solitude-filled destinations on Sulphur Ridge and Lick Branch, as well as historic Fenwick Mines and hikes in the Rich Patch Mountains. This includes the incredible waterfalls and rock formations of Roaring Run, along with the Hoop Hole National Recreation Trails, a set of paths with waterfalls and everywhere-you-look Appalachian beauty.

Catawba contains the "triple crown" hikes along the Appalachian Trail near Roanoke: view-filled McAfee Knob, geologically challenging and fascinating Dragons Tooth, and eye-popping Tinker

Cliffs. You can also visit the Audie Murphy Monument or find Hay Rock. **Peaks of Otter** includes several hikes along the Blue Ridge Parkway north of Roanoke. They visit not only mountaintops but also waterfalls and historic sights.

Roanoke and Smith Mountain Lake encompasses preserves such as Read Mountain, Explore Park, and Mill Mountain Park, as well as destinations along the immediate Blue Ridge Parkway and hikes at Smith Mountain Lake, Roanoke's favorite stillwater destination. Finally, **The South** includes treks near the town of Rocky Mount, as well as two preserves and a pair of trail adventures on the Blue Ridge Parkway south of Roanoke and Blacksburg.

Altogether, the trail-laced geographic regions of Roanoke and the New River Valley create a mosaic of natural splendor that will please the most discriminating hiker.

How to Use This Guidebook

The following section walks you through this book's organization, making it easy and convenient to plan great hikes.

The Overview Map, Overview Map Key, and Legend

The overview map on the inside front cover shows the primary trailheads for all 40 hikes. The numbers on the overview map pair with the map key on the facing page. A legend explaining the map symbols used throughout the book appears on the inside back cover.

Trail Maps

In addition to the overview map on the inside cover, a detailed map of each hike's route appears with its profile. On each of these maps, symbols indicate the trailhead, the complete route, significant features, facilities, and topographic landmarks such as creeks, overlooks, and peaks.

To produce the highly accurate maps in this book, I used a handheld GPS unit to gather data while hiking each route, then sent that data to Menasha Ridge Press's expert cartographers. Be aware, though, that your GPS device is no substitute for sound, sensible navigation that takes into account the conditions that you observe while hiking.

Elevation Profile

Each hike includes this graphical element in addition to a trail map. Each entry's key information also lists the elevation at the trailhead and at the hike's high point.

The elevation diagram represents the rises and falls of the trail as viewed from the side, over the complete distance (in miles) of that trail. On the diagram's vertical axis, or height scale, the number of feet indicated between each tick mark lets you visualize the climb. To avoid making flat hikes look steep and steep hikes appear flat, varying height scales provide an accurate image of each hike's climbing challenge.

The Hike Profile

This book contains a concise and informative narrative that describes each hike from beginning to end. The text will get you from a well-known road or highway to the trailhead, through the twists and turns of the hike route, back to the trailhead, and to notable nearby attractions, if there are any.

At the beginning of each hike profile's full description are its star ratings and its key at-a-glance information. Here's a sample from Hike 20, McAfee Knob (page 128), plus an explanation of each element:

STAR RATINGS

The hikes in *Five-Star Trails: Roanoke and the New River Valley* were carefully chosen to give the hiker a stellar experience overall and represent the diversity of trails found in the region. Each hike was assigned a one- to five-star rating in each of the following categories: scenery, trail condition, suitability for children, level of difficulty, and degree of solitude. While one hike may merit five stars for its stunning scenery, that same trail may rank as a two-star trail for children. Similarly, another hike might receive two stars for difficulty but earn

Continued on page 6

20 Sample Profile: McAfee Knob

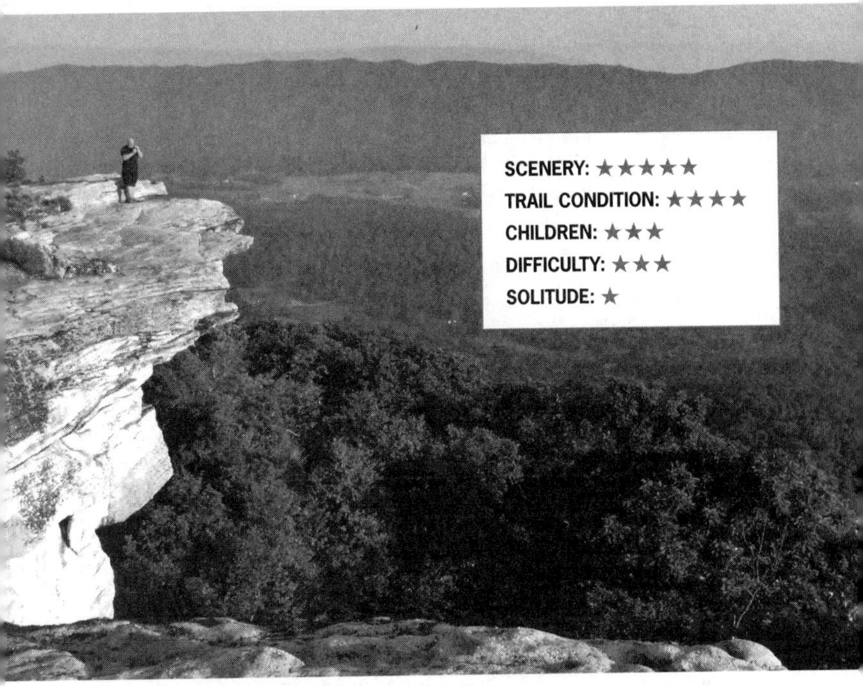

SCENERY: ★★★★★
TRAIL CONDITION: ★★★★
CHILDREN: ★★★
DIFFICULTY: ★★★
SOLITUDE: ★

McAFEE KNOB IS PERHAPS THE MOST PHOTOGRAPHED OVERLOOK ON THE ENTIRE APPALACHIAN TRAIL.

GPS TRAILHEAD COORDINATES: N37° 22.812' W80° 5.360'

DISTANCE & CONFIGURATION: 7.8-mile out-and-back

HIKING TIME: 4.5 hours

OUTSTANDING FEATURES: Views from the most photographed trailside vista in Virginia

ELEVATION: 1,950 at trailhead, 3,150 feet at high point

ACCESS: No fees or permits required

MAPS: National Geographic #788, *Covington/Alleghany Highlands;* USGS *Catawba*

FACILITIES: None

WHEELCHAIR ACCESS: None

INFO: George Washington National Forest, Eastern Divide Ranger District, 110 Southpark Drive, Blacksburg, VA 24060; 540-552-4641, www.fs.usda.gov/gwj

five stars for solitude. A few trails max out at four stars in a particular category; nevertheless, all trails stand out in at least one category, if not others. Here's how the star ratings for each of the five categories break down:

FOR SCENERY:

★★★★★	Unique, picturesque panoramas
★★★★	Diverse vistas
★★★	Pleasant views
★★	Unchanging landscape
★	Not selected for scenery

FOR TRAIL CONDITION:

★★★★★	Consistently well maintained
★★★★	Stable, with no surprises
★★★	Average terrain to negotiate
★★	Inconsistent, with good and poor areas
★	Rocky, overgrown, or often muddy

FOR CHILDREN:

★★★★★	Babes in strollers are welcome
★★★★	Fun for anyone past the toddler stage
★★★	Good for young hikers with proven stamina
★★	Not enjoyable for children
★	Not advisable for children

FOR DIFFICULTY:

★★★★★	Grueling
★★★★	Strenuous
★★★	Moderate: won't beat you up, but you'll know you've been hiking
★★	Easy with patches of moderate
★	Good for a relaxing stroll

FOR SOLITUDE:

★★★★★	Positively tranquil
★★★★	Spurts of isolation
★★★	Moderately secluded
★★	Crowded on weekends and holidays
★	Steady stream of individuals and/or groups

GPS TRAILHEAD COORDINATES

As noted in "Trail Maps," page 3, I used a handheld GPS unit to obtain geographic data and sent the information to Menasha Ridge's cartographers. In the at-a-glance information for each hike profile, I've provided the intersection of the latitude (north) and longitude (west) coordinates to orient you at the trailhead. In some cases, you can drive within viewing distance of a trailhead. Other hikes require a short walk to reach the trailhead from a parking area. Either way, the trailhead coordinates are given from the trail's actual head—its point of origin.

This guidebook expresses GPS coordinates in degree–decimal minute format. The latitude–longitude grid system is likely quite familiar to you, but here's a refresher, pertinent to visualizing the coordinates:

Imaginary lines of latitude—called *parallels* and approximately 69 miles apart from each other—run horizontally around the globe. The equator is established to be 0°, and each parallel is indicated by degrees from the equator: up to 90°N at the North Pole and down to 90°S at the South Pole.

Imaginary lines of longitude—called *meridians*—run perpendicular to latitude lines. Longitude lines are likewise indicated by degrees. Starting from 0° at the Prime Meridian in Greenwich, England, they continue to the east and west until they meet 180° later at the International Date Line in the Pacific Ocean. At the equator, longitude lines also are approximately 69 miles apart, but that distance narrows as the meridians converge toward the North and South Poles.

To convert GPS coordinates given in degrees, minutes, and seconds to the format shown above in degrees–decimal minutes, the seconds are divided by 60. For more on GPS technology, visit usgs.gov.

DISTANCE AND CONFIGURATION

"Distance" notes the length of the hike round-trip, from start to finish. If the hike description includes options to shorten or extend the hike, those round-trip distances are also included here. "Configuration" defines the type of route—for example, an out-and-back (which takes you in and out the same way), a point-to-point (or one-way route), a figure-eight, or a balloon.

HIKING TIME

Two miles per hour is a general rule of thumb for the hiking times noted in this guidebook. That pace typically allows time for taking photos, for dawdling and admiring views, and for alternating stretches of hills and descents. When deciding whether or not to follow a particular trail in this guidebook, consider the weather as well as your own pace, general physical condition, and energy level on a given day.

OUTSTANDING FEATURES

Lists highlights that draw hikers to the trail: mountain or forest views, water features, historic sites, and the like.

ELEVATION

The at-a-glance information also includes the elevation at the trailhead and another figure for the peak height on the route. The full hike profile also includes a complete elevation profile (see page 4).

ACCESS

Fees or permits required to hike the trail are listed here, if they apply.

MAPS

Resources for maps, in addition to those in this guidebook, are listed here. As noted earlier, we recommend that you carry more than one map—and that you consult those maps before heading out on the trail.

FACILITIES

Includes visitor centers, restrooms, water, picnic tables, and other basics at or near the trailhead.

WHEELCHAIR ACCESS

Notes paved sections or other areas where one can safely use a wheelchair.

INFO

Listed here are phone numbers and websites for checking trail conditions, trail-access hours and seasons, and other day-to-day information before you head out.

Overview, Route Details, Nearby Attractions, and Directions

These four elements compose the heart of the hike. "Overview" gives you a quick summary of what to expect on that trail; "Route Details" guides you on the hike, from start to finish; and "Nearby Attractions" suggests appealing adjacent sites, such as restaurants, museums, and other trails and recreational sites. "Directions" will get you to the trailhead from a well-known road or highway.

Weather

Each of the four seasons distinctly lay their hands on Western Virginia. Summer is generally mild but humid in the mountains of the South. However, the lower parts of the New River Valley, the Roanoke Valley, and the Piedmont can and will have uncomfortable hot spells during the summer. Thunderstorms can pop up in the afternoons. Storm possibilities increase with elevation. Hikers get a little extra pep in their step when fall's first northerly fronts sweep cool, clear air across Roanoke and the New River Valley. Mountaintop vistas are best enjoyed during this time. Crisp mornings give way to warm afternoons. Fall is the driest of all seasons. Winter can bring subfreezing days and chilling rains—and copious snow in the high country. We're talking more than 36 inches per year above 4,000 feet. However, a brisk hiking pace will keep you warm. Each cold month will have a few days of mild weather. However, be apprised that if it's mild in the lowlands, it may still be frigid in the nearby highlands. Spring will be more variable. A warm day can be followed by a cold one. Extensive spring rains bring regrowth but also keep hikers indoors. Moreover, spring rains can mean spring snow in the

Monthly Weather Averages for Roanoke, Virginia						
	JAN	FEB	MAR	APR	MAY	JUN
High	46°F	49°F	58°F	68°F	76°F	83°F
Low	27°F	30°F	37°F	45°F	53°F	62°F
Precipitation	2.9"	2.9"	3.5"	3.4"	4.1"	3.8"
	JUL	AUG	SEP	OCT	NOV	DEC
High	87°F	86°F	78°F	69°F	59°F	48°F
Low	66°F	65°F	58°F	47°F	38°F	30°F
Precipitation	4.1"	3.5"	3.5"	2.8"	3.4"	2.9"

highlands. On average, March dumps the most snow on the region. Roanoke's annual average is 18 inches, though adjacent highlands can receive much more. Nevertheless, you'll find more good hiking days than you'll have time to hike in spring and every other season.

Water

A hiker walking steadily in 90-degree heat needs about 10 quarts of fluid per day. That's 2.5 gallons—the equivalent of 12 large water bottles or 16 small ones. A good rule of thumb is to hydrate before your hike, carry (and drink) 6 ounces of water for every mile you plan to hike, and hydrate again after the hike.

For most people, the pleasures of hiking make carrying water a relatively minor burden, so pack more water than you anticipate needing, even for short hikes. If you don't like drinking tepid water on a hot day, freeze a couple of bottles overnight. It's also a good idea to carry a bottle of sports drink such as Gatorade; the electrolytes replace essential salts that you sweat out.

If you find yourself tempted to drink "found water," proceed with extreme caution. Many ponds and lakes you'll encounter are fairly stagnant, and the water tastes terrible. Drinking such water presents inherent risks for thirsty trekkers. Giardia parasites contaminate many water sources and cause the absolutely awful intestinal ailment giardiasis, which can last for weeks after onset. For more information, visit the Centers for Disease Control and Prevention website: cdc.gov/parasites/giardia.

In any case, effective treatment is essential before you use any water source found along the trail. Boiling water for 2–3 minutes is always a safe measure for camping, but day hikers can consider iodine tablets, approved chemical mixes, filtration units rated for giardia, and ultraviolet filtration. Some of these methods (for example, filtration with an added carbon filter) remove bad tastes typical in stagnant water, while others add their own taste. Carry a means of purification to help in a pinch.

Clothing

Weather, unexpected trail conditions, fatigue, extended hiking duration, and wrong turns can individually or collectively turn a great outing into a very uncomfortable one at best—and a life-threatening one at worst. Thus, proper attire plays a key role in staying comfortable and, sometimes, staying alive. Here are some helpful guidelines:

★ Choose silk, wool, or synthetics for maximum comfort in all of your hiking attire—from hats to socks and in between. Cotton is fine if the weather remains dry and stable, not so much if that material gets wet.

★ Always wear a hat, or at least tuck one into your day pack or hitch it to your belt. Hats offer all-weather sun and wind protection as well as warmth if it turns cold.

★ Be ready to layer up or down as the day progresses and the mercury rises or falls. Today's outdoor wear makes layering easy, with such designs as jackets that convert to vests and zip-off or button-up legs.

★ Wear hiking boots or sturdy hiking sandals with toe protection. Flip-flopping on a paved path in an urban botanical garden is one thing, but never hike mountain trails in open sandals or casual sneakers. (The AT, for example, can be very rocky.) Your bones and arches need support, and your skin needs protection.

- ★ Pair that footwear with good socks. If you prefer not to sheathe your feet when wearing hiking sandals, tuck the socks into your day pack; you may need them if the weather plummets or if you hit rocky turf and pebbles begin to irritate your feet. And, in an emergency, if you have lost your gloves, you can use the socks as mittens.
- ★ Don't leave rainwear behind, even if the day dawns clear and sunny. Tuck into your day pack, or tie around your waist, a jacket that is breathable and either water-resistant or waterproof. Investigate different choices at your local outdoors retailer. If you're a frequent hiker, ideally you'll have more than one rainwear weight, material, and style in your closet to protect you in all seasons in your regional climate and hiking microclimates.

Essential Gear

Today you can buy outdoor vests that have up to 20 pockets shaped and sized to carry everything from toothpicks to binoculars. Or, if you don't aspire to feel like a burro, you can neatly stow all of the following items in your day pack or backpack:

- ★ *Extra clothes:* raingear, a change of socks and shirt, and, depending on the season, a warm hat and gloves.
- ★ *Extra food:* trail mix, granola bars, or other high-energy snacks.
- ★ *Flashlight or headlamp* with extra bulb and batteries, for getting back to the trailhead if you take longer than expected.
- ★ *Insect repellent.* When you want it, you really want it. Bring a small bottle of a product with DEET in it.
- ★ *Maps and a high-quality compass.* Even if you know the terrain from previous hikes, don't leave home without these tools. And, as previously noted, bring maps in addition to those in this guidebook, and consult your maps prior to the hike. If you own a GPS unit, bring that too, but don't rely on it as your sole navigational tool—batteries can die.

  A smartphone not only enables you to call for help but also has built-in GPS hardware and software that can help with orientation. (Don't call for help, though, unless you're truly in need—remember that your phone's battery can die, too.) Smartphones are also valuable for downloading maps to use on the trail, although it's always better to download a map *before* your hike rather than trying to on the fly. In the mountainous terrain around Roanoke—especially isolated valleys—coverage can be spotty.

- ★ *Pocketknife and/or multitool.*
- ★ *Sun protection:* sunglasses with UV tinting, a sunhat with a wide brim, and sunscreen. (*Tip:* Check the expiration date on the tube or bottle.)
- ★ *Water.* Again, bring more than you think you'll drink. Depending on your destination, you may want to bring a container and iodine or a filter for purifying water in case you run out.
- ★ *Whistle.* It could become your best friend in an emergency.
- ★ *Windproof matches and/or a lighter,* for real emergencies—please don't start a forest fire.

First-Aid Kit

In addition to the preceding items, those that follow may seem daunting to carry along for a day hike. But any paramedic will tell you that the products listed here—again, in alphabetical order, because all are important—are just the basics. The reality of hiking is that you can be out for a week of backpacking and acquire only a mosquito bite. Or you can hike for an hour, slip, and suffer a cut or broken bone. Fortunately, the items listed pack into a very small space. You may also purchase convenient prepackaged kits at your pharmacy or online.

- ★ Adhesive bandages
- ★ Antibiotic ointment (such as Neosporin)
- ★ Aspirin, acetaminophen (Tylenol), or ibuprofen (Advil)
- ★ Athletic tape
- ★ Blister kit (moleskin or an adhesive variety such as Spenco 2nd Skin)
- ★ Butterfly-closure bandages
- ★ Diphenhydramine (Benadryl), in case of allergic reactions
- ★ Elastic bandages (such as Ace) or joint wraps (such as Spenco)
- ★ Epinephrine in a prefilled syringe (EpiPen), typically by prescription only, for people known to have severe allergic reactions to hiking mishaps such as bee stings

- Gauze (one roll and a half-dozen 4-by-4-inch pads)
- Hydrogen peroxide or iodine

Note: Consider your intended terrain and the number of hikers in your party before you exclude any article listed above. A short stroll may not inspire you to carry a complete kit, but anything beyond that warrants precaution. When hiking alone, you should always be prepared for a medical need. And if you're a twosome or with a group, one or more people in your party should be equipped with first-aid supplies.

General Safety

Here are a few tips to make your hike safer and easier:

- *Always let someone know where you'll be hiking and how long you expect to be gone.* It's a good idea to give that person a copy of your route, particularly if you're headed into an isolated area. Let him or her know when you return.
- *Always sign in and out of any trail registers provided.* Don't hesitate to comment on the trail condition if space is provided; that's your opportunity to alert others to any problems you encounter.
- *Don't count on a mobile phone for your safety.* Reception may be spotty or nonexistent on the trail.
- *Always carry food and water, even for a short hike.* And bring more water than you think you'll need.
- *Ask questions.* Public-land employees are on hand to help. It's a lot easier to solicit advice before a problem occurs, and it will help you avoid a mishap away from civilization when it's too late to amend an error.
- *Stay on designated trails.* Even on the most clearly marked trails, you usually reach a point where you have to stop and consider in which direction to head. If you become disoriented, don't panic. As soon as you think you may be off-track, stop, assess your current direction, and then retrace your steps to the point where you went astray. Using a map (paper or digital), a compass, a GPS unit or smartphone, and this book, and keeping in mind what you've passed thus far, reorient

yourself, and trust your judgment on which way to continue. If you become absolutely unsure of how to continue, return to your vehicle the way you came in. Should you become completely lost and have no idea how to find the trailhead, remaining in place along the trail and waiting for help is most often the best option for adults and always the best option for children.

★ *Always carry a whistle.* It may become a lifesaver if you get lost or hurt.

★ *Be especially careful when crossing streams.* Whether you're fording the stream or crossing on a log, make every step count. If you have any doubt about maintaining your balance on a log, ford the stream instead: Use a trekking pole or stout stick for balance and *face upstream as you cross.* If a stream seems too deep to ford, turn back. Whatever is on the other side isn't worth risking your life for.

★ *Be careful at overlooks.* While these areas may provide spectacular views, they are potentially hazardous. Stay back from the edge of outcrops, and make absolutely sure of your footing—a misstep can mean a nasty and possibly fatal fall.

★ *Standing dead trees and storm-damaged living trees pose a significant hazard to hikers.* These trees may have loose or broken limbs that could fall at any time. While walking beneath trees, and when choosing a spot to rest or enjoy your snack, *look up.*

★ *Know the symptoms of subnormal body temperature, or hypothermia.* Shivering and forgetfulness are the two most common indicators of this stealthy killer. Hypothermia can occur at any elevation, even in the summer, especially if you're wearing lightweight cotton clothing. If symptoms develop, get to shelter, hot liquids, and dry clothes as soon as possible.

★ *Likewise, know the symptoms of heat exhaustion, or hyperthermia.* Here's how to recognize and handle three types of heat emergencies:

Heat cramps are painful cramps in the leg and abdomen, accompanied by heavy sweating and feeling faint. Caused by excessive salt loss, heat cramps must be handled by getting to a cool place and sipping water or an electrolyte solution (such as Gatorade).

Dizziness, headache, irregular pulse, disorientation, and nausea are all symptoms of **heat exhaustion,** which occurs as blood vessels dilate and attempt to move heat from the inner body to the skin. Find a cool place, drink cool water, and get a friend to fan you, which can help cool you off more quickly.

Dilated pupils; dry, hot, flushed skin; a rapid pulse; high fever; and abnormal breathing are all symptoms of **heatstroke,** a life-threatening condition that can cause convulsions, unconsciousness, or even death. If you should be sweating and you're not, that's the signature warning sign. If you or a hiking partner is experiencing heatstroke, do whatever you can to cool down and find help.

★ *Most importantly, take along your brain.* A cool, calculating mind is the single most important asset on the trail. Think before you act. Watch your step. Plan ahead. Avoiding accidents before they happen is the best way to ensure a rewarding and relaxing hike.

Animal, Insect, and Plant Hazards

Black Bears

Though attacks by black bears are very rare, they have happened in Virginia's mountains. The sight or approach of a bear can give anyone a start. If you encounter a bear while hiking, remain calm and don't run away. Make loud noises to scare off the bear, and back away slowly. In primitive and remote areas, assume bears are present. In more-developed sites, check on the current bear situation prior to hiking. Most encounters are food-related—a fact of greater concern to backpackers and campers than day hikers—but remain aware and alert nevertheless, especially at shelters along the AT and other popular national forest destinations.

Snakes

Rattlesnakes, cottonmouths, copperheads, and corals are among the most common venomous snakes in the United States, and their hibernation season is typically October–April. In the Southern Appalachians, you'll possibly encounter the timber rattler or copperhead. However, the snakes you are most likely to see while hiking are nonvenomous species and subspecies. The best rule is to leave all snakes alone, give them a wide berth as you hike past, and make sure any hiking companions (including dogs) do the same.

Photo: Jane Huber

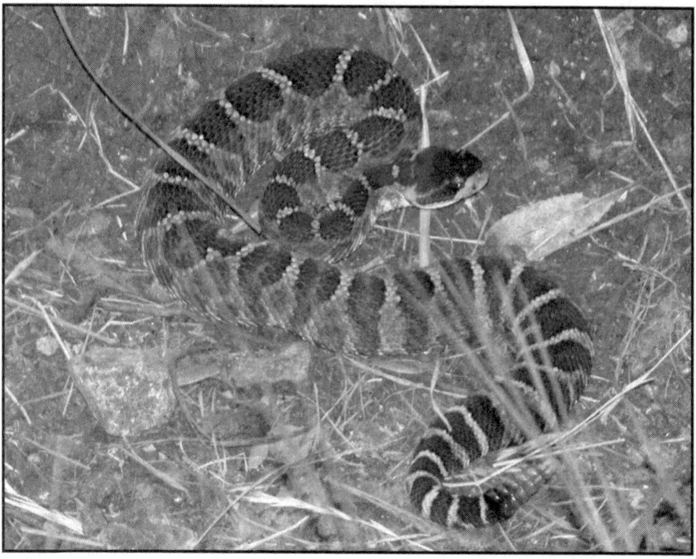

When hiking, stick to well-used trails and wear over-the-ankle boots and loose-fitting long pants. Rattlesnakes like to bask in the sun and won't bite unless threatened. Do not step or put your hands where you cannot see, and avoid wandering around in the dark. Step onto logs and rocks, never over them, and be especially careful when climbing rocks. Always avoid walking through dense brush or willow thickets. Copperheads are most often found along streams, looking for a sunny spot atop a rock.

Mosquitoes

These little naggers are usually found in urban areas but also sparingly in the hillier Southern Appalachians, though they can be a nuisance in open agricultural valleys in the mountains. Insect repellent and repellent-impregnated clothing are the only simple methods to ward off these pests. In some areas, mosquitoes are known to carry the West Nile virus, so take every precaution to avoid their bites.

Ticks

Generally speaking, ticks are rare in the Southern Appalachians but are sometimes found on brush and tall grass, waiting to hitch a ride on a warm-blooded passerby. Adult ticks are most active April into May and again October into November. Primarily of two varieties—deer ticks (the primary carriers of Lyme disease) and dog ticks—they may settle in shoes, socks, or hats, and they may take several hours to actually latch on. Wear light-colored clothing, so ticks can be spotted before they make it to your skin. Moreover, be sure to visually check your hair, the back of your neck, your armpits, and socks at the end of the hike, and when you take a posthike shower, do an even more thorough check of your entire body. Remove ticks that are already embedded using tweezers made for this purpose. Treat the bite with disinfectant solution.

Poison Ivy, Oak, and Sumac

Recognizing and avoiding poison ivy, oak, and sumac are the most effective ways to prevent the painful, itchy rashes associated with these plants. Poison ivy occurs as a vine or ground cover, 3 leaflets

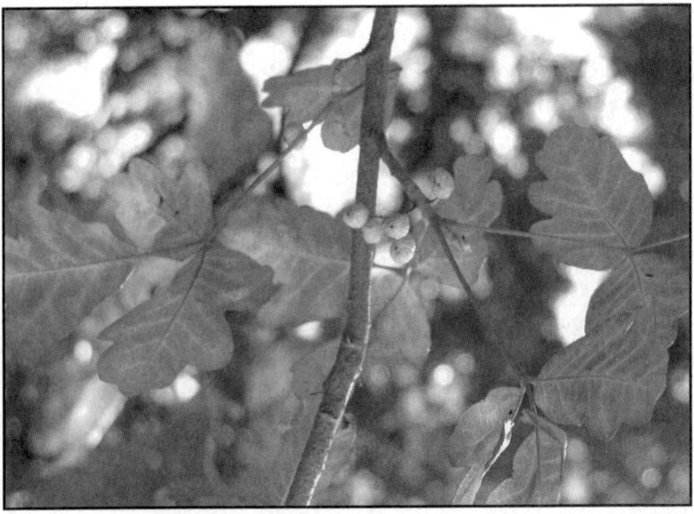

Photo: Jane Huber

to a leaf; poison oak *(see photo on previous page)* occurs as either a vine or shrub, also with 3 leaflets; and poison sumac flourishes in swampland, each leaf having 7–13 leaflets. Urushiol, the oil in the sap of these plants, is responsible for the rash. Within 14 hours of exposure, raised lines and/or blisters will appear on the affected area, accompanied by a terrible itch. Try to refrain from scratching if at all possible, though, as bacteria under your fingernails can cause an infection. Wash and dry the affected area thoroughly, applying a calamine lotion to help dry out the rash. If itching or blistering is severe, seek medical attention. To keep from spreading the misery to someone else, wash not only any exposed parts of your body but also any oil-contaminated clothes, hiking gear, and pets. Long pants and a long-sleeved shirt may offer the best protection.

Hunting

Separate rules, regulations, and licenses govern the various hunting types and related seasons. Hikers may wish to forgo venturing out during the big-game seasons, usually in November and December, when the woods suddenly seem filled with orange and camouflage. You'll encounter hunters primarily in the Jefferson National Forest.

Tips on Enjoying Hiking Roanoke and the New River Valley

Before you go, read the hike descriptions in this book and visit the websites of the land-management agencies. Call ahead to check hours/conditions or if you have further questions. This will help you get oriented to the forthcoming hike.

Here are a few more tips for enjoying your time on the trails:

★ *Investigate different destinations.* The hikes in this guide traverse terrain spanning more than 3,000 feet in elevation while exploring ridges, rivers, lakes, and geological and historic sights. Take a chance and make a new adventure instead of trying to re-create the same one over and over. You'll be pleasantly surprised to see so many distinct landscapes in this region.

- *Take your time along the trails.* Pace yourself. The landscapes along area trails are filled with wonders both big and small. Don't rush past a tiny salamander to get to that overlook. Stop and smell the wildflowers. Go ahead and take a seat on a trailside rock. Peer into a stream to find secretive fish. Take pictures. Make memories. Don't miss the trees for the forest.
- *Hike during the week,* when crowds are lighter. Likewise, trails that are packed in the summer are often clear during the colder months. If you're hiking on a busy day, go early in the morning; it will enhance your chances of seeing wildlife. The trails really clear out during rainy times; avoid hiking during a thunderstorm, however.

Trail Etiquette

Always treat trails, wildlife, and fellow hikers with respect. Here are some reminders.

- *Plan ahead in order to be self-sufficient at all times.* For example, carry necessary supplies for changes in weather or other conditions. A well-planned trip brings satisfaction to you and to others.
- *Hike on open trails only.*
- *Check conditions before you head out* if you think road or trail closures may be a possibility (use the websites or phone numbers listed in the "Info" section at the beginning of each hike profile). And don't try to circumvent such closures.
- *Don't trespass on private land,* and obtain all permits and authorization as required. Leave gates as you found them or as directed by signage.
- *Be courteous to other hikers,* bikers, equestrians, and others you encounter on the trails.
- *Never spook wild animals or pets.* An unannounced approach, a sudden movement, or a loud noise startles most critters, and a surprised animal can be dangerous to you, to others, and to itself. Give animals plenty of space.
- *Observe any* YIELD *signs* you encounter. Typically they advise hikers to yield to horses, and bikers to yield to both horses and hikers. Observing common courtesy on hills, hikers and bikers yield to any uphill traffic. When encountering mounted riders or horsepackers, hikers can courteously step off the trail, on the downhill side if

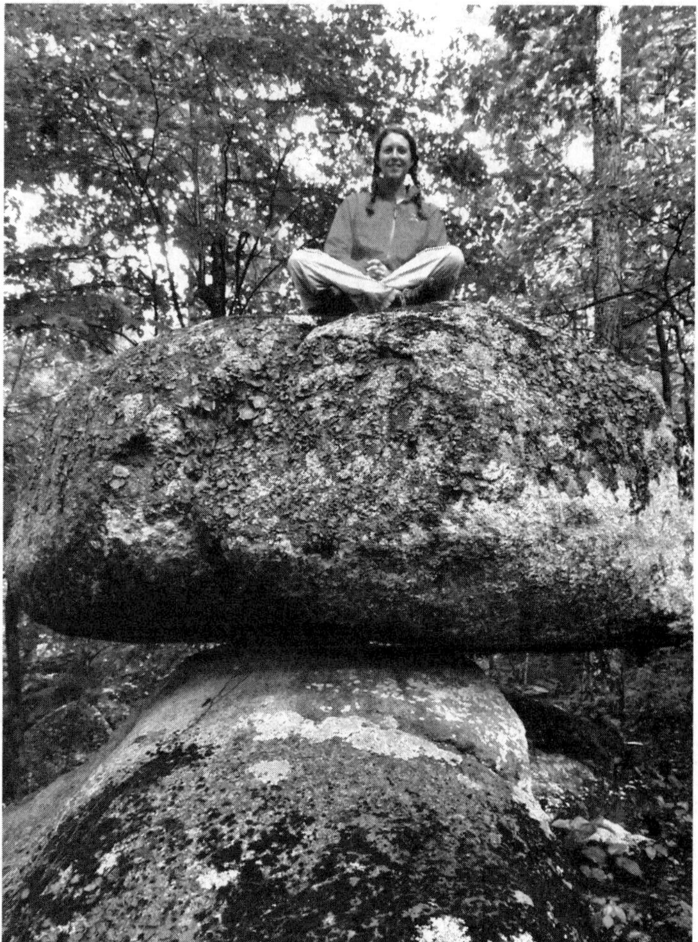

A HIKER STRIKES A CONTEMPLATIVE POSE ATOP BALANCE ROCK.
(See Hike 27, Johnson Farm via Harkening Hill, page 167.)

possible. Calmly greet riders before they reach you, and don't dart behind trees. (You're less spooky if the horse can see and hear you.) Don't pet a horse unless you're invited to do so.

★ *Practice **Leave No Trace** principles.* Leave the trail in the same shape you found it in, if not better. Visit lnt.org for more information.

New River Valley

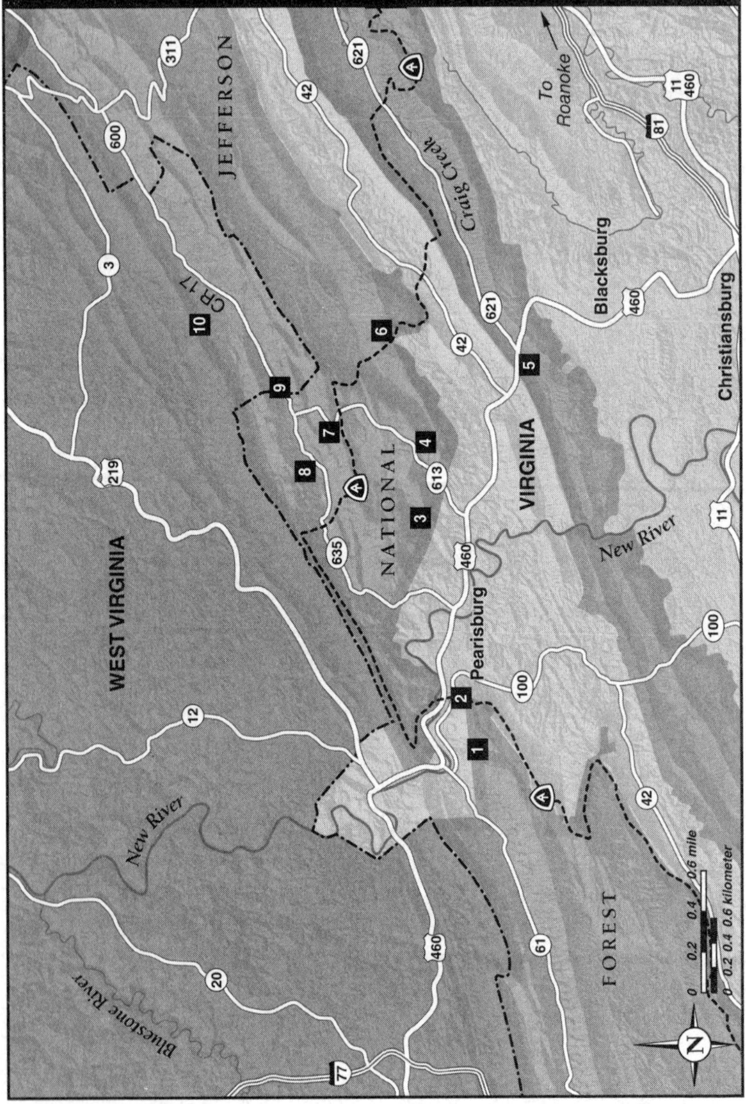

New River Valley

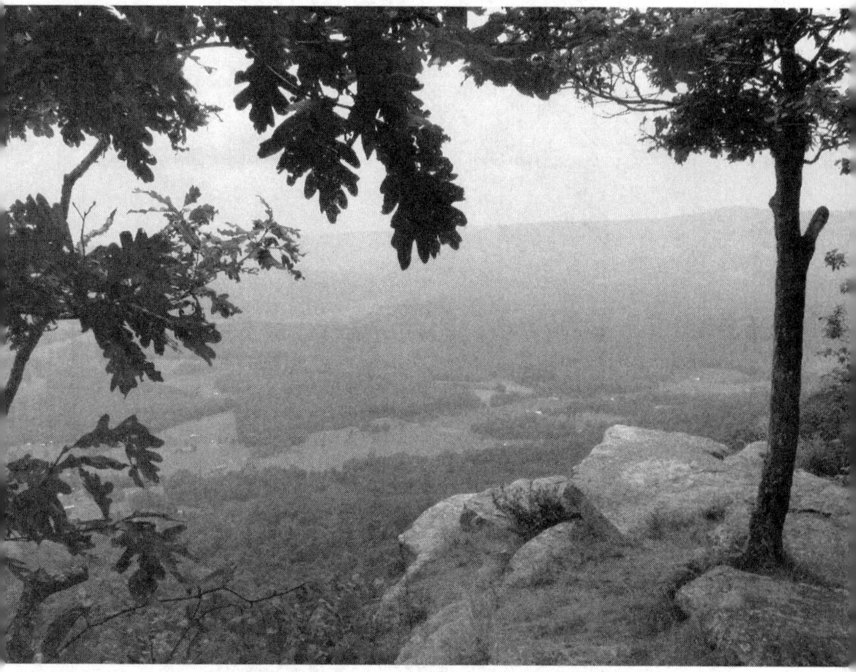

THE CLIMB FROM PEARISBURG YIELDS THIS PANORAMA OF WILBURN VALLEY.
(See Hike 2, Angels Rest, page 30.)

1 Sentinel Point and Falls of Mill Creek

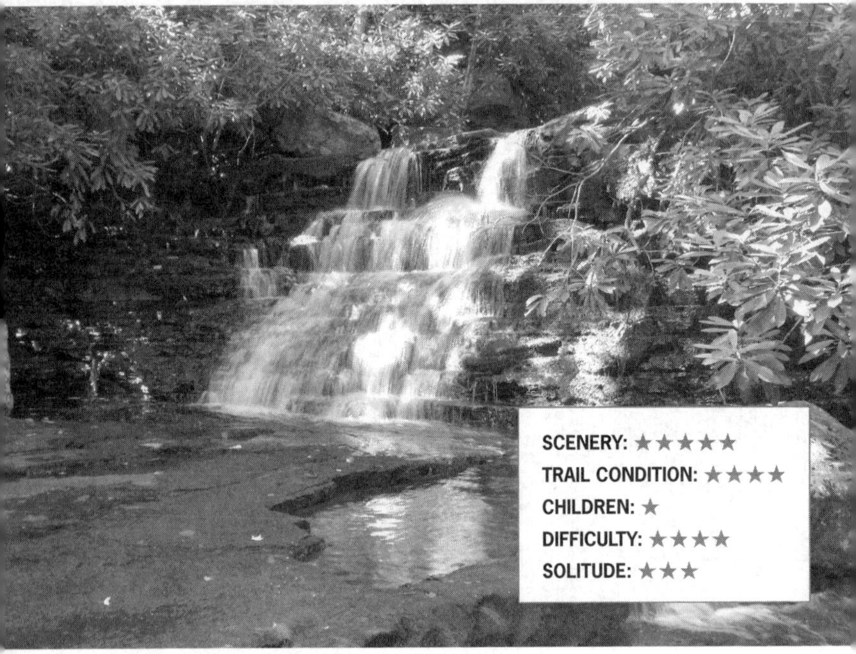

SCENERY: ★★★★★
TRAIL CONDITION: ★★★★
CHILDREN: ★
DIFFICULTY: ★★★★
SOLITUDE: ★★★

THIS FROTHY SPILLER IS BUT ONE OF MANY FALLS ON MILL CREEK.

GPS TRAILHEAD COORDINATES: N37° 19.016' W80° 47.626'

DISTANCE & CONFIGURATION: 6.8-mile out-and-back

HIKING TIME: 4 hours

OUTSTANDING FEATURES: Views, waterfalls, old reservoir

ELEVATION: 1,890 feet at trailhead, 3,430 feet at high point

ACCESS: No fees or permits required

MAPS: Mill Creek Nature Park, USGS *Narrows*

FACILITIES: Picnic shelter, restroom

WHEELCHAIR ACCESS: None

INFO: Mill Creek Nature Park, Town of Narrows, 210 Main St., Narrows, VA 24124; townofnarrows.org. George Washington & Jefferson National Forests, Eastern Divide Ranger District, 110 Southpark Drive, Blacksburg, VA 24060; 540-552-4641, www.fs.usda.gov/gwj.

In Brief

This hike leaves the town of Narrows, then climbs along Mill Creek, where waterfalls await. Make your way to the high country and Sentinel Point. From here, gain a commanding view of the New River as it slices between East River Mountain and Peters Mountain into West Virginia. A second view can be had from the west side of Sentinel Point as well.

Route Details

The town of Narrows has taken advantage of the mountain lands rising above it, creating a park along Mill Creek where a network of trails course through the town's 145-acre preserve, then upward to Pearis Mountain and ultimately to aptly named Sentinel Point, among other destinations in the adjacent Jefferson National Forest.

Starting on the correct trail is key to your hike. Leave the parking area and pass near the picnic shelter in a small field on the Wheezer Trail. Enter woods and join a wide track, with Mill Creek flowing to your right. Don't take the trail that crosses over Mill Creek by bridge—it links to the Upper Loop and Lower Loop Trails. Don't take the gravel road leading uphill to a water tank, either. Mill Creek is tumbling clear among boulders and rocks. Buckeyes, black birches, maples, and other hardwoods shade the gorge.

At 0.4 mile, a short spur leads right to a three-sided wooden trail shelter and picnic area in a small flat. Nearby are the dam and pool of the old Narrows Reservoir, where the town once stored its water. This is an alluring spot that would be nice for a picnic. Continue up the trail to reach another intersection. Here, the Wheezer Trail goes left, but you stay right, joining the Waterfalls Trail. Enter the Jefferson National Forest and ascend a rocky defile with bluffs rising above. Cut across boulder fields. Mill Creek flows below through a sea of rhododendron.

At 1.0 mile, stay right, joining the Catwalk Trail. Shortly come to Mercy Branch at 1.1 miles. Here, Mercy Branch tumbles in cascades

Sentinel Point and Falls of Mill Creek

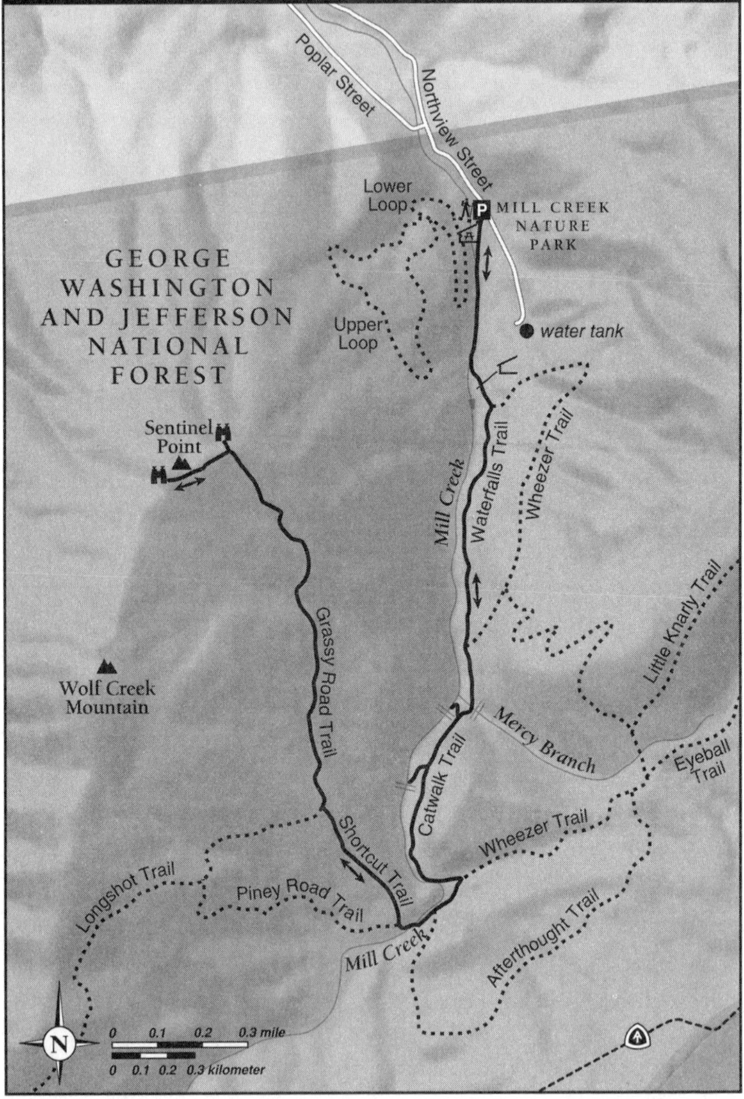

both above and below the stream crossing—bonus falls. Just ahead, reach the first signed waterfall spur to a waterfall. Turn right here and descend to Mill Creek. Emerge onto a rock slab in a stone cathedral. Upstream, Mill Creek splashes white 15 feet over a dark layered ledge, then flows beside the slab upon which you stand, then drops 10 feet more below the slab into a pool.

Resume the steepening Catwalk Trail. Come to another signed spur trail at 1.3 miles. This longer spur takes you through rhododendron to the lower end of a long angled cataract starting 80 or more feet above you. There, the narrow spiller dashes in stages, then caroms through a massive boulder garden and continues a little below your viewing spot to slow in stony shoals. What a spot! Beyond this fall, the ascent eases and you enter a perched valley, where now-timid Mill Creek gently gurgles under a canopy of evergreens.

Reach a trail intersection at 1.8 miles. Here, the Wheezer Trail comes in on your left, but you stay right, joining the Piney Road Trail. Continue up the smaller, intimate Mill Creek vale. Pass the Afterthought Trail at 1.9 miles. Walk over wet-weather drainages, then rock-hop Mill Creek at 2.0 miles. Trace a pine needle–carpeted track to quickly meet the Shortcut Trail. Take this path right, uphill. It is an official trail and leads through pine-dominated forest, mixed with

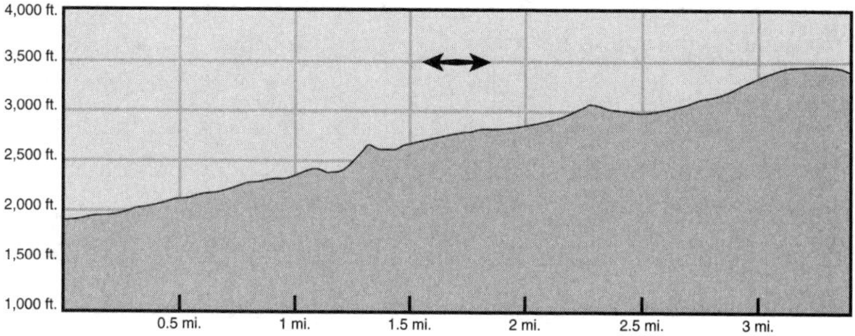

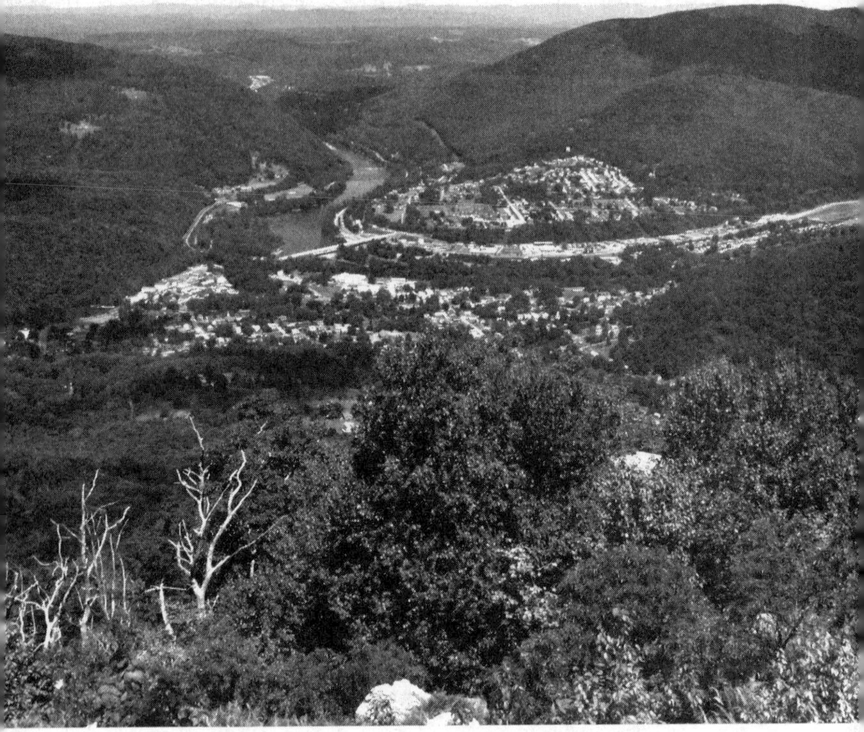

THE TOWN OF NARROWS, THE NEW RIVER, AND THE STATE OF WEST VIRGINIA ALL CAN BE SEEN FROM SENTINEL POINT.

club moss and mountain laurel, that makes for pleasant walking. The Mill Creek Valley falls sharply to the right.

Meet the Grassy Road Trail at 2.3 miles. You are expecting to climb more, and you will, but for the moment turn right on the Grassy Road Trail, heading downhill along the east slope of Wolf Creek Mountain. Bottom out at 2.6 miles, then continue the ascent as expected. Open onto a power line at 2.8 miles. Here, the trail works uphill along the power-line corridor, among low-slung pines and mountain laurel. Although this isn't the most scenic route, the sun-splashed path is expedient. Top out at 3.1 miles, below a transmission-line tower at the north end of Wolf Creek Mountain. Here, an open view extends north. The town of Narrows forms a cluster of civilization below, just before the New River cuts through the actual narrows bordered by

Peters Mountain on the right and East River Mountain on the left. Beyond, the state of West Virginia and its Appalachian ranges and valleys stretch north and west.

You aren't finished yet: Adventurous vista-seekers can enter the woods west from the transmission-line clearing, crossing the forested flat to a rock outcrop on the west side of Sentinel Point. The path to the outcrop is faint, so search around. Here, you can gaze up the Wolf Creek Valley and across to East River Mountain, which forms the West Virginia–Virginia state line. Consider making your return trip via other trails that comprise this network of paths emanating from Mill Creek Nature Park.

Nearby Attractions

The New River is a nationally renowned fishing and paddling destination. There are multiple put-ins and takeouts near the town of Narrows.

Directions

From Blacksburg, drive 27 miles on US 460 West to the town of Narrows, exiting US 460 at Fleshman Street. Follow Fleshman Street a short distance to turn left onto VA 61 and bridge the New River. After 0.5 mile on VA 61, turn left on VA 100 South in downtown Narrows. Follow VA 100 South 0.4 mile, then turn right onto Northview Street. Follow Northview Street past houses 1.2 miles to dead-end at Mill Creek Nature Park. Parking is on the left.

2 Angels Rest

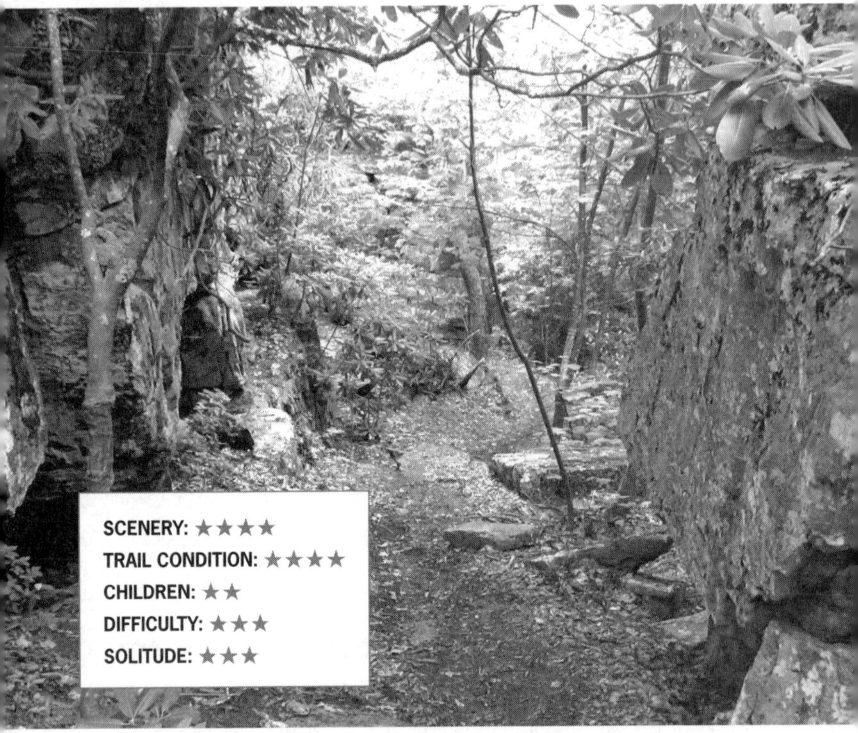

SCENERY: ★★★★
TRAIL CONDITION: ★★★★
CHILDREN: ★★
DIFFICULTY: ★★★
SOLITUDE: ★★★

THE APPALACHIAN TRAIL BREAKS THROUGH A BOULDER CLUSTER EN ROUTE TO ANGELS REST.

GPS TRAILHEAD COORDINATES: N37° 19.757' W80° 45.063'

DISTANCE & CONFIGURATION: 5.0-mile out-and-back

HIKING TIME: 3 hours

OUTSTANDING FEATURES: Multiple vistas, challenging climb

ELEVATION: 2,005 feet at trailhead, 3,680 feet at high point

ACCESS: No fees or permits required

MAPS: National Geographic #787, *Blacksburg/New River Valley;* USGS *Narrows*

FACILITIES: None

WHEELCHAIR ACCESS: None

INFO: George Washington National Forest, Eastern Divide Ranger District, 110 Southpark Drive, Blacksburg, VA 24060; 540-552-4641, www.fs.usda.gov/gwj

In Brief

This trek on the Appalachian Trail climbs the northeast shoulder of Pearis Mountain to three vistas. Start near Pearisburg, then trace a series of switchbacks up a thickly wooded ridge. Once on the crest, enter a boulder garden to emerge at Angels Rest and its view of the New River Valley. From there, head south along Pearis Mountain, passing a lesser view before reaching Wilburn Valley Overlook, which presents bucolic Virginia countryside set between long ridges.

Route Details

This is a classic mountain climb to a view—or three views in this case. You will earn your reward as the hike ascends nearly 1,700 feet from the trailhead. However, bear in mind that the trail is well maintained and well graded and does not have any insanely steep segments, making it doable by your average hiker at a leisurely pace.

From Cross Avenue, join the AT southbound as it quests for the crest of Pearis Mountain. Switchback on a steep slope cloaked in hardwoods. The trail curves in and out of drainages cutting down the north slope of Pearis Mountain. Mossy boulders are scattered in the woods. Cross a trickling branch at 0.5 mile, still ascending. Briefly join an old logging road at 0.7 mile. Stay with the white blazes, avoiding the erosive paths created by hikers who shortcut the switchbacks.

At 1.1 miles, the path crosses a rocky wet-weather drainage, then passes by an impressive oak on the right at 1.2 miles. Break the 3,000-foot barrier by 1.4 miles. You have climbed 1,000 feet with less than 700 to go. At 1.5 miles, the trail leads you across a rock garden, but at least it is on a level stretch. At 1.7 miles, tunnel into a rhododendron thicket.

Upon reaching a cluster of truck-sized boulders at 1.8 miles, you have made the crest of Pearis Mountain. While amid the gray giants, watch for the spur trail leading right to Angels Rest. It leads to an outcrop and a view. The scene is a mix of land and water, civilization and wilderness. Here, you can look down on the New River, as

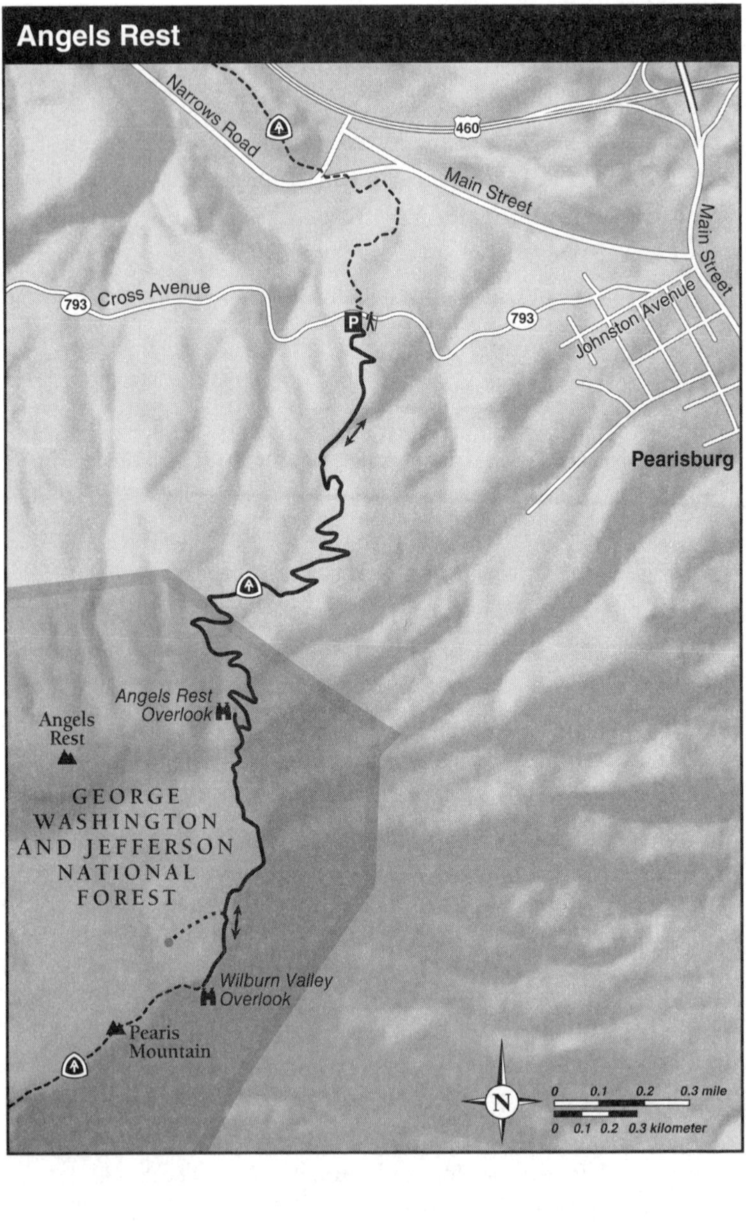
Angels Rest
Narrows Road
460
Main Street
Main Street
793
Cross Avenue
793
Johnston Avenue
P
Pearisburg
Angels Rest Overlook
Angels Rest
GEORGE WASHINGTON AND JEFFERSON NATIONAL FOREST
Wilburn Valley Overlook
Pearis Mountain
N
0 0.1 0.2 0.3 mile
0 0.1 0.2 0.3 kilometer

well as the towns of Narrows and Pearisburg. Sturdy Peters Mountain guards the rear. It's amazing how the New River—a truly big waterway at this point—looks so small from such a perch.

Funny thing about the New River, purportedly the second-oldest river on the planet: How did it get that name? While Virginia was still an English colony, a man named Abraham Wood sent two men west to what was then terra incognita. The two explorers—Thomas Batts and Robert Fallam—came upon this large, previously unknown waterway. When drawing a map of the newly explored territory, they wrote "new river" on the map that they had drawn, then promptly forgot about it. Later, Batts and Fallam turned in their map to a cartographer and the "new river" became the "New River," an accident of history. That is fodder for an AT hiker looking out from Angels Rest.

After soaking in the vista, even resting perhaps, backtrack to the AT, and resume your southbound course. The trail slices between more boulders then levels off. Enjoy your well-earned walk, from here a nearly level course winding through oaks and mountain laurel. Parallel the southeast edge of the ridge, getting glimpses of lands below. At 2.2 miles, a short path leads left to an outcrop and a warm-up view of the Wilburn Valley. Beyond here, the walking remains glorious. At 2.4 miles, a blue-blazed spur trail leads right to a spring. However,

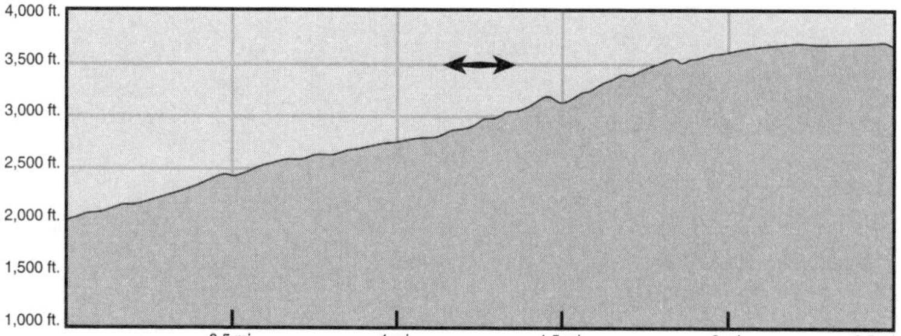

this spring is known to dry up in late summer and early fall. A little more walking brings you to the rocky brow of Pearis Mountain. At 2.5 miles, a short spur leads left to a flat, open rock and an easterly panorama of Wilburn Valley, part of the great Walker Creek watershed that you see below. This scene is decidedly more agricultural than the view from Angels Rest. Patterns of farm fields dot the lowlands, while Wooded Walker Mountain rises as a backdrop. Relax and enjoy the panorama that was well worth the climb.

Nearby Attractions

The New River offers paddling and angling opportunities galore. Multiple launch points and outfitters make a float trip on the river a breeze. Historic downtown Pearisburg, very near the trailhead, is also worth exploring.

Directions

From Exit 117 on I-81 near Christiansburg, take US 460 West to the second exit for Pearisburg (VA 100/US 460 Business East). Follow this exit as it heads into Pearisburg. After traveling 0.2 mile, turn right on Johnston Avenue, a residential street, just past the right turn to VA 100 North. Follow Johnston Avenue just a short distance, then veer right onto Morris Avenue. Morris Avenue turns into Cross Avenue. Drive 0.7 mile to the AT crossing from US 460 Business East. Do not park at the exact trail crossing, which is on a curve. Rather, park on the left about 150 feet after the AT trail crossing. Space is limited, so be courteous.

3 Cascade Falls

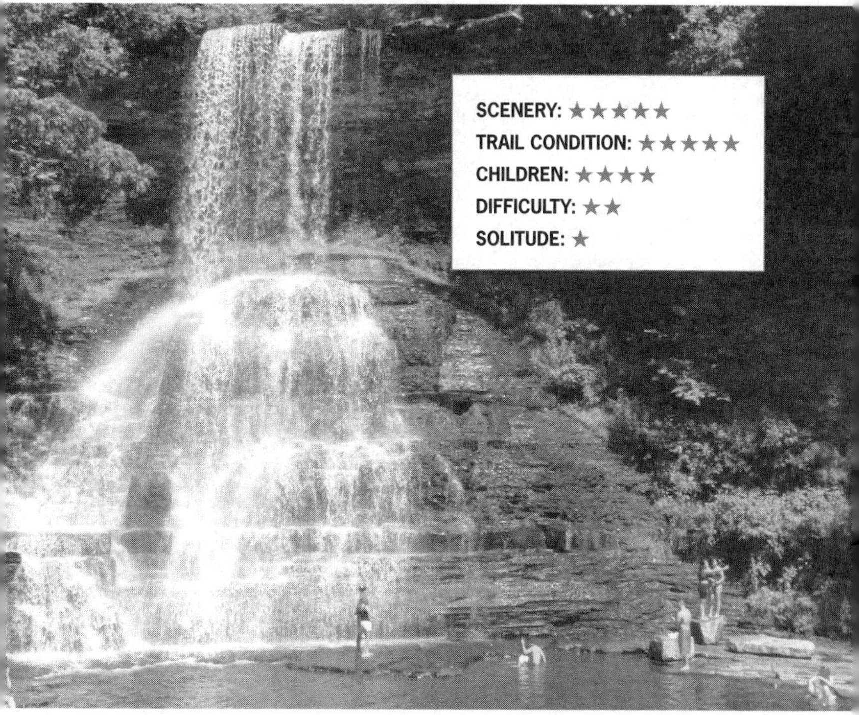

SCENERY: ★★★★★
TRAIL CONDITION: ★★★★★
CHILDREN: ★★★★
DIFFICULTY: ★★
SOLITUDE: ★

THE 60-FOOT PLUNGE OF CASCADE FALLS COOLS A POPULAR SUMMERTIME SWIMMING HOLE.

GPS TRAILHEAD COORDINATES: N37° 21.217' W80° 35.935'

DISTANCE & CONFIGURATION: 4.0-mile loop

HIKING TIME: 2.5 hours

OUTSTANDING FEATURES: Cascade Falls, Little Stony Creek Gorge

ELEVATION: 2,140 feet at trailhead, 2,900 feet at high point

ACCESS: $3 day-use fee

MAPS: National Geographic #787, *Blacksburg/New River Valley;* USGS *Eggleston*

FACILITIES: Restrooms, drinking water, picnic area

WHEELCHAIR ACCESS: None

INFO: George Washington & Jefferson National Forests, Eastern Divide Ranger District, 110 Southpark Drive, Blacksburg, VA 24060; 540-552-4641, www.fs.usda.gov/gwj

Cascade Falls

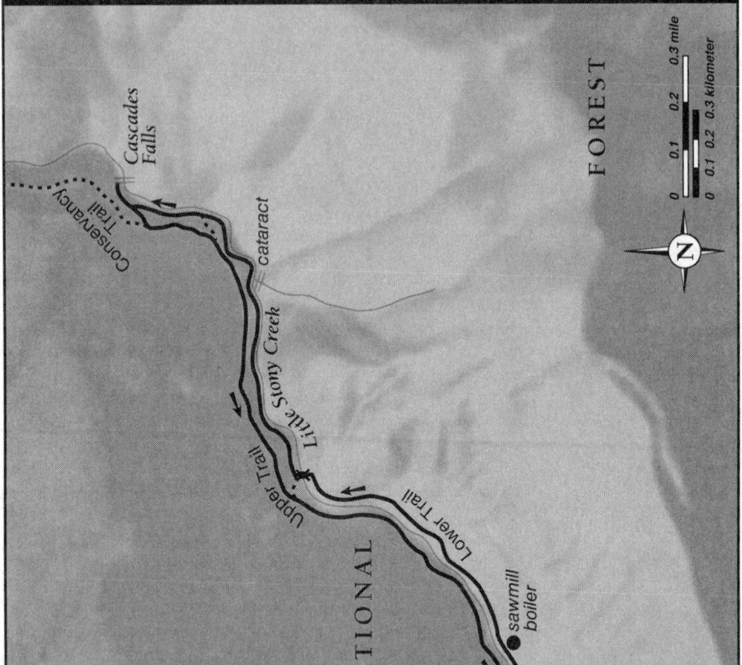

In Brief

This hike leads to Cascade Falls, the centerpiece of a nicely developed Jefferson National Forest day-use area near the town of Pembroke. A loop hike heads directly up Little Stony Creek Gorge, visiting rock walls, boulders, pools, and rapids. Navigate up the creek, and then reach big Cascade Falls and a huge pool. Return via a wider, easier track you will appreciate after experiencing Little Stony Creek Gorge.

Route Details

A network of interconnected trails leads up to Cascade Falls. It is a net 700-foot ascent from the trailhead to the falls. The trails range from challenging, narrow, and undulating to a wide, well-graded track that makes for the easiest route. No matter which way you go, it's 2.0 miles by foot to the waterfall. I recommend taking the scenic and exciting Lower Trail first. Carved stone signs located at trail intersections keep you on track. Using stone steps and rock walkways integrated into the incredible landscape, the waterside trails literally get into the heart of the Little Stony Creek Valley. And there are boulder gardens, cliffs, cataracts, and an everywhere-you-look beauty that cannot be denied. Be forewarned: Cascade Recreation Area can

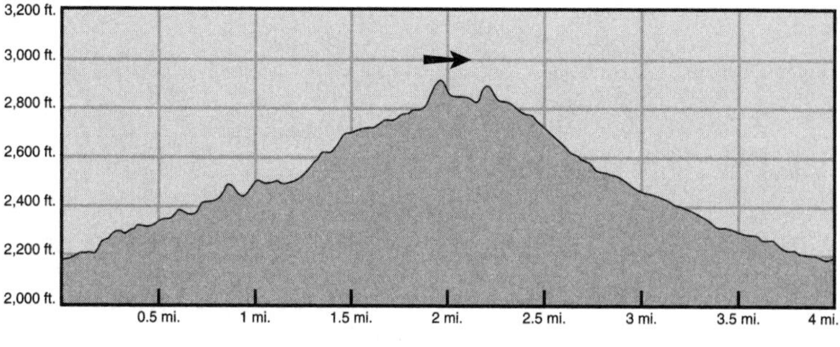

be very crowded on nice-weather weekends. Solitude seekers should plan their visit for off times.

Begin the hike near the recreation area restrooms. By the way, the recreation area features a shady waterside picnic area. Pass a kiosk and enter woods, quickly meeting up with another path coming from the picnic area. The wide, heavily used trail reaches an intersection at 0.2 mile. Head right on the Lower Trail, bridging Little Stony Creek. Begin coursing your way up the incredible gorge of Little Stony Creek. The path is fascinating, too, when you consider the extensive construction that went into working it up the rock-walled, boulder-strewn canyon. Stone steps and inlaid stone walkways achieve passage beyond still, deep pools and fast-moving cataracts, past fern clusters and rhododendron thickets. Little Stony Creek is shaded by black birch, yellow birch, and buckeye. The wildflowers can be grand in spring.

At 0.5 mile, view the trailside metal boiler, used to provide steam power for a mobile sawmill that once operated in the valley. The richness of the forest belies its denuded past. You may encounter anglers vying for native brook trout, especially in the bigger pools of this lower section. Most swimmers wait until they reach the big pool at Cascade Falls.

At 1.1 miles, come to Bridge 2. Here, the Lower Trail crosses over to the left bank of Little Stony Creek. A shortcut leads left to the Upper Trail. Stay right and continue up the gorge. Bridges span the sheer sides of the canyon. Stone walls, walkways, and other means squeeze you past otherwise impassable terrain. The trail work here is amazing in its own right, yet it doesn't exceed the God-given mosaic of variegated rock, moving water, and diverse vegetation, all enhanced by sunlight piercing the gorge.

At 1.6 miles, an incoming tributary across the creek creates its own 40-foot cataract while adding its flow to Little Stony Creek. At 1.8 miles, another shortcut leads left to the Upper Trail. Stay on the Lower Trail—you're almost to the star attraction.

Cascade Falls, at 2.0 miles, creates quite a setting. Here, the 60-foot cataract pours over a stone cliff into a huge pool framed by rock walls. Rock houses are overhung by ledges. Multiple viewing platforms provide different vantage points. A dead-end trail cruises near the top of the falls. In summer, visitors play around the fall's base, swim in the enormous pool, and hang out on nearby rock slabs. I've had the privilege of seeing Cascade Falls at high water and can tell you that the roar, spray, and raw power are amazing.

After exploring the falls and viewing it from multiple angles, take the Upper Trail away from the falls. Climb the side of the gorge to reach a wide track and a trail intersection. Here, at 2.2 miles, the Conservancy Trail leads right, up toward Barneys Wall. This hike heads left to join the doubletrack Upper Trail. This is essentially a rescue road used by medical personnel to rapidly reach injured visitors at Cascade Falls. (Mix thousands of annual visitors and a big waterfall, and you end up with occasional accidents.)

Hikers will appreciate the wide, easy nature of the road after the serpentine, irregular Lower Trail. And it's downhill just about the whole way. Ahead, pass the uppermost shortcut. Watch for a conspicuous overhanging bluff at 2.5 miles. Reach the shortcut to Bridge 2 at 2.9 miles. Continue downhill in a widening valley. Pass Bridge 1 at 3.8 miles. You have completed the loop. Backtrack 0.2 mile to finish the hike.

Nearby Attractions

The New River is a nationally renowned fishing and paddling destination. There are multiple put-ins and takeouts near the town of Pembroke, plus outfitters nearby for boat rentals and shuttles.

Directions

From Blacksburg, take US 460 West to the town of Pembroke. Turn right on Cascade Drive (VA 623) and follow it 3.3 miles to dead-end at the trailhead.

4 Bald Knob and Bear Cliffs

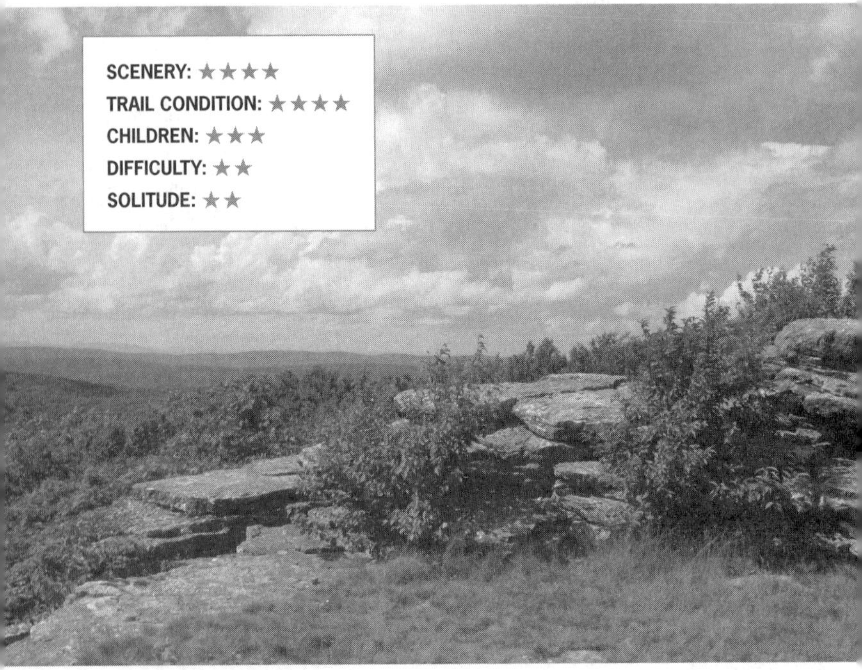

SCENERY: ★★★★
TRAIL CONDITION: ★★★★
CHILDREN: ★★★
DIFFICULTY: ★★
SOLITUDE: ★★

STELLAR VIEWS FROM BALD KNOB EXTEND INTO THE APPALACHIANS OF THE OLD DOMINION.

GPS TRAILHEAD COORDINATES: N37° 21.300' W80° 32.289'

DISTANCE & CONFIGURATION: 3.6-mile loop

HIKING TIME: 2 hours

OUTSTANDING FEATURES: Views from Bald Knob and Bear Cliffs, high country

ELEVATION: 3,900 feet at trailhead, 4,365 feet at high point

ACCESS: No fees or permits required; donation appreciated

MAPS: Mountain Lake Conservancy Trail Map; USGS *Eggleston*

FACILITIES: Outfitter at trailhead, lodge and cottages nearby

WHEELCHAIR ACCESS: None

INFO: Mountain Lake Conservancy, 115 Hotel Circle, Pembroke, VA 24136; 540-626-7121, mtnlakeconservancy.com

In Brief

This hike takes place at majestic Mountain Lake, near a historic lodge on protected lands. First, make the short but steep climb to Bald Knob, a rocky promontory with outstanding views. Next, head out on Salt Pond Mountain in high-country splendor to Bear Cliffs Overlook, which boasts a southerly panorama. Finally, return to the trailhead, coming near Mountain Lake.

Route Details

Mountain Lake, one of only two natural lakes in Virginia and the highest lake east of the Mississippi, is one of the Old Dominion's finest physical features. Since the 1800s, the lake and surrounding highlands have beckoned visitors and recreationists, formerly to escape hot summers, but nowadays to enjoy the nature of the mountains year-round, including winter sports. At first, a small hotel and summer cottages dotted the locale, but in the 1930s an impressive stone lodge was built by William Lewis Moody Jr. His heirs acquired the property that is now run by an endowment commissioned to "provide a place for people to connect with nature for future generations."

And so Mountain Lake stands today, with its historic structures and recreation facilities offering lodging and outdoor activities, including hiking. You will see some of the facilities at the hike's beginning and can explore others or even overnight there. However, neither fires nor camping is allowed on the property.

Stop by Mountain Outfitters to donate to the Mountain Lake Conservancy and grab a trail map. From there, cross paved VA 613 and walk up the steps to the Chesterfield Cabin, then angle left across the cabin lawn to reach a footpath. Head right on the Bald Knob Trail, quickly passing under a power line, then come to Bald Knob Road, a gravel track open only to personnel attending transmission towers atop Bald Knob. The road is twice as long (1 mile) but half as steep for those going to Bald Knob. Being intrepid hikers, we stay straight on the hiker-only Bald Knob Trail. It sharply angles up the north slope

Bald Knob and Bear Cliffs

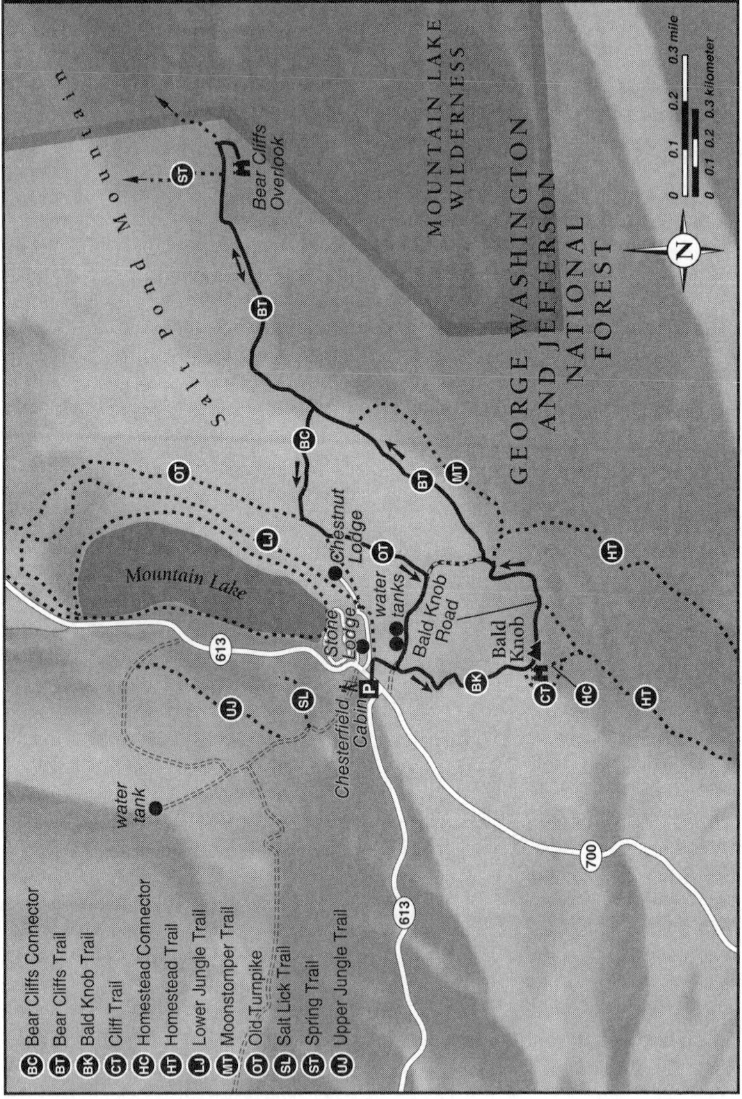

of Bald Knob under hardwood canopy dotted with ferns, moss, and boulders. By 0.4 mile, you are in a lichen-covered boulder field. Just ahead, the Cliff Trail goes right and heads under the rock promontories of Bald Knob. You, however, stay straight on the Bald Knob Trail and scramble up stone steps in more rock than soil. Shortly emerge at Bald Knob, at 4,365 feet. Here stands an array of rock outcrops, each one beckoning your presence. Stunted woods border the clearing, and transmission antennas rise from the knob's high point. Stellar views extends west, into and across the New River and the New River Valley; south toward Blacksburg; and north into Butt Mountain, Peters Mountain, and the Jefferson National Forest. More mountains range into the yon. What a panorama!

After taking your time atop Bald Knob, pass the Homestead Connector and join Bald Knob Road, the gravel doubletrack. Walk downhill. At 0.6 mile, pass the Homestead Trail leaving right. Continue descending, still above 4,000 feet in altitude. At 0.8 mile, pass the other end of the Homestead Trail, also leaving right. Keep on the gravel Bald Knob Road, then at 0.9 mile meet the Bear Cliffs Trail. Note the alluring stone bench at the intersection. Join the singletrack Bear Cliffs Trail, heading northeast along Salt Pond Mountain. Gently climb in rocky woods rife with stunted witch hazel trees to

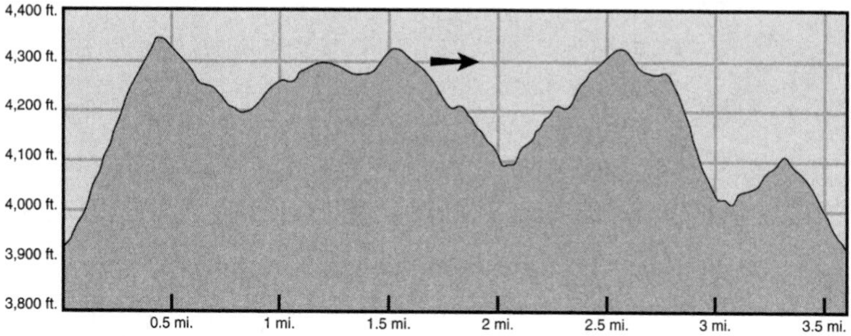

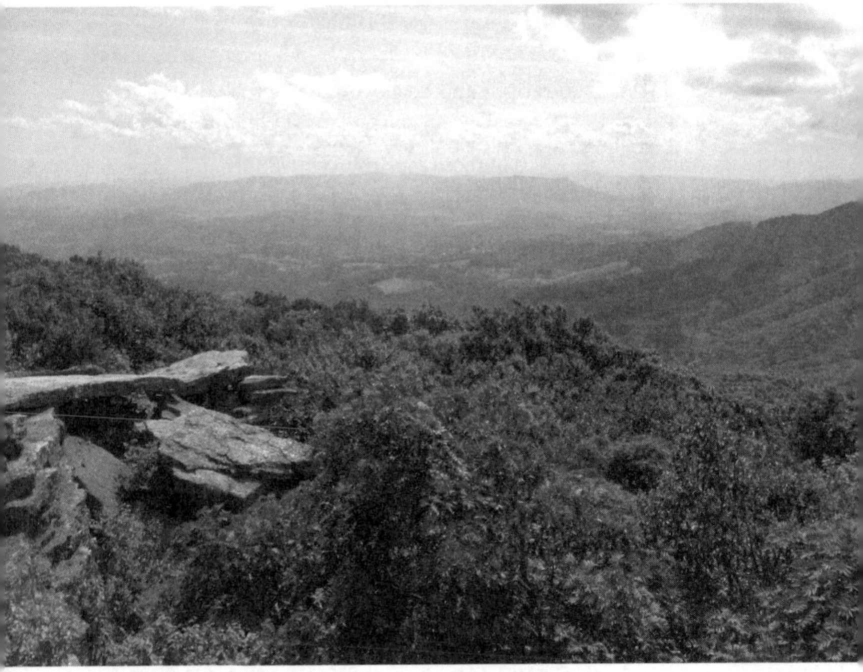

PEERING INTO THE NEW RIVER VALLEY FROM BALD KNOB

meet the Moonstomper Trail at 1.2 miles. Keep straight with the Bear Cliffs Trail, reveling in more high-country rambling to find the Bear Cliffs Connector at 1.3 miles. For now, keep straight with the Bear Cliffs Trail, still undulating above 4,000 feet among boulder gardens and young chestnut trees. Cool breezes blow even in summer in these majestic highlands.

At 1.9 miles, meet the Spring Trail. It leads left into the adjacent national forest land to reach the UVA Mountain Lake Biological Station, the employees of which study this precious parcel of the Old Dominion. Our hike slips off the east slope of Salt Pond Mountain, coming onto a huge stone fissure, with drop-offs on both sides of you. An unnamed spur leaves left for the bio station, but to reach the overlook, keep right above the fissure, looking into a geological marvel of a mini-chasm to your right (north) and the primary drop-off to your left (south). Reach the Bear Cliffs Overlook, elevation 4,100 feet, at 2.0 miles. Here, a small, flat stone slab opens to an easterly view to Blacksburg and beyond. Trees hem in the vista somewhat, especially compared to Bald Knob. Nevertheless, the destination is worth the walk.

Backtrack from the vista to turn right on the Bear Cliffs Connector at 2.8 miles. Drop quickly to meet the Old Turnpike at 3.0 miles. It's hard to imagine that this was the original route of VA 613. Turn left here on the Old Turnpike, quickly passing a connector leading right to the Chestnut Lodge, one of many overnighting options here. At 3.3 miles, turn right onto Bald Knob Road. Make an easy descent on gravel doubletrack, passing water reservoirs, then meet the Bald Knob Trail at 3.5 miles. Turn right and backtrack, reaching the trailhead at 3.6 miles.

Nearby Attractions

Mountain Lake offers lodging, guided activities, disc golf, canopy tours, and more.

Directions

From Exit 117 on I-81 near Christiansburg, take US 460 West 19 miles to VA 700 (Mountain Lake Road). Turn right onto VA 700 East toward Mountain Lake and drive 7.3 miles. Park at the intersection of VA 700 and VA 613 at the day-visitor/Mountain Lake Outfitters gravel lot.

5 Pandapas Pond Walk

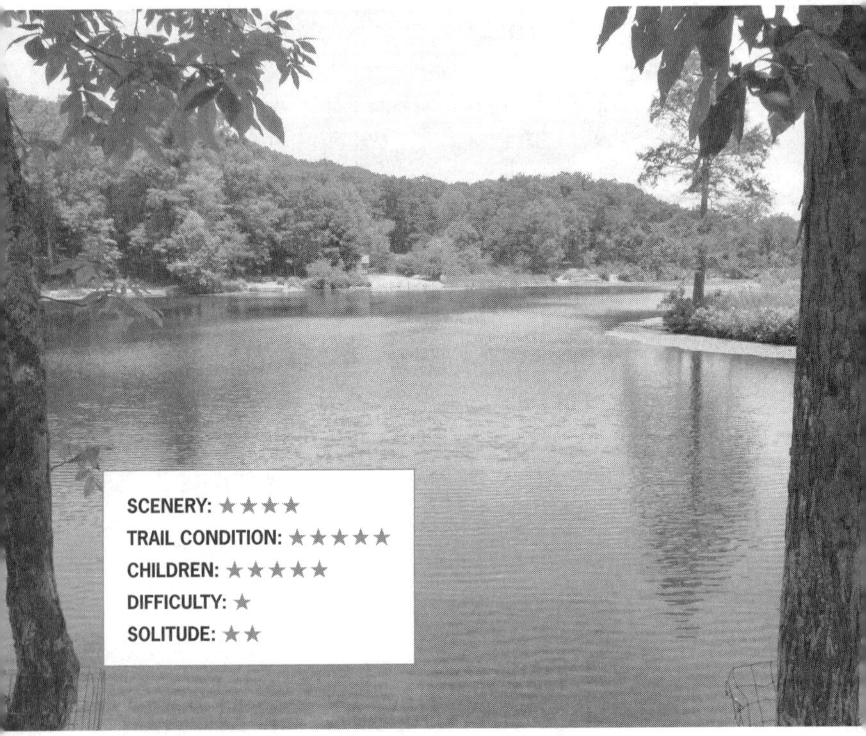

SCENERY: ★★★★
TRAIL CONDITION: ★★★★★
CHILDREN: ★★★★★
DIFFICULTY: ★
SOLITUDE: ★★

HIKERS OF ALL ABILITIES AND AGES WILL ENJOY THE WALK AROUND PANDAPAS POND.

GPS TRAILHEAD COORDINATES: N37° 16.975' W80° 28.194'

DISTANCE & CONFIGURATION: 2.6-mile double loop

HIKING TIME: 1.5 hours

OUTSTANDING FEATURES: All-access trails, pond, wetland, wildlife, pollinator gardens

ELEVATION: 2,200 feet at trailhead, 2,310 feet at high point

ACCESS: No fees or permits required

MAPS: National Geographic #787, *Covington/Alleghany Highlands;* USGS *Newport*

FACILITIES: Restroom, picnic tables along trail

WHEELCHAIR ACCESS: None

INFO: George Washington & Jefferson National Forests, Eastern Divide Ranger District, 110 Southpark Drive, Blacksburg, VA 24060; 540-552-4641, www.fs.usda.gov/gwj

In Brief

This is an excellent adventure for hikers of all ages. Circle wildlife-rich Pandapas Pond, viewing the 8-acre impoundment and the surrounding environment. Stay with the all-access path around the wetland and pond, or make a miniloop through the rhododendron using the Lady Slipper and Larkspur Trails. Visit a pollinator garden and wildlife blind as an added bonus.

Route Details

Pandapas Pond is the legacy of James Pandapas, prominent Blacksburg businessman who originally established the recreation area for his employees by damming Poverty Creek, creating an 8-acre pond on 500 acres of land. At that time, he ran the manufacturing concern known as Electro-Tec. In 1953, Pandapas sold his interest in Electro-Tec and founded a new company known as Poly Scientific. The employees of his new company had the same privileges at Pandapas Pond.

In 1968, Pandapas opened the recreation area to the public but was dismayed by how poorly it was treated, regularly sending crews out to clean the grounds around the pond. Finally, he sold the pond and acreage to the Jefferson National Forest, stipulating that they improve the site. The US Forest Service held up their end of the bargain, making the waterside trails handicap-accessible; putting two bridges over the pond; and adding restrooms, parking areas, a fishing pier, and a slew of mountain biking trails. Today, Pandapas Pond is a much-appreciated destination for nearby Blacksburg and area residents, whether they walk, mountain-bike, fish, picnic, or just have an all-around appreciation for nature. The network of trails is usable for hikers of all ages. Moreover, the trails around the pond are designated hiker-only—no need to worry about being run over by a mountain biker. So get out there and have a good time.

For a full exploration of the pond, leave the lower parking area on the pea gravel all-access path leading toward the impoundment. The only other trail leaving here—the Woods & Field Trail—heads to

Pandapas Pond Walk

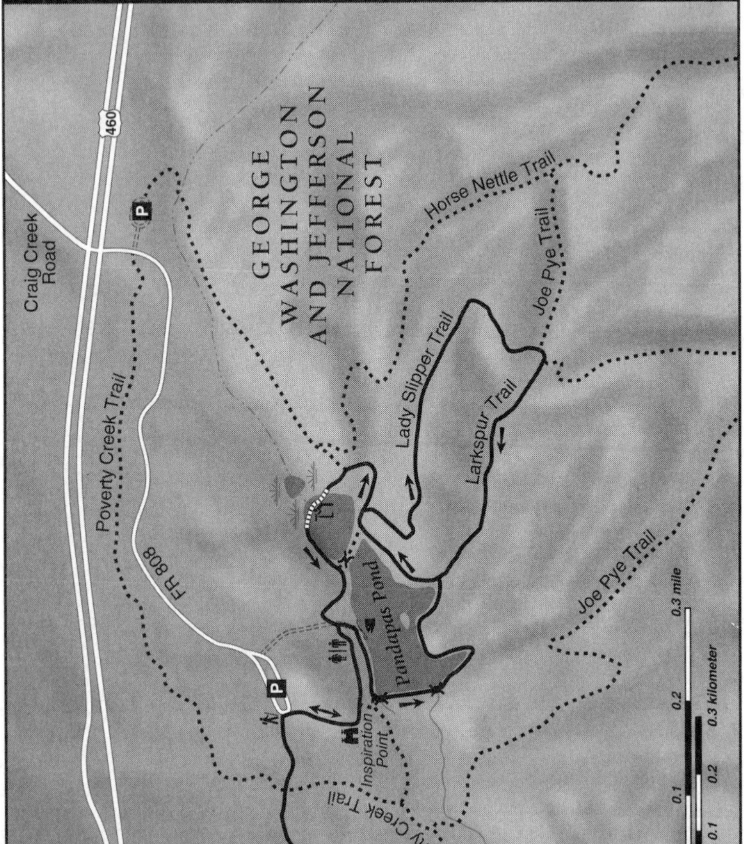

the Pollinator Garden; you can do that trail last. Quickly pass Inspiration Point, named in honor of Pandapas in 2005 after he passed away in 2003, and then come to his namesake pond. Here, a spur trail heads to the mountain biker–oriented Poverty Creek Trail, but you stay with the main path, curving to reach a trailhead, restrooms, and the pond itself after 0.2 mile. Here a spur trail leads back to the parking area. Come along the water at a fishing pier and begin circling around the impoundment counterclockwise. The all-access path crosses the dam and the outflow of Poverty Creek at 0.4 mile. Continue ringing the pond. Note that the trees' lower trunks are wrapped in wire; this is to prevent beavers from toppling them.

At 0.6 mile, the Larkspur Trail comes in on your right. Save that for later. For now, keep along the pond, cruising a level trail amid trees, brush, shade benches, and water accesses. At 0.7 mile, a dam/trail separates the lower open pond from the upper pond/wetland. Stay right, quickly coming to the natural-surface Lady Slipper Trail. If you and your crew can tackle irregular natural-surface trails, head right on the Lady Slipper Trail. If you have disabled or very old or young hikers with you, stay on the loop around the pond. It is about a mile walk around the pond and back to the parking area. The Lady Slipper Trail climbs past pines, rhododendrons, and mountain laurel.

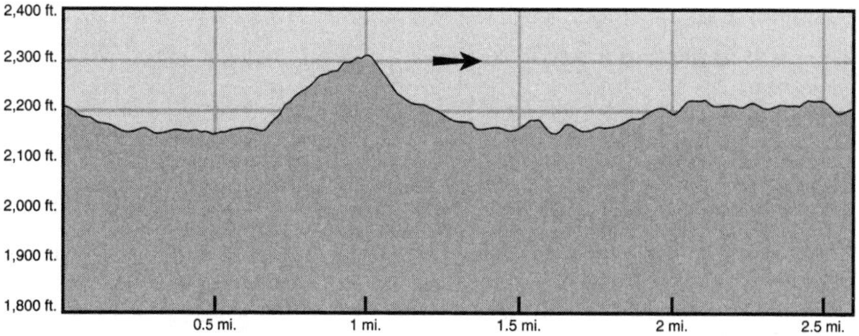

At 1 mile, stay right to meet the Larkspur Trail and the Joe Pye mountain bike trail. Cross a small branch and descend through deep rhododendron thickets along a creek. Crisscross the creek, and return to Pandapas Pond at 1.4 miles.

Continue the circuit around the impoundment to pass the spur going right to the Horse Nettle Trail and upper parking lot. Stay left, crossing the wetland of Pandapas Pond on a long boardwalk. Complete the pond loop at 1.8 miles. A spur going right heads to the upper end of the lower parking area. Return to the lower parking lot the way you came, reaching it at 2.0 miles.

For a bonus hike, take the Woods & Field Trail, a wide gravel track heading west from the lower parking area. Shortly intersect and cross the Poverty Creek mountain bike trail. At 0.3 mile from the parking area, emerge at the Pollinator Garden, managed by volunteers. Here, flowers and plants are raised to attract butterflies, bees, and other pollinating insects. Make sure to head to the wildlife blind to see if you might spot a deer or other animal in the nearby field. Even if you cannot see wildlife, the view of Brush Mountain isn't bad. From there, backtrack to the trailhead, completing the adventure at Pandapas Pond.

Nearby Attractions

Pandapas Pond not only features the above walk using hiker-only trails, but it also has an extensive network of mountain bike trails emanating from the upper parking lot near Pandapas Pond entrance road.

Directions

From Exit 117 on I-81 near Christiansburg, take US 460 West 15 miles to the signed Pandapas Pond on your left, just across from Craig Creek Road, 3 miles west of the Blacksburg exit on US 460. Follow the entrance road to the lower parking area. (The upper parking area is for mountain bikers.)

6 Kelly Knob

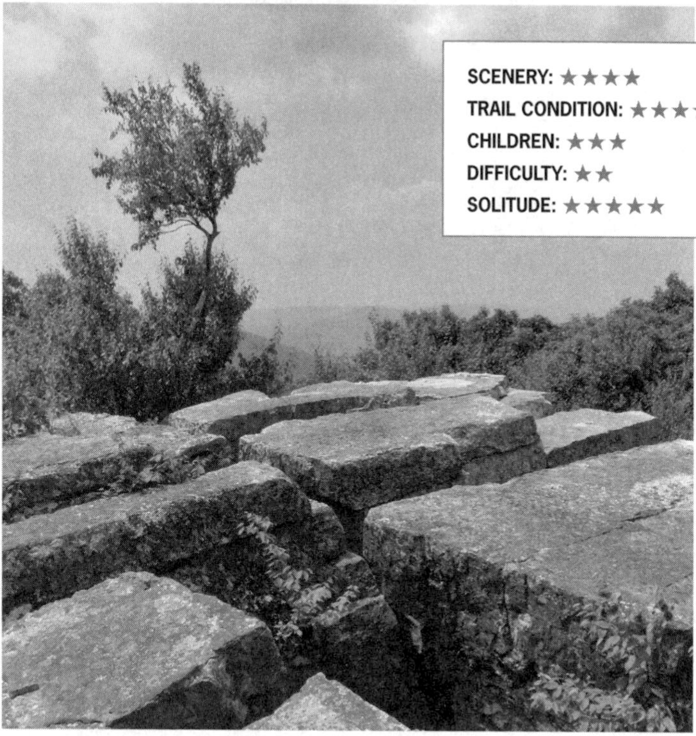

SCENERY: ★★★★
TRAIL CONDITION: ★★★★
CHILDREN: ★★★
DIFFICULTY: ★★
SOLITUDE: ★★★★★

THIS VIEW FROM KELLY KNOB OFFERS SOLITUDE ALONG THE APPALACHIAN TRAIL.

GPS TRAILHEAD COORDINATES: N37° 22.379' W80° 26.800'

DISTANCE & CONFIGURATION: 4.0-mile out-and-back

HIKING TIME: 2.5 hours

OUTSTANDING FEATURES: Solitude, high country, view

ELEVATION: 3,260 feet at trailhead, 3,800 feet at high point

ACCESS: No fees or permits required

MAPS: National Geographic #787, *Blacksburg/New River Valley;* USGS *Newport*

FACILITIES: None

WHEELCHAIR ACCESS: None

INFO: George Washington National Forest, Eastern Divide Ranger District, 110 Southpark Drive, Blacksburg, VA 24060; 540-552-4641, www.fs.usda.gov/gwj

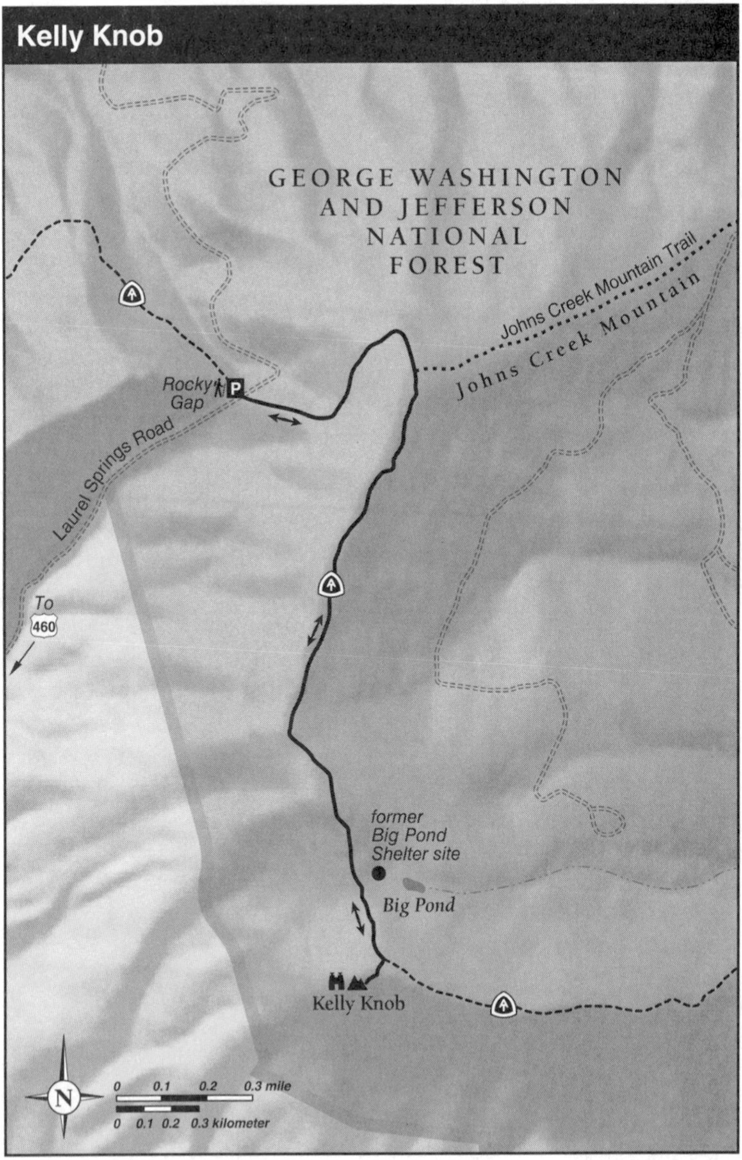
Kelly Knob
GEORGE WASHINGTON
AND JEFFERSON
NATIONAL
FOREST
Johns Creek Mountain Trail
Johns Creek Mountain
Rocky Gap
Laurel Springs Road
To
460
former
Big Pond
Shelter site
Big Pond
Kelly Knob
N
0 0.1 0.2 0.3 mile
0 0.1 0.2 0.3 kilometer

In Brief

This fairly easy hike to a view offers solitude aplenty, sometimes hard to find on the Appalachian Trail. Start your hike at remote Rocky Gap, north of Blacksburg, and make a quick but short climb to the crest of Johns Creek Mountain. From there, it is an easy walk to Kelly Knob, where a spur leads to an outcrop and views of the New River Valley and adjoining mountains.

Route Details

Rocky Gap is little used as a trailhead, judging by the limited parking spaces. It is not difficult to reach, yet it seems to be off the radar for most AT hikers. From the direction you drove, the AT goes either right or left. Head right, northbound on the AT. Here, the AT follows an old jeep road easterly and uphill. You are already at 3,200 feet in elevation, so the weather should be cooler than the lowlands below. Oak, mountain laurel, and maple flank the uphill path. A practiced eye will be able to spot bush-sized regenerating chestnut trees. Look for the chestnut's long, serrated leaves.

The American chestnut tree was the once dominant giant of the Southern Appalachians. This tree formerly ranged from Maine to

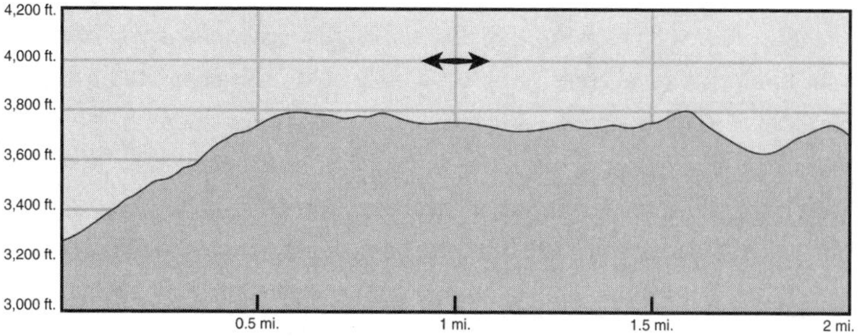

Mississippi, growing to massive proportions in Virginia. Its fruit was very important; chestnut acorns fed everything from bears to birds. Humans ate them, too: Remember the words from "The Christmas Song," "chestnuts roasting on an open fire." The tree also provided excellent wood for everyday use by pioneers; the wood was also coveted by timber companies, which harvested the titans.

The day of the mighty chestnut is gone—for now. In the early 1900s, Asian chestnut trees were imported to the United States, bringing a fungus with them. The Asian trees had developed immunity to the fungus, but the American chestnut was helpless. Before long, chestnuts were dying in the Northeast, and the blight worked its way south, reaching Virginia in the 1920s. Two decades later, all the giant chestnuts were lost. But there is hope. To this day, chestnut trees such as those beside the trail sprout from the roots of the ancients, growing up but always succumbing to the blight. Hopefully, these chestnuts are building a resistance to the blight and will one day tower over the mountains again, long after we are gone. Scientists are expediting the process, and experiments are under way to crossbreed American chestnut trees with the Asian chestnuts in an effort to develop a blight-resistant American chestnut.

At 0.3 mile, walk next to a trailside boulder that has become a resting bench. Pass an outcrop to your left at 0.4 mile with partial views. The trail levels off at 0.5 mile. Congratulations! You just climbed 500 feet. Just ahead, intersect the Johns Creek Mountain Trail. It leaves left for VA 658. The walking is easy now as you head south along a level crest. Drop off a little bouldery spot at 0.9 mile, and then resume easy walking over small, flat stones resembling tile. Descend a little to reach a gap at 1.7 miles. Here, a faint trail leaves left a short distance to the site of the Big Pond trail shelter, now dismantled. There is still a seldom-used campsite at this small flat.

It is but a small climb to Kelly Knob, which you reach at 1.9 miles. A sign indicates a blue-blazed path leaving right. Follow the spur southwest and downhill to reach a narrow stone brow. Turn right here and soon emerge at an open outcrop, elevation 3,700 feet. The stone base of the outcrop is fissured, so you have to hop over cracks to explore. Stepping out to the main overlook, the Sinking Creek Valley, flanked by Johns Creek Mountain and Clover Hollow Mountain, stretches to the west. The New River, into which Sinking Creek flows, is down there too. To the north, the high plateau of Salt Pond Mountain rises wide. And you will likely share this view with nothing but the wind. Solitude is one of the primary lures of this hike.

Nearby Attractions

Along the way to the trailhead, you will pass the **Sinking Creek Covered Bridge.** There is a small park and wayside near the bridge on your right. The bridge was built in 1916 and is owned and maintained by Giles County. The 70-foot-long span was left in place after another bridge was built nearby in 1949.

Directions

From Exit 117 on I-81 near Christiansburg, take US 460 West 17 miles and turn right onto VA 42 East toward Newport. Follow VA 42 East as it winds through Newport 1 mile to turn left onto VA 601 (Clover Hollow Road). Stay with Clover Hollow Road for 5 miles. Here, paved Clover Hollow Road leaves left and turns into VA 602, but you stay straight, joining gravel Laurel Springs Road. Stay with Laurel Springs Road 1.6 miles to reach Rocky Gap. There are just a few parking spots, so be courteous with your spacing.

7 Mountain Lake Wilderness

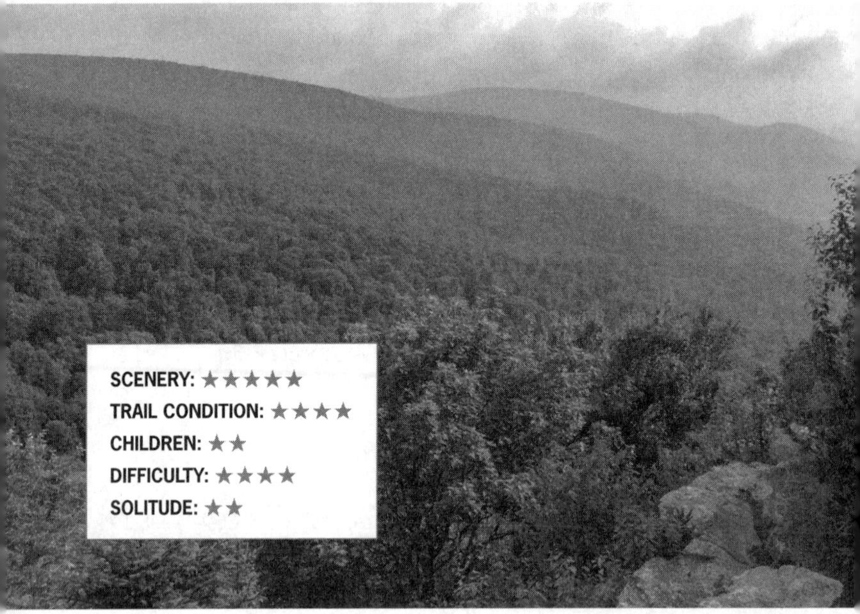

SCENERY: ★★★★★
TRAIL CONDITION: ★★★★
CHILDREN: ★★
DIFFICULTY: ★★★★
SOLITUDE: ★★

FROM WAR SPUR LOOKOUT, YOU CAN SEE SALT POND MOUNTAIN RISING ABOVE WAR SPUR BRANCH.

GPS TRAILHEAD COORDINATES: N37° 24.725' W80° 31.367'

DISTANCE & CONFIGURATION: 10.5-mile out-and-back, 0.5-mile out-and-back, or 9.0-mile loop using forest road

HIKING TIME: 6 hours, 0.5 hour, or 5 hours

OUTSTANDING FEATURES: Two views, wilderness, spruce highland plateau, varied hike possibilities

ELEVATION: 3,970 feet at trailhead, 3,420 feet at low point

ACCESS: No fees or permits required

MAPS: National Geographic #787, *Blacksburg/New River Valley;* USGS *Interior, Waiteville*

FACILITIES: None

WHEELCHAIR ACCESS: None

INFO: George Washington National Forest, Eastern Divide Ranger District, 110 Southpark Drive, Blacksburg, VA 24060; 540-552-4641, www.fs.usda.gov/gwj

In Brief

This hike enters Mountain Lake Wilderness and quickly reaches Wind Rock Lookout and extensive views. Then the Appalachian Trail traverses a high plateau in a forest recalling New England. The hike splits off and heads for War Spur Lookout and more vistas. From there, you can backtrack or make a loop using the forest road upon which you drove to the trailhead. A third possibility is a short walk to Wind Rock and back.

Route Details

This hike starts in the unnamed gap between Big Mountain to the west and Potts Mountain to the east. Join the AT, northbound, and head east toward Wind Rock Lookout. Enter the Mountain Lake Wilderness. The trail is well trammeled here. A slight uptick through northern hardwoods leads to Wind Rock Lookout at 0.25 mile. Split left from the AT and reach the crag of Wind Rock. Rocky Mountain and Fork Mountain stand in the fore, while Peters Mountain forms a long ridge and the boundary of West Virginia and Virginia. To the south, Big Mountain creates runs south. From Wind Rock Lookout, less-hardy hikers can turn back to the trailhead, and judging by the AT as you continue on, most hikers do turn back.

The AT continues east along Potts Mountain. Begin to look for occasional spruce trees that survive on this cold, elevated plateau that also harbors short, squat hardwoods carpeted with ferns. At 1.6 miles, come near an intermittent stream and campsite. Keep east in this highland wilderness. At 2.0 miles, the AT abruptly turns right (south) and begins rolling on the elevated plateau of Salt Pond Mountain. The walking is glorious. Enjoy the wilderness while scoping for spruce trees, not to be confused with hemlocks, which can also be found among the hardwoods here.

At 2.7 miles, the AT drops off the slope of Salt Pond Mountain. At 3.2 miles, reach an intersection with the War Spur Trail, ending your descent—turn right onto the War Spur Trail. This path proceeds to regain the lost elevation. You are back on the nearly level shoulder

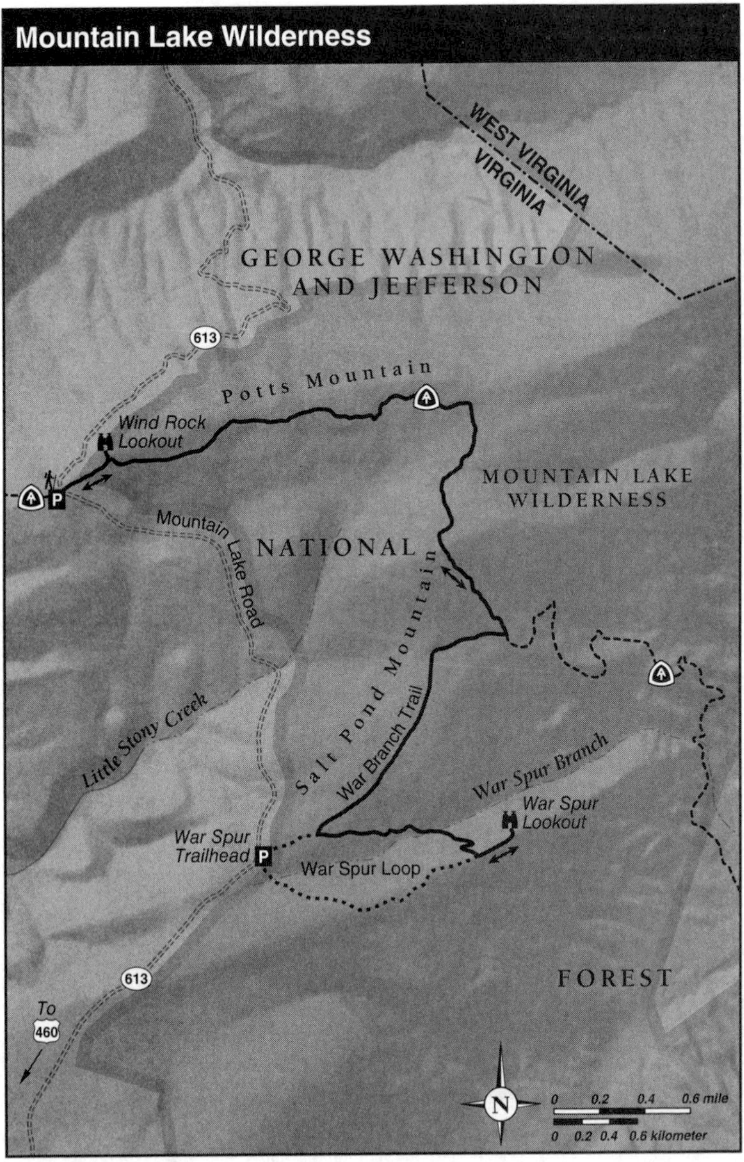
Mountain Lake Wilderness
WEST VIRGINIA
VIRGINIA
GEORGE WASHINGTON AND JEFFERSON
NATIONAL
FOREST
613
Potts Mountain
Wind Rock Lookout
MOUNTAIN LAKE WILDERNESS
Mountain Lake Road
Salt Pond Mountain
War Branch Trail
Little Stony Creek
War Spur Branch
War Spur Lookout
War Spur Trailhead
War Spur Loop
613
To 460
N
0 0.2 0.4 0.6 mile
0 0.2 0.4 0.6 kilometer

of Salt Pond Mountain by 3.5 miles. At 3.6 miles, look for a silted pond on the right. Turn southwest and relish more easy highland wilderness walking, a rare combination. Pass a second filled-in pond at 4.3 miles. At 4.4 miles, meet the War Spur Loop. Head left, then descend into the War Spur Branch valley. The path finagles through rocks and rhododendron thickets while crossing War Spur Branch at 4.9 miles. This little valley stays cold to cool year-round, judging by the preponderance of spruces. This is the low point of the hike, at a little over 3,400 feet. Note the tea-colored water. Ascend from War Spur Branch and reach an intersection at 5.3 miles. Head left to the War Spur Lookout, descending in woods. At 5.5 miles, the trail emerges onto a cliff, the War Spur Lookout. Here, Salt Pond Mountain looms across War Spur Branch. Potts Mountain extends to the horizon. Glimpse down to the Johns Creek Valley in the distance. The view is a fitting reward for a hike through the 10,753-acre wilderness that the Old Dominion shares with West Virginia.

What is wilderness anyway? After 18,600 pages of testimony and the consolidation of 65 bills, the Wilderness Act of 1964 was passed by Congress. The legal definition of wilderness, spelled out in the bill, is as follows: "A wilderness, in contrast with those areas where man and his works dominate the landscape, is hereby recognized as

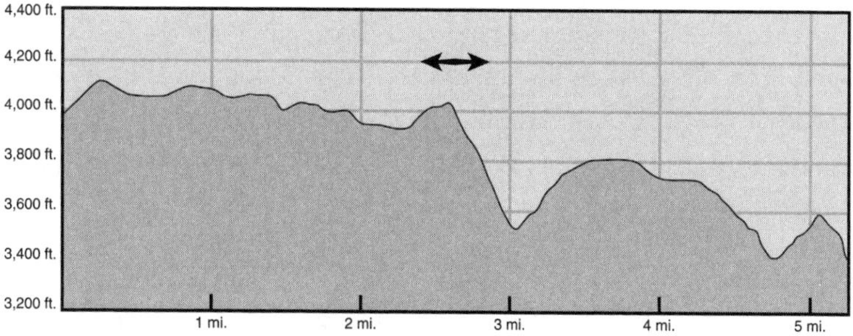

an area where the earth and its community of life are untrammeled by man, where man . . . is a visitor and does not remain." Ranging from 6 to more than 9 million acres in size, wilderness areas have multiple uses, such as hiking, hunting, canoeing, climbing, fishing, and camping. Virginia has 24 wildernesses, mostly located in the mountains. Mountain Lake Wilderness was established in 1984.

At this point, you have two choices. The first choice is a simple backtrack, and that will get you back to the trailhead after 5.5 more miles. The other alternative is to take the War Spur Loop out to Mountain Lake Road, then follow the gravel road into the Little Stony Creek drainage and up to the parking area near Wind Rock Overlook. If you do this, you will reach the road at 6.7 miles, bridge Little Stony Creek at 7.4 miles, and then return to the trailhead at 9.0 miles.

Nearby Attractions

You will pass **Mountain Lake Lodge** on the way to the trailhead. Situated on a natural highland tarn—one of only two natural lakes in Virginia—it has been the site of hotels and summer visitors since the early 1800s. The resort is surrounded by a large nature preserve that offers more trails of its own. For more information, visit mtnlakelodge.com.

Directions

From Exit 117 on I-81 near Christiansburg, take US 460 West 19 miles to VA 700 (Mountain Lake Road). Turn right onto VA 700 East and drive 7.3 miles to Mountain Lake. Here, Mountain Lake Road becomes VA 613. Stay with it another 4.6 miles for a total of 11.9 miles from US 460 to the AT crossing. The parking area is on the left just before the crossing.

8 Flat Peter Loop

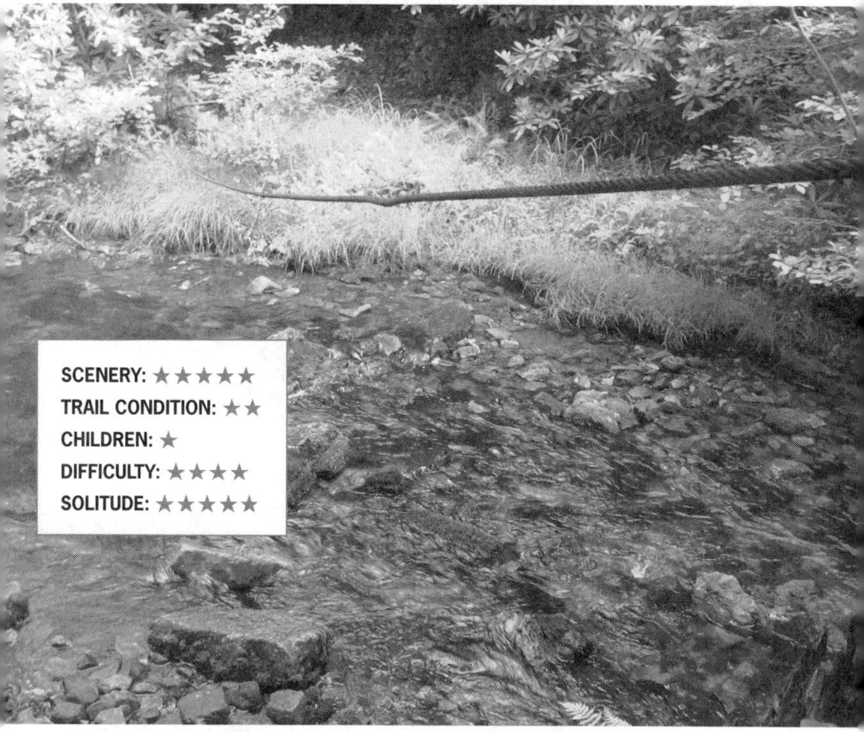

SCENERY: ★★★★★
TRAIL CONDITION: ★★
CHILDREN: ★
DIFFICULTY: ★★★★
SOLITUDE: ★★★★★

THIS CLASSIC LOOP HIKE FEATURES CREEK CROSSINGS AND OTHER CHALLENGES.

GPS TRAILHEAD COORDINATES: N37° 25.603' W80° 33.329'

DISTANCE & CONFIGURATION: 8.7-mile loop

HIKING TIME: 5 hours

OUTSTANDING FEATURES: Wilderness, streams, remoteness, solitude

ELEVATION: 2,590 feet at trailhead, 3,520 feet at high point

ACCESS: No fees or permits required

MAPS: National Geographic #788, *Covington/Alleghany Highlands;* USGS *Interior*

FACILITIES: None

WHEELCHAIR ACCESS: None

INFO: George Washington & Jefferson National Forests, Eastern Divide Ranger District, 110 Southpark Drive, Blacksburg, VA 24060; 540-552-4641, www.fs.usda.gov/gwj

Flat Peter Loop

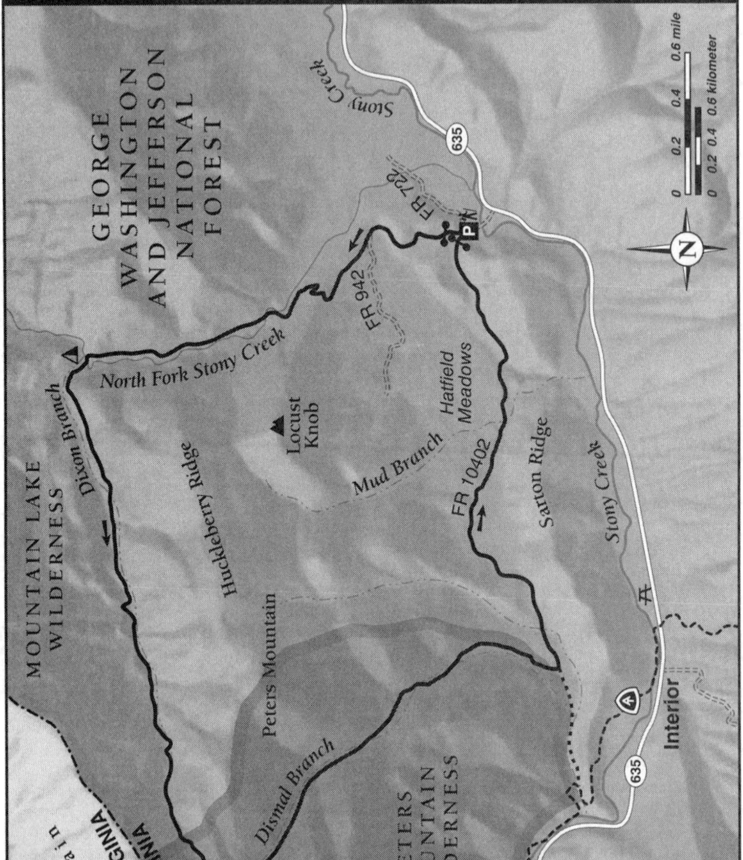

In Brief

This challenging circuit hike presents a variety of scenery and trail conditions to sate hardened mountain hikers. The loops ascends rugged North Fork Stony Creek, turns up rhododendron-heavy Dixon Branch to enter Mountain Lake Wilderness, and then descends rocky and rough Dismal Branch. Finally, meander fields and forest through the Hatfield Meadows, where highland panoramas await. Be apprised that trail markings are faint in places, so you'll have to do some route tracking.

Route Details

This is a classic rugged national forest hike. For starters, the circuit traverses craggy terrain as it circles Huckleberry Ridge then passes through Peters Mountain Wilderness. This ruggedness includes densely forested creek valleys pocked with boulders and rock outcrops, compact rhododendron thickets where daytime is as dark as dusk, and fern gardens obscuring an already faint trailbed. This rich mountain woodland also delivers everywhere-you-look beauty and a true sense of being in the back of beyond. Yet the final part of the hike leads through the mostly level Hatfield Meadows, where wetlands and fire-managed forest border grassy clearings where surrounding

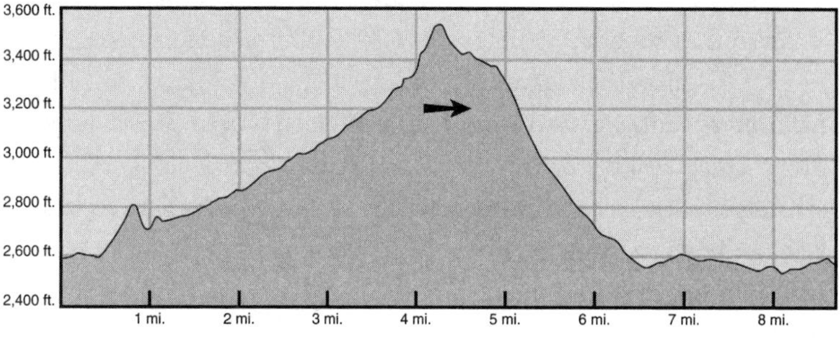

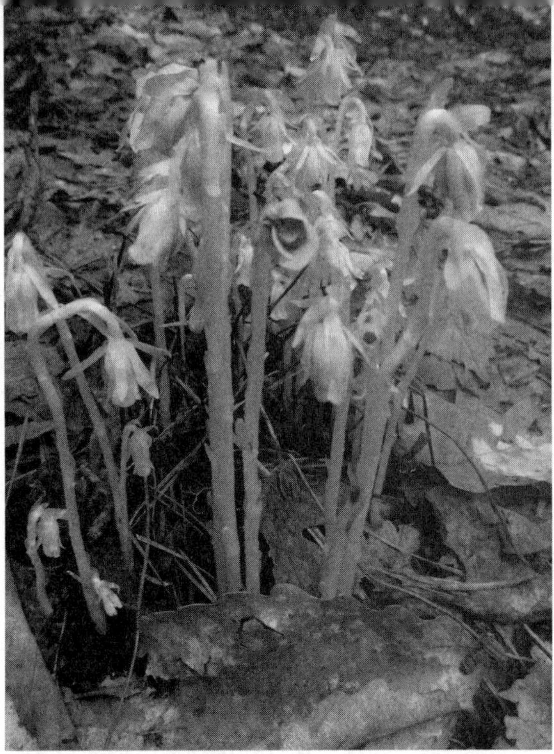

INDIAN GHOST PIPE RISES FROM THE SUMMERTIME FOREST FLOOR.

ridges rise to create a highland panorama. Lace up your boots and be prepared to earn your visual rewards on this trek that also goes by the name Dixon Branch Loop.

Start the hike by passing around a pole gate of Forest Road 942. This gate will be open during big-game hunt seasons in the fall. Your return route will come out near gated FR 10402. Trace doubletrack FR 942 for 0.4 mile, then leave right on a singletrack path marked with paint blazes and plastic diamonds. Ascend woods, with North Fork Stony Creek well below to your right. Recreation area signs on the right refer to the Glen Alton farm below. At 0.8 mile, the path curves right and descends toward North Fork, reaching it at 0.9 mile. Head left upstream in thick rhododendron and black birch. The trail rises over a bluff, then returns to noisy, tea-colored North Fork, which you cross at 1.2 miles. A metal cable and stepping-stones aid your crossing. Keep up the scenic vale, stepping over small tributaries.

At 2.0 miles, come to a second crossing of North Fork. There has been a bridge here in the past and may be in the future. Once across, come to a small campsite. The Flat Peter Loop turns left (west) to cross small Dixon Branch just above its confluence with North Fork and an alluring pool. The trail turns up the Dixon Branch valley, where rhododendron thickets cause hikers to lean over at times. In other places the trailbed is faint—look for paint blazes. Make the first of numerous hop-overs of Dixon Branch at 2.7 miles. The valley begins running out of water as you rise the vale bordered by Huckleberry Ridge on your left and Peters Mountain—forming the Virginia–West Virginia boundary—on your right. Make the last Dixon Branch crossing at 3.9 miles. Continue climbing a shallow valley where ferns rise waist-high in summer.

Cut through a gap at 4.2 miles, entering the Peters Mountain Wilderness. You may see a wilderness sign here. Descend into the uppermost Dismal Branch valley, keeping west. Stay with the blazes and reach a campsite at 4.6 miles. Here, the trail arcs south and crosses Dismal Branch in yellow birch. In places, the trail and forest are extremely rocky. Hop over increasing-in-size Dismal Branch at 4.9 miles, then fight your way down the heavily vegetated valley. At 5.0 miles, pass a rock ledge and cave on your left. Return to the creek, but don't cross it, instead working along boulders and thick brush—and a faint trailbed on a very steep slope.

Continue descending to saner terrain and cross Dismal Branch at 5.3 miles. You're now on the right-hand bank. The trailbed is more obvious by now but can be washed out and irregular in places. Look in this area for metal relics and a stone foundation from what appears to be a former logging camp. Cross Dismal Branch again at 5.5, 5.9, and 6.0 miles. The valley has opened and you are on the left bank in pine-, oak-, and laurel-dominated woods.

Reach a major intersection at 6.6 miles. You've dropped 1,000 feet from the gap above Dismal Branch. Head left—the right turn leads west to the Appalachian Trail and VA 635. The Flat Peter Loop really is flat from here on out. At 6.7 miles, step over an intermittent stream on a partly washed-out bridge. Just ahead, enter what is an almost continuous stretch of meadows and linear wildlife clearings, collectively known as the Hatfield Meadows. Follow the trail east through these clearings. You can see Sarton Ridge, Locust Knob, and more-distant mountains above the clearings. Fire-managed woodlands border the clearings, adding more ecotone to the hike. Bridge Mud Branch by culvert at 7.8 miles. The farther east you go, the more the trail morphs into a gravel jeep track labeled FR 10402 near the trailhead. At 8.6 miles, emerge onto FR 942 after passing around the pole gate of FR 10402. The parking area is just to your left.

Nearby Attractions

Glen Alton Farm provides a level walking experience through a historic farm and on to a wetland of Stony Creek. Visit glenaltonfarm.com for more information.

Directions

From Exit 117 on I-81 near Christiansburg, take US 460 West 19 miles to VA 700 (Mountain Lake Road). Turn right onto VA 700 and drive 7.3 miles to Mountain Lake. Here, Mountain Lake Road becomes VA 613. Stay with it another 6.4 miles (along the way the road becomes gravel), going over Potts Mountain to reach a stop sign. Turn right, staying with VA 613. Continue 1.1 miles, passing White Rocks Campground to reach a T-intersection. Turn left on paved VA 635 and drive west 2.6 miles to Glen Alton Road (VA 622). Follow VA 622 for 0.1 mile. At this point, the road to Glen Alton veers right—stay straight on FR 942 and follow it just a short distance to curve right to a small parking area and gate, just beyond gated FR 10402. *Note:* During fall big-game hunts, the gate on FR 942 will be open.

9 Potts Valley Rail Trail

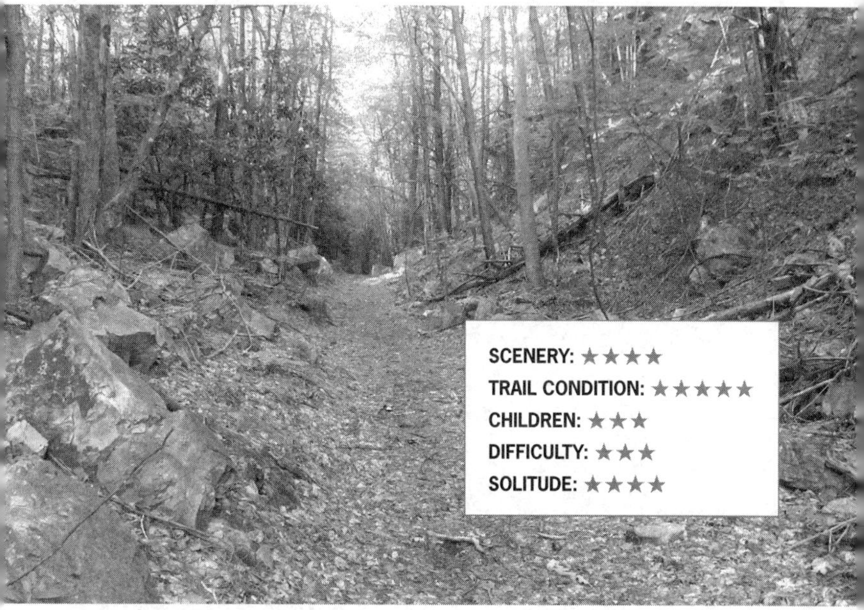

SCENERY: ★★★★
TRAIL CONDITION: ★★★★★
CHILDREN: ★★★
DIFFICULTY: ★★★
SOLITUDE: ★★★★

THIS FORMER RAILROAD GRADE IS NOW A QUIET, UNDERUTILIZED MOUNTAIN TRAIL.

GPS TRAILHEAD COORDINATES: N37° 26.850' W80° 29.570'

DISTANCE & CONFIGURATION: 6.6-mile out-and-back

HIKING TIME: 3.5 hours

OUTSTANDING FEATURES: Level rail-trail through mountainous terrain, stone construction

ELEVATION: 2,810 feet at trailhead, 2,550 feet at low point

ACCESS: No fees or permits required

MAPS: National Geographic #788, *Covington/Alleghany Highlands;* USGS *Waiteville*

FACILITIES: None

WHEELCHAIR ACCESS: None

INFO: George Washington & Jefferson National Forests, Eastern Divide Ranger District, 110 Southpark Drive, Blacksburg, VA 24060; 540-552-4641, www.fs.usda.gov/gwj

Potts Valley Rail Trail

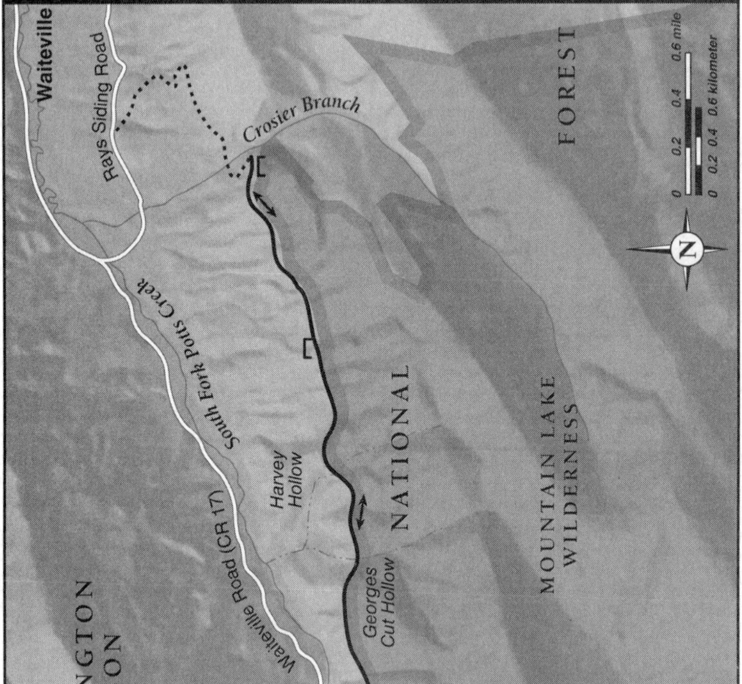

In Brief

This is your chance to enjoy marvelous mountain scenery on a nearly level rail-trail that courses through the Appalachians just inside the West Virginia boundary. The lesser-used former rail line slices through the slope of Little Mountain in the upper South Fork Potts Creek Valley. Pass through old railroad cuts and along level slopes before turning around at the site of a large but now dismantled trestle.

Route Details

The Potts Creek Valley of the year 1900 was upturned when a rail line was extended from the New River Valley east into Monroe County, West Virginia, and onward to Paint Bank, Virginia. It was difficult getting the track over the divide between the New River Valley and Potts Creek Valley, but the lure of iron ore, manganese, and seemingly limitless forests to be cut provided adequate impetus for the Norfolk and Western Railway to find a route. Though many landowners were so excited to sell their lumber that they were already bringing it into the proposed rail stop at Waiteville before the railroad was finished, some area farmers were unwilling to part with their land to have the railway built. Condemnation fights slowed the progress of the railroad, but it

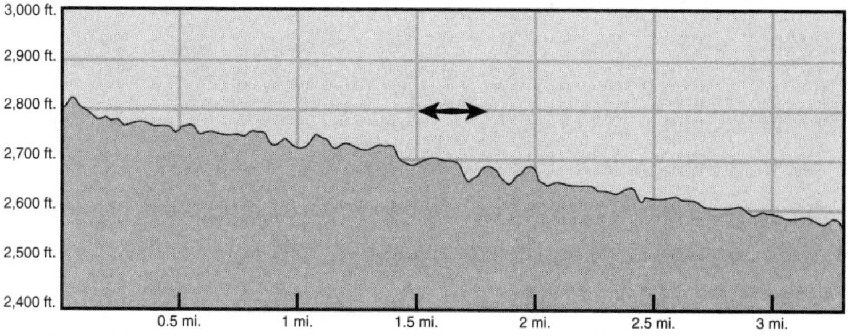

was eventually running by 1909. Initially the line moved mostly ore, but by 1920 the mining materials had played out and the line moved forest products, along with some passengers and limited goods. The first automobiles were shipped into the Potts Creek Valley during this period. They were too big to fit fully assembled on the railroad cars and thus were assembled once they arrived at their destination.

Despite finding different ways to use the line, by 1932 the Potts Valley Branch ceased to operate. The trestles were dismantled and the tracks pulled up, leaving only the railroad grade. Eventually, the slope of Little Mountain was purchased by the Forest Service, which turned the old railroad grade into a rail-trail.

Our hike starts at the west end of the rail-trail, just a quarter-mile into West Virginia. The rail-trail is shared with bicycles (no horses or ATVs), but it is underused by both hikers and those who like to travel trails by pedal power. Pass around a pole gate and join the old grade of the railroad line. The surface is grass in the summer and cinders in the winter. Begin the hike by passing through one of the many cuts the grade makes to stay level in this mountain fastness. Here, land was blasted and removed, allowing the railway to cleave what would have been a hill. Conversely, additional soil was used to build up little valleys, which would have otherwise been too steep for the rail line to dip into and come out of. Thus, you end up with a nearly level trail coursing through mountain terrain. The path makes a great way to experience mountain hiking without excessive effort. The trail drops less than 250 feet in 3.3 miles, making your return trip easy.

Old timbering roads spur off the main route, but the correct way remains obvious. Mountain Lake Wilderness rises to your right. The trail forms the wilderness boundary here. At 0.2 mile, work around a short eroded section of the grade. Rhododendrons, tulip trees, maples, and other hardwoods border and shade the track. At 0.6 mile, a fence reroutes hikers briefly off the grade. Pass a bench on your left at 0.9 mile. Continue northeast, occasionally bridging small tributaries of Potts Creek. At 1.1 miles, traverse a wet stretch of trail, where a spring trickles across the path. The slope dropping to your left sharpens.

At 1.5 miles, the stream of Georges Cut Hollow flows under the path. Ahead, bisect boulder-strewn Georges Cut. At 1.9 miles, bridge the stream of Harvey Hollow by culvert. The grade enters drier woods of sourwood, black gum, and scads of oak and mountain laurel. At 2.4 miles, on a long straightaway, take a short spur to a bench and view of a culvert exhibiting stonework of yesteryear. Leave the wilderness boundary behind.

Curve into Crosier Branch, passing through a sharp cut and finding a bench and interpretive information at 3.3 miles. This is a good place to relax then turn around to see where a 600-foot trestle once crossed the valley ahead. The rail-trail continues by leaving then rejoining the grade before dropping to end at Rays Siding Road after another mile. Soak in more mountain scenery on your return trip.

Nearby Attractions

White Rocks Campground provides lesser-used wooded camps. Restrooms and water are available in season. Lots of hiking and fishing are within easy driving distance.

Directions

From Exit 117 on I-81 near Christiansburg, take US 460 West 19 miles to VA 700 (Mountain Lake Road). Turn right onto VA 700 East and drive 7.3 miles to Mountain Lake. Here, Mountain Lake Road becomes VA 613. Stay with it another 6.4 miles (along the way the road becomes gravel), going over Potts Mountain to reach a stop sign. Turn right, staying with VA 613. Continue 1.1 miles, passing White Rocks Campground to reach a T-intersection. Here, turn right on paved VA 635. Drive east 1.2 miles to enter Monroe County, West Virginia, and WV 17 East. A quarter-mile into West Virginia, turn right at the sign for the Potts Valley Rail Trail and quickly dead-end at the parking area.

10 Hanging Rock

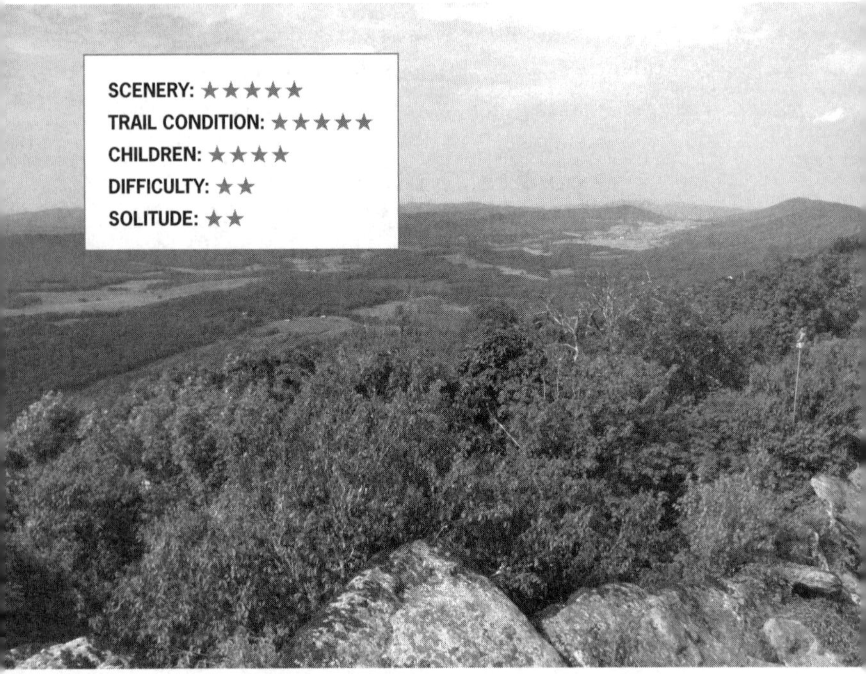

SCENERY: ★★★★★
TRAIL CONDITION: ★★★★★
CHILDREN: ★★★★
DIFFICULTY: ★★
SOLITUDE: ★★

HANGING ROCK NOT ONLY DELIVERS SPECTACULAR VIEWS BUT IS ALSO AN IMPORTANT RAPTOR-MIGRATION SURVEY POINT.

GPS TRAILHEAD COORDINATES: N37° 30.584' W80° 26.271'

DISTANCE & CONFIGURATION: 2.0-mile out-and-back

HIKING TIME: 1 hour

OUTSTANDING FEATURES: Views from tower, raptor migration, Allegheny Trail

ELEVATION: 3,470 feet at trailhead, 3,810 feet at high point

ACCESS: No fees or permits required

MAPS: National Geographic #788, *Covington/Alleghany Highlands;* USGS *Gap Mills*

FACILITIES: None

WHEELCHAIR ACCESS: None

INFO: George Washington & Jefferson National Forests, Eastern Divide Ranger District, 110 Southpark Drive, Blacksburg, VA 24060; 540-552-4641, www.fs.usda.gov/gwj, hangingrocktower.org

In Brief

This short trek starts high and gets higher, topping out on an upthrust outcrop and observation tower made famous as a raptor-migration monitoring station. You leave a gap on Peters Mountain, then take the long-distance Allegheny Trail along the ridgeline to the open outcrop upon which stands a tower offering 360-degree views guaranteed to make the trip worthwhile.

Route Details

Hanging Rock is an emergent outcrop on the crest of Peters Mountain in Monroe County, West Virginia. This natural stone promontory allows for incredible views southeast into the Potts Creek Valley and onward over the waves of mountains into the Old Dominion. To the northwest, you can peer over the Greenbrier River Valley and a host of mountains and valleys in West Virginia. The New River Valley stretches to the northwest.

The view was improved in 1956 when the state of West Virginia built a tower atop Hanging Rock to use as a fire lookout. For 16 years the tower was seasonally occupied by rangers scanning the ridges and valleys below, looking for conflagrations. The tower was abandoned for a period then refurbished in 1984 after the land became part of the Jefferson National Forest in 1983. However, in 1996 the tower burned down. It was subsequently rebuilt using the original plans.

Today the tower is a destination where visitors can gain 360-degree views of the surrounding landscape—and watch some serious raptor migration in the fall. The tower is accessed by the Allegheny Trail, West Virginia's master path that extends 330 miles from its southern terminus with the Appalachian Trail, just 12 miles south of Hanging Rock, north to the Mason–Dixon Line and the Pennsylvania border near Bruceton Mills. The Allegheny Trail travels through some of the finest scenery in the Mountain State and is a rewarding long-distance backpacking pathway.

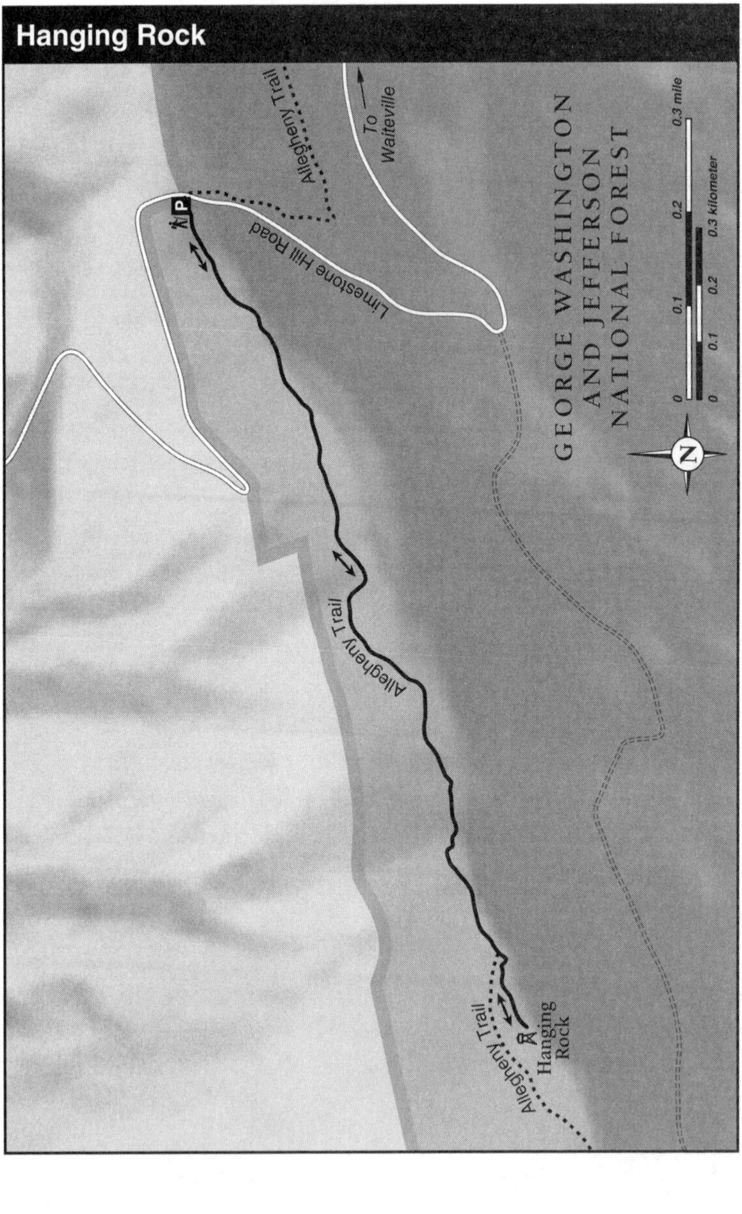
Hanging Rock
Allegheny Trail
To Waiteville
Limestone Hill Road
P
Allegheny Trail
Allegheny Trail
Hanging Rock
GEORGE WASHINGTON
AND JEFFERSON
NATIONAL FOREST
0 0.1 0.2 0.3 mile
0 0.1 0.2 0.3 kilometer
N

We enjoy just a mile of the Allegheny Trail en route to Hanging Rock. Leave west from the parking area in the gap on Peters Mountain, joining a singletrack path blazed in yellow—the Allegheny Trail. Gently climb from the gap into hardwoods rising above a rocky forest floor where ferns thrive in the summertime. The walking is easy. and you cut under a power-line clearing after a quarter-mile.

The trail becomes rocky then drops into a gap after a half-mile. Look for the old wire fence to the left of the trail, from days when livestock grazed Peters Mountain. The woods have grown up since then. Resume climbing, passing beneath huge boulder gardens above the trail.

At 0.9 mile, take the spur trail leading left toward the Hanging Rock observation tower. The Allegheny Trail keeps right, below the rock. The trailbed becomes much fainter on its journey to meet the Appalachian Trail a dozen miles distant. The spur path rises to the base of Hanging Rock, which really does overhang here and might even provide shelter from a storm. The trail cuts through a break in the stone then climbs just a bit farther to reach the top of Hanging Rock and the observation tower.

Commanding views can be had from the linear tilted outcrop extending along Peters Mountain, but the tower view is just a little bit higher. Inside the small structure stands a sitting table and lots of

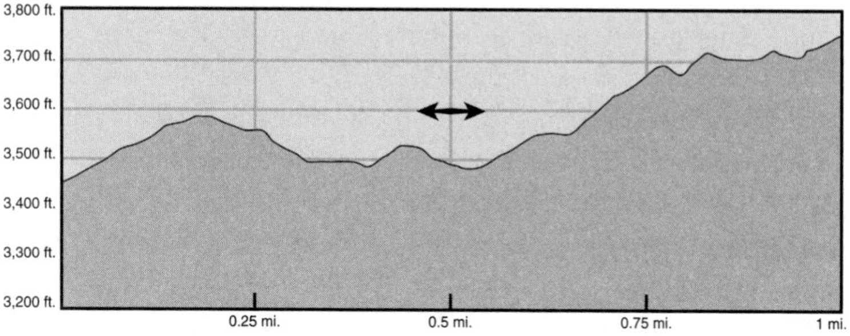

information about raptor counts, which have been undertaken annually from Hanging Rock since 1952. The migration counts are generally in mid-September, and 52-mile-long Peters Mountain is ideal for traveling hawks, eagles, osprey, and other birds of prey as the thermal air currents astride the long ridge help migrating birds expend less energy as they fly.

The view along Peters Mountain is every bit as worthy as that beyond the peak. Shoot for a clear day, and you'll be amply rewarded for your efforts reaching Hanging Rock.

Nearby Attractions

White Rocks Campground provides lesser-used wooded camps. Restrooms and water are available in season. Lots of hiking and fishing are within easy driving distance. The **Potts Valley Rail Trail** (page 67) is just a few miles from the hike to Hanging Rock.

Directions

From Exit 117 on I-81 near Christiansburg, take US 460 West 19 miles to VA 700 (Mountain Lake Road). Turn right onto VA 700 East and drive eat 7.3 miles to Mountain Lake. Here, Mountain Lake Road becomes VA 613. Stay with it another 6.4 miles (along the way the road becomes gravel), going over Potts Mountain to reach a stop sign. Turn right, staying with VA 613. Continue 1.1 miles, passing White Rocks Campground to reach a T-intersection. Turn right on paved VA 635. Drive east 1.2 miles to enter Monroe County, West Virginia, and join WV 17 East. Continue east to reach Waiteville, West Virginia, 5 miles after entering West Virginia. Turn left on Bert Williams Road (WV 15/3). Follow Bert Williams Road as it turns to gravel after 1.2 miles. At 2.6 miles, at a T-intersection, turn left onto paved Limestone Hill Road. Follow Limestone Hill 2 miles to the gap in Peters Mountain and the sign for Hanging Rock. Park here.

Alternative directions from Roanoke: From Exit 141 on I-81 just south of Roanoke, take VA 419 North 0.3 mile, then turn right on

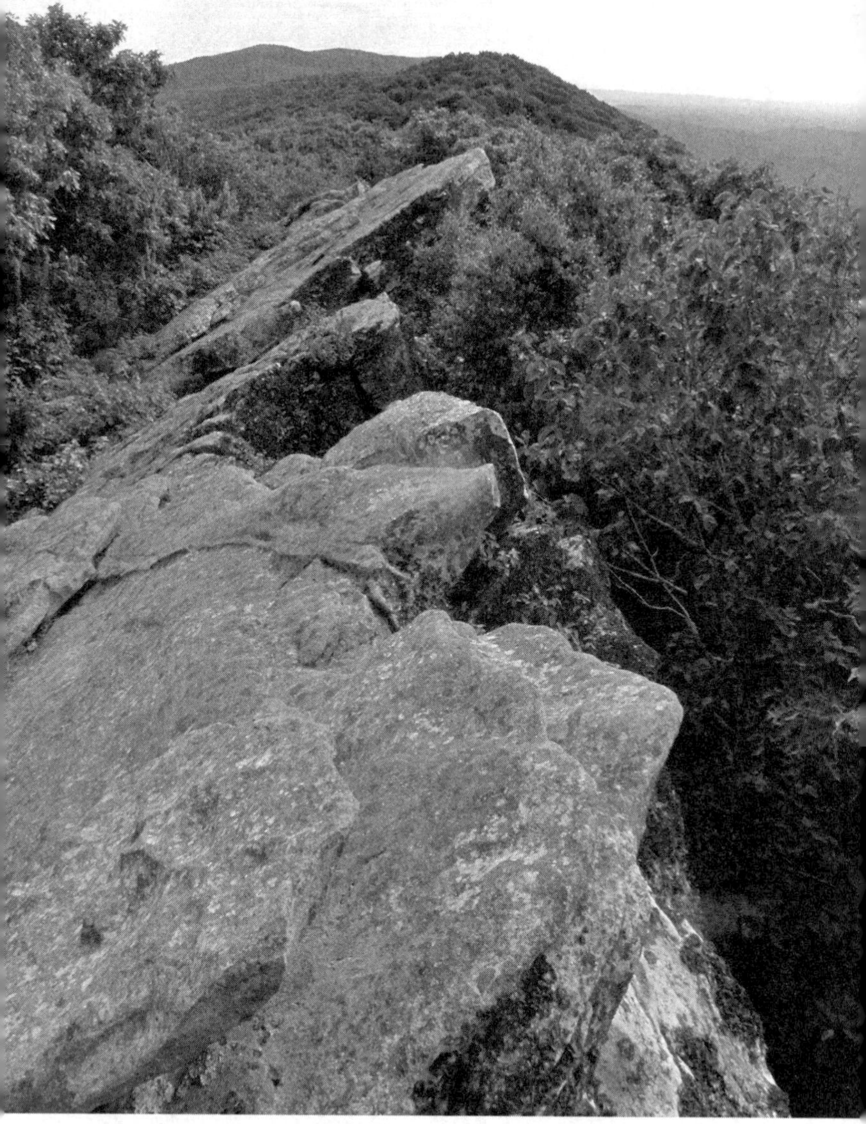

HANGING ROCK JUTS ABOVE THE CREST OF PETERS MOUNTAIN.

VA 311 North and follow it 35 miles to Paint Bank, Virginia. From there, take VA 600 West (Waiteville Road) into West Virginia for a total of 11.6 miles to reach Bert Williams Road; then follow the directions on the previous page.

Lower Craig Creek Valley

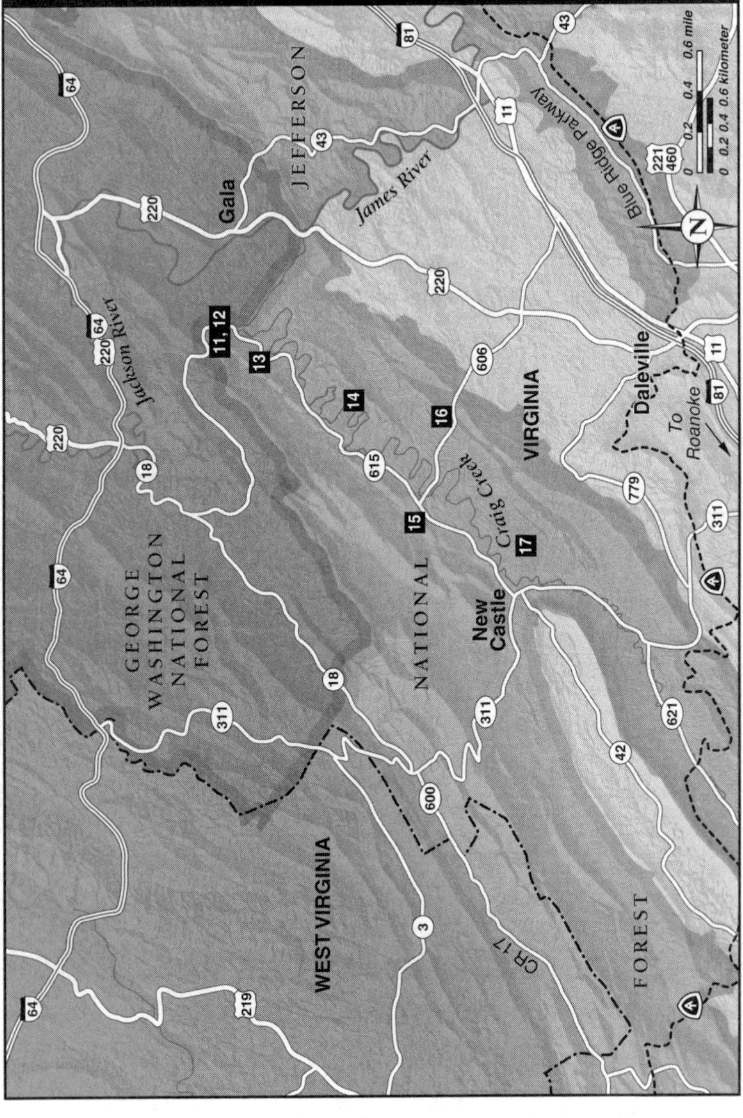

Lower Craig Creek Valley

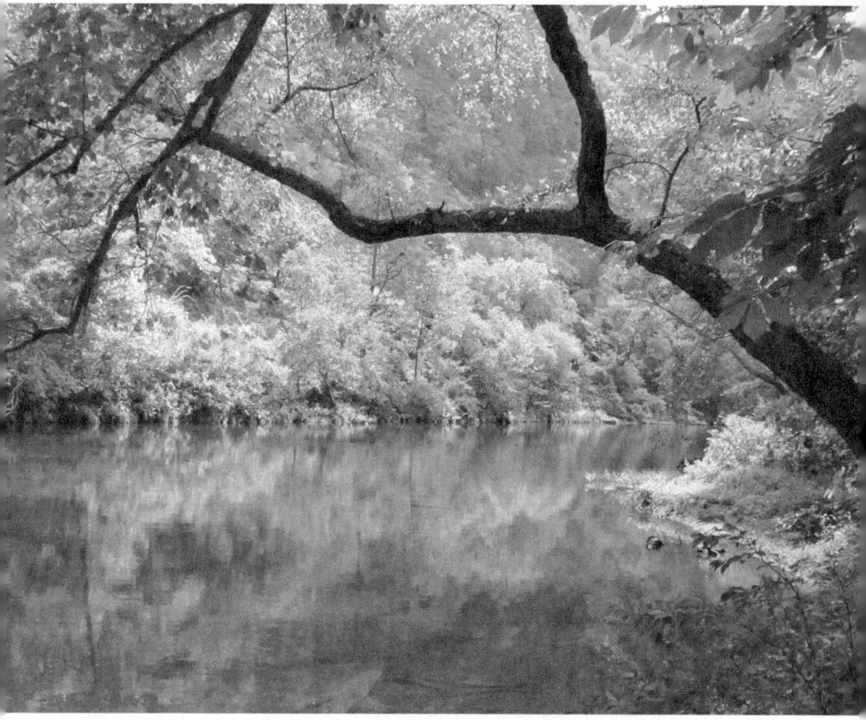

CRAIG CREEK IS ONE OF THE MOST SCENIC WATERSHEDS IN WESTERN VIRGINIA.
(See Hike 14, Craig Creek Loop Trail, page 95.)

11 Roaring Run Falls and Furnace

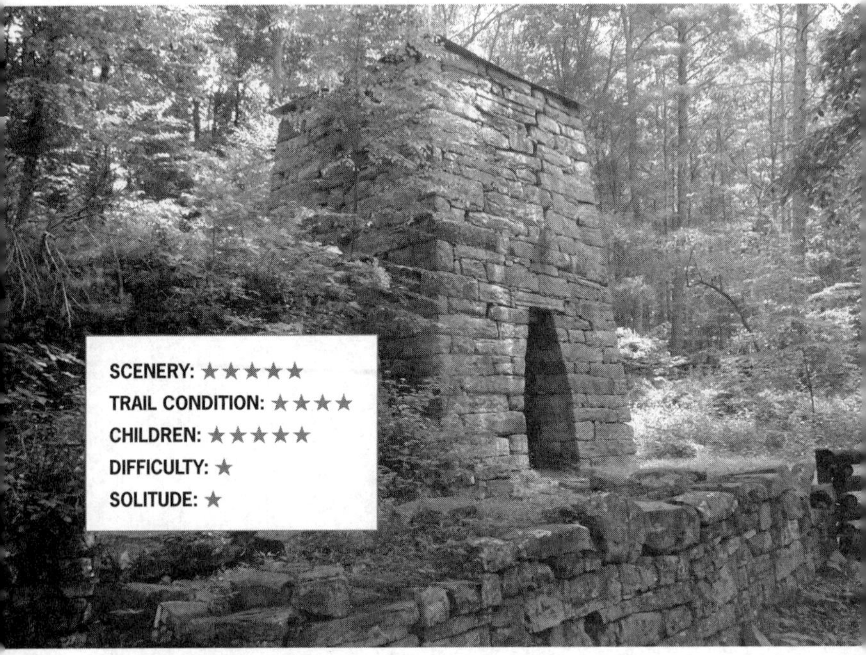

SCENERY: ★★★★★
TRAIL CONDITION: ★★★★
CHILDREN: ★★★★★
DIFFICULTY: ★
SOLITUDE: ★

ROARING RUN FURNACE HAS BEEN STANDING SINCE THE 1830S.

GPS TRAILHEAD COORDINATES: N37° 42.396' W79° 53.592'

DISTANCE & CONFIGURATION: 1.6-mile loop

HIKING TIME: 1 hour

OUTSTANDING FEATURES: Roaring Run Falls and other falls, intact iron ore furnace, picnicking

ELEVATION: 1,150 feet at trailhead, 1,450 feet at high point

ACCESS: No fees or permits required

MAPS: National Geographic #788, *Covington/Alleghany Highlands;* USGS *Strom*

FACILITIES: Picnic tables, vault toilets

WHEELCHAIR ACCESS: Along picnic area trail

INFO: George Washington & Jefferson National Forests, Eastern Divide Ranger District, 110 Southpark Drive, Blacksburg, VA 24060; 540-552-4641, www.fs.usda.gov/gwj

In Brief

This hike packs a lot into a short distance. First, revel in the stonework of the trailhead picnic area, and then visit Roaring Run Furnace, a stone edifice from the 1830s that once fashioned iron. Next, work your way through woods to a view, and visit a series of cascades capped by Roaring Run Falls. Finally, descend past more cataracts as you traverse the Roaring Run gorge.

Route Details

After seeing the numerous noisy cataracts along this hike, you'll agree that Roaring Run is aptly named. This tributary of Craig Creek cuts through the Rich Patch Mountains then dives through a gorge where it truly does roar—and creates falls aplenty—before emptying its waters into Craig Creek.

Back in the 1830s, John Garth and Benjamin Scruggs saw the energy potential of such falling water and purchased a 9,000-acre tract to build an iron ore furnace. These furnaces, essentially giant ovens made of stone, needed five things: stone, iron ore, limestone, rich forests, and water. The stone was needed to build the furnace. The iron ore and limestone were needed to make the final product. The forest was needed to make charcoal to fire the furnace. Water was needed to power the giant bellows used to raise temperatures inside the furnace to a point where iron could be made.

The valley of Roaring Run had all five. First, the furnace was built from cut stone quarried a mile away. Then a water diversion was dug from Roaring Run to power a waterwheel that in turn powered the bellows. The forests grew rich and magnificent in the Roaring Run Valley. Roaring Run Iron Works was incorporated, and the 36-foot-high furnace was built. By 1839, the furnace was operating, and over the next three decades furnace tenders smelted iron, allowing it to flow into molds. These molds were known as pigs, hence the term "pig iron."

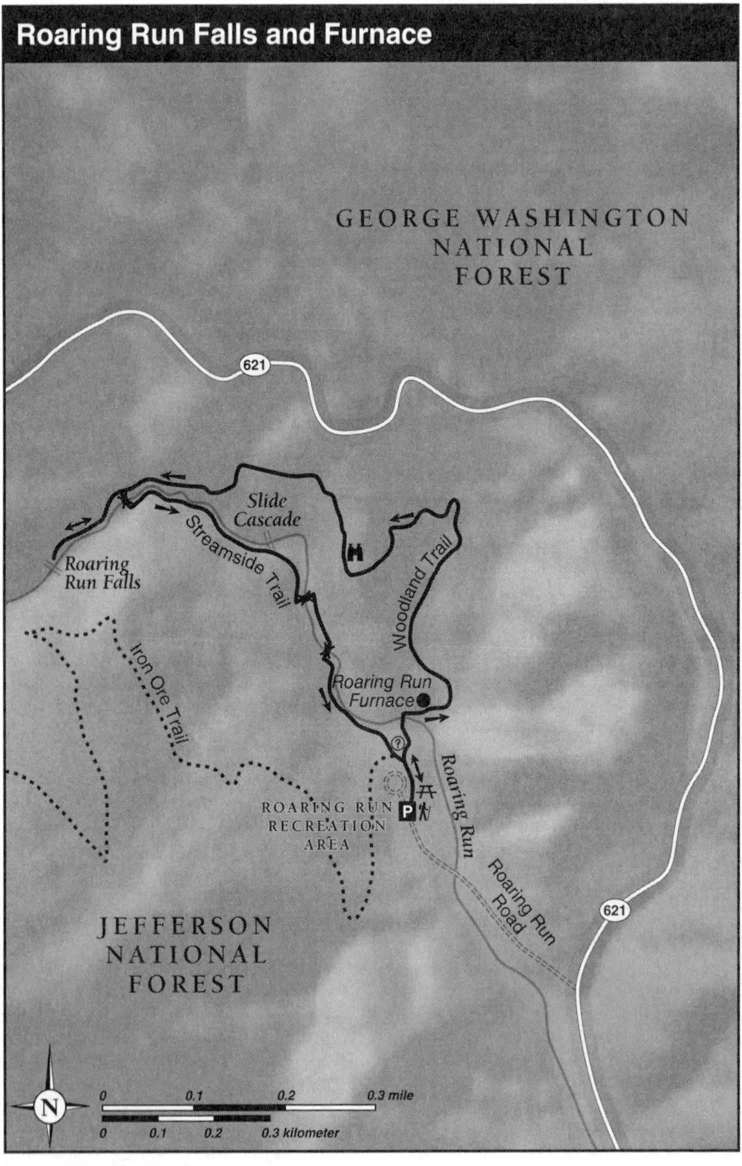
Roaring Run Falls and Furnace
GEORGE WASHINGTON NATIONAL FOREST
621
Slide Cascade
Roaring Run Falls
Streamside Trail
Woodland Trail
Iron Ore Trail
Roaring Run Furnace
ROARING RUN RECREATION AREA
Roaring Run
Roaring Run Road
621
JEFFERSON NATIONAL FOREST
N
0 0.1 0.2 0.3 mile
0 0.1 0.2 0.3 kilometer

Roaring Run Furnace went through several owners and was rebuilt in 1847. However, by 1855, the furnace cooled for the final time, and most of the equipment was sold at auction. In the 1880s, a New York financier began to reopen the furnace and did some nearby test digs for iron ore, but the plan fell through. Eventually, the property fell into the hands of the US Forest Service, which turned it into a recreation area. Today we have a trail system that complements the natural beauty that is Roaring Run.

Leave the parking area, passing around the attractive stone. Roaring Run and the picnic area are to your right. Quickly reach a trail intersection. Here, the Iron Ore Trail leaves left for the high country. The Streamside Trail heads straight up Roaring Run. Our loop turns right on the Woodland Trail to quickly pass a connector to the picnic area then bridge Roaring Run. Shortly reach Roaring Run Furnace standing tall and proud. Interpretive information adds context to the edifice. Curve around the former iron processing site, viewing it from different angles. Look for the blue-green slag on the forest floor.

The hike then curves away from the stream and furnace, meandering through woods that were surely cleared to power the furnace when it roared. Look for unnatural mounds of soil, test pits from the ore-searching days. Pines and oaks rise now above the piles. Climb up a draw, curve around a rib ridge, and open to a view above the

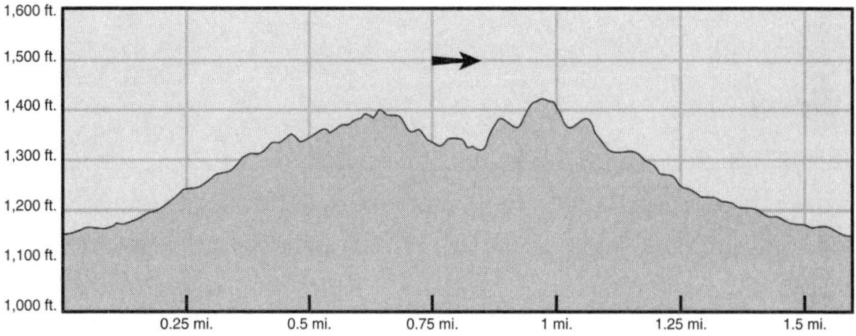

Roaring Run gorge at 0.6 mile. Shoemaker Knob rises across the chasm, as do the Rich Patch Mountains. Mud Run Mountain stands in the distance, while Roaring Run roars below.

Continue on the Woodland Trail, dropping to Roaring Run. Hike along a cliff, and reach a trail intersection at 0.9 mile. Turn right up this spur along Roaring Run. Lesser falls are already putting on a show as you climb past them. A 35-foot slide cascade dropping in four stages provides a warm-up. Wooden stairs and stone steps aid your climb in this jagged spot. Pass another fall with a huge swimming hole. Reach Roaring Run Falls at 1.0 mile. Here, the falls drop 35 feet over a vegetated rock face. Wide stone slabs border the cataract. Boulders lie in repose. It is truly a beauty spot.

Backtrack and then bridge Roaring Run on the Streamside Trail. Rock walls, boulders, and crashing water meld with forest to make "gorge-ous" scenes. Take your time descending this wild watershed. Pass a notable slide cascade at 1.3 miles, then bridge Roaring Run at 1.4 miles and 1.5 miles. You are now on the right-hand bank. Shortly complete the loop portion of the hike, then make a quick backtrack, completing the circuit.

Nearby Attractions

Access the **Hoop Hole National Recreation Trail** system either at Roaring Run Recreation Area or at an alternate trailhead a short distance down VA 615 toward the hamlet of Oriskany.

Directions

From Exit 150B on I-81, take US 220 North 8 miles to Fincastle and continue on US 220 for 12 more miles to VA 615 (Craig Creek Road) near Eagle Rock. Turn left on VA 615 and follow it 5.5 miles, then turn right on Roaring Run Road (VA 621). Follow Roaring Run Road 0.9 mile, then turn left into the Roaring Run Recreation Area, following it 0.3 mile to dead-end at the trailhead.

12 Upper Hoop Hole Hike

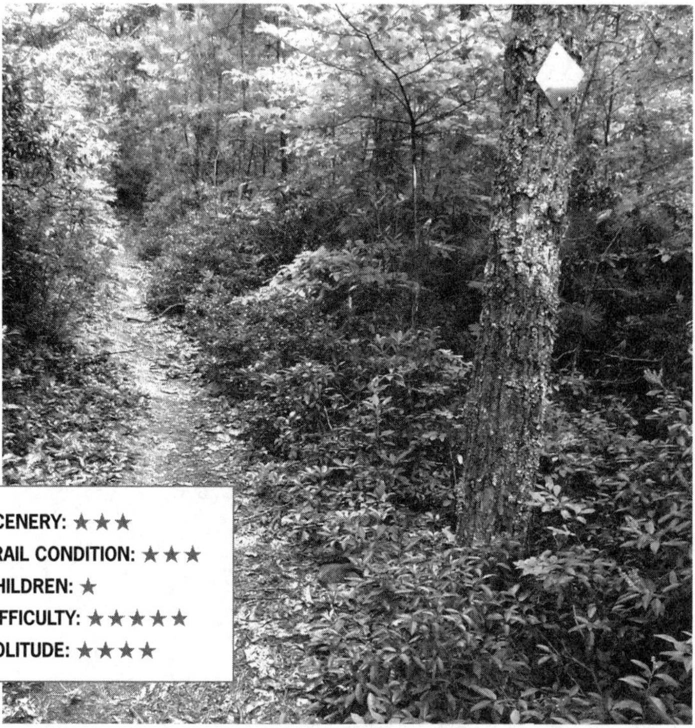

SCENERY: ★★★
TRAIL CONDITION: ★★★
CHILDREN: ★
DIFFICULTY: ★★★★★
SOLITUDE: ★★★★

ENJOY SOLITUDE AND TRAILSIDE SCENERY LIKE THIS ON THE UPPER HOOP HOLE TRAIL.

GPS TRAILHEAD COORDINATES: N37° 42.396' W79° 53.592'

DISTANCE & CONFIGURATION: 10.8-mile balloon loop

HIKING TIME: 6 hours

OUTSTANDING FEATURES: Solitude, some views, challenge

ELEVATION: 1,150 feet at trailhead, 3,340 feet at high point

ACCESS: No fees or permits required

MAPS: National Geographic #788, *Covington/Alleghany Highlands;* USGS *Strom*

FACILITIES: Picnic tables, vault toilets at trailhead

WHEELCHAIR ACCESS: Along picnic area trail at trailhead

INFO: George Washington & Jefferson National Forests, Eastern Divide Ranger District, 110 Southpark Drive, Blacksburg, VA 24060; 540-552-4641, www.fs.usda.gov/gwj

Upper Hoop Hole Hike

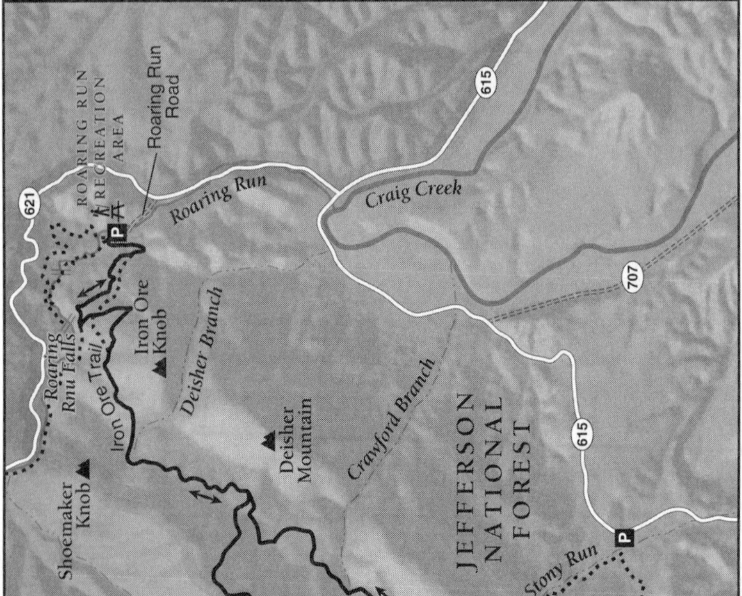

In Brief

Solitude lovers will enjoy this long and challenging but rewarding hike on a federally designated national recreation trail. Start by climbing from Roaring Run Recreation Area on the Iron Ore Trail. Ascend the Rich Patch Mountains, rising along stone outcrops and woods overlooking the Craig Creek Valley. Climb 2,200 feet before working your way back, crossing stony tributaries of Craig Creek. Be apprised that parts of this trail can be brushy during the warm season.

Route Details

The Hoop Hole National Recreation Trail system is overshadowed by the much shorter circuit hike traveling to Roaring Run Falls and Roaring Run Furnace, which starts at the same trailhead as this hike. That leaves the Hoop Hole area for adventurous hikers ready to tackle a lesser known destination. If you are looking for solitude and trial, this is the hike for you. You will be rewarded with partial views along the way. *Note:* During the warm season, long pants are recommended due to trailside brush and stinging nettle.

Leave the Roaring Run Recreation Area parking lot on a pea gravel track, passing the picnic area on your right. Shortly reach

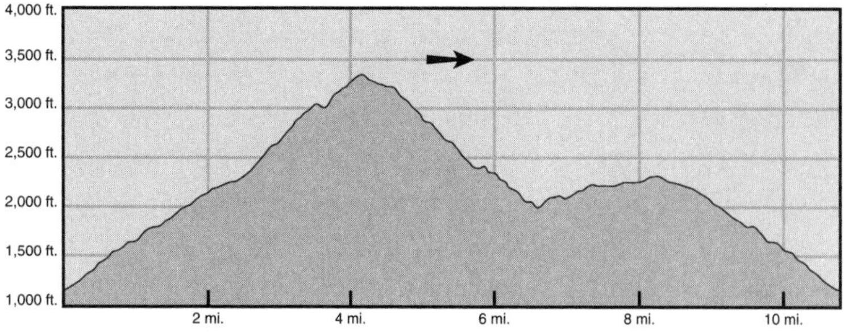

restrooms and the loop trail to Roaring Run Falls. Head left on the doubletrack Iron Ore Trail, named for Iron Ore Knob, which it nears. Trace a doubletrack path through pines and oaks, switchbacking up the east slope of Iron Ore Knob. Crisscross under a power line. At 0.7 mile, the path leads above Roaring Run Falls. You can hear the cataract, but it remains out of view. At 0.9 mile, the trail, blazed with plastic rectangles, leaves the roadbed and makes a gradual climb through oaks managed using prescribed fire. Rejoin the old roadbed at 1.2 miles, aiming for the upper reaches of Deisher Branch, which you cross at 1.8 miles. The branch may be dry. Look for a building foundation here.

Keep rising, alternating between gnarled xeric pine–mountain laurel woods and taller, straighter cove hardwoods. At 2.5 miles, reach a gap and trail intersection lying between Pine Mountain to the west and Deisher Mountain to the east. Leave right on the Upper Hoop Hole Trail, hiking uphill on a much narrower and fainter yet well-marked trail bordered in blueberries, pines, and chestnut oaks and pocked with reddish-mauve iron ore outcrops. Ascend the shoulder of Pine Mountain, working parallel to a linear rock outcrop. Partial views of the Craig Creek Valley and Patterson Mountain open south. Top out on the crest of Pine Mountain at 4.0 miles. You've climbed 2,200 feet. Glance north into the upper Roaring Run watershed and Alleghany County. Catch your breath.

The Upper Hoop Hole Trail leaves Pine Mountain, then stays below the crest of the crest of Rich Patch Mountain. Here begins the infamous section where stinging nettle thrives in summer. Enjoy a brief respite at 4.6 miles as you pass through a grassy gap with Bald Knob to your left. Descend through rocky woods, stepping over the uppermost tributaries of Hipes Branch—brushy spots in summer. At 5.4 miles, make a sharp switchback to the right, leaving the stinging nettle behind and coming alongside über-rocky Hipes Branch. Rock-hop the clear, moving stream at 5.7 miles. Hipes Branch dives into a gorge of its own making just below this crossing.

Keep downhill, meeting the west leg of the Lower Hoop Hole Trail at 6.4 miles. Stay left here, joining a much more worn-down trail tread. Hop over upper Stony Run, and meet the east leg of the Lower Hoop Hole Trail at 6.6 miles. Stay left, as the Lower Hoop Hole Trail leads right 1.2 miles through the Stony Run gorge to the parking area on Craig Creek Road. Our hike keeps left (northeast) once again on lesser used trailbed among pine, blueberry, and mountain laurel. Step over another tributary of Hipes Branch at 6.9 miles, then turn straight up a dry drainage.

At 7.3 miles, the Upper Hoop Hole Trail splits a gap with an unnamed knob rising to your right, then dips to cross the tiny upper reaches of Crawford Branch. Keep working northeast, curving around a couple of high coves to complete the Upper Hoop Hole Trail at 8.3 miles. From here, it's a 2.5-mile backtrack on the Iron Ore Trail. You will appreciate the wider trailbed and downward slope of the path on your reprise trip.

Nearby Attractions

From this same trailhead, you can visit Roaring Run Furnace, a stone edifice from the 1830s that once fashioned iron; hike to Roaring Run Falls and return via the Roaring Run gorge; enjoy a fine picnic area; and fish for trout.

Directions

From Exit 150B on I-81, take US 220 North 8 miles to Fincastle and continue on US 220 for 12 more miles to VA 615 (Craig Creek Road) near Eagle Rock. Turn left on VA 615 and follow it 5.5 miles to turn right on Roaring Run Road (VA 621). Follow Roaring Run Road 0.9 mile and turn left into the Roaring Run Recreation Area, following it 0.3 mile to dead-end at the trailhead.

13 Lower Hoop Hole Hike

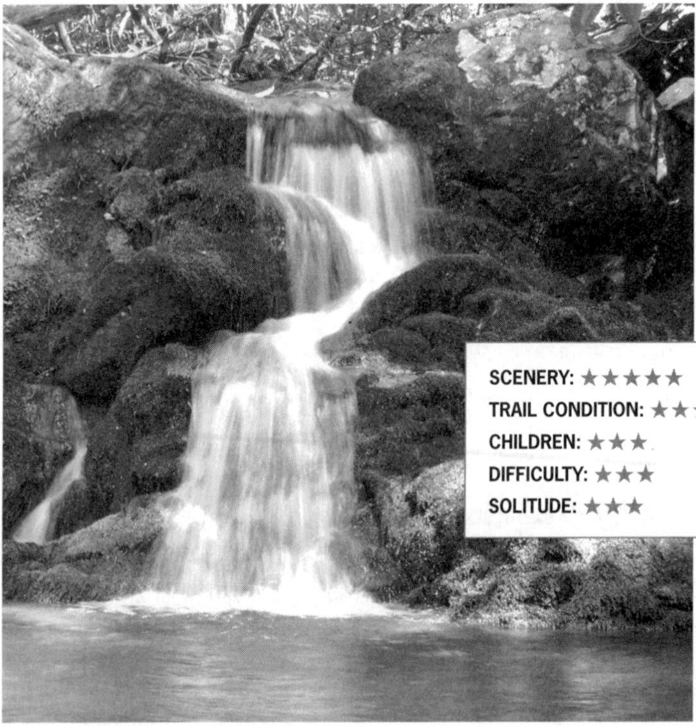

SCENERY: ★★★★★
TRAIL CONDITION: ★★★
CHILDREN: ★★★
DIFFICULTY: ★★★
SOLITUDE: ★★★

HIPES BRANCH TUMBLES WHITE INTO A COOL POOL.

GPS TRAILHEAD COORDINATES: N37° 40.369' W79° 55.062'

DISTANCE & CONFIGURATION: 3.3-mile loop

HIKING TIME: 2 hours

OUTSTANDING FEATURES: Rocky gorges, waterfall, pools

ELEVATION: 1,305 feet at trailhead, 2,035 feet at high point

ACCESS: No fees or permits required

MAPS: National Geographic #788, *Covington/Alleghany Highlands;* USGS *Strom*

FACILITIES: None

WHEELCHAIR ACCESS: None

INFO: George Washington & Jefferson National Forests, Eastern Divide Ranger District, 110 Southpark Drive, Blacksburg, VA 24060; 540-552-4641, www.fs.usda.gov/gwj

In Brief

This hike is truly deserving of its National Recreation Trail designation. Start the adventure by entering the Stony Run canyon, crisscrossing the alternating cascade-and-pool-filled stream 11 times while ascending through a world of geological amazement where cliffs, boulders, and crags fashion a rocky picture. Next, stroll a pleasant upland vale before dropping along Hipes Branch, where more pools and falls await.

Route Details

This hike, which explores the area between Craig Creek and Bald Knob, traverses a pair of gorges cutting their way from the heights of Bald Knob in the Rich Patch Mountains north of Roanoke to their mother stream, Craig Creek. You'll be surprised at the exposed geology of these watersheds, as water and time have carved narrow passages between craggy cliffs, a sea of boulders, rocks, and pebbles contrasting in their stillness with the ever-descending crystalline streams.

Be forewarned that your ascent through the Stony Run gorge requires 11 bridgeless stream crossings, but under normal flows they will all be simple rock-hops you can do dry-footed. Moreover, if the water is very low, as it can be during late summer and autumn, then you can go ahead and scoff at the warning.

Leave the Hoop Hole parking area, passing an informative trail kiosk. Drop to quickly reach Stony Run, which gently courses over rock beds, belying its altogether different nature upstream. Just after the crossing, reach the loop portion of the Lower Hoop Hole Trail. Stay right, heading up Stony Run in gently sloping, rocky woods—former pastureland. The path comes alongside the stream. By 0.4 mile, the valley narrows and you enter the gorge. Sycamores rise along the stream.

The singletrack path steepens. Make your first crossing of Stony Run at 0.6 mile. Rock bluffs rise on either side of the path. Rhododendron finds its place in the cool vale. The crossings come

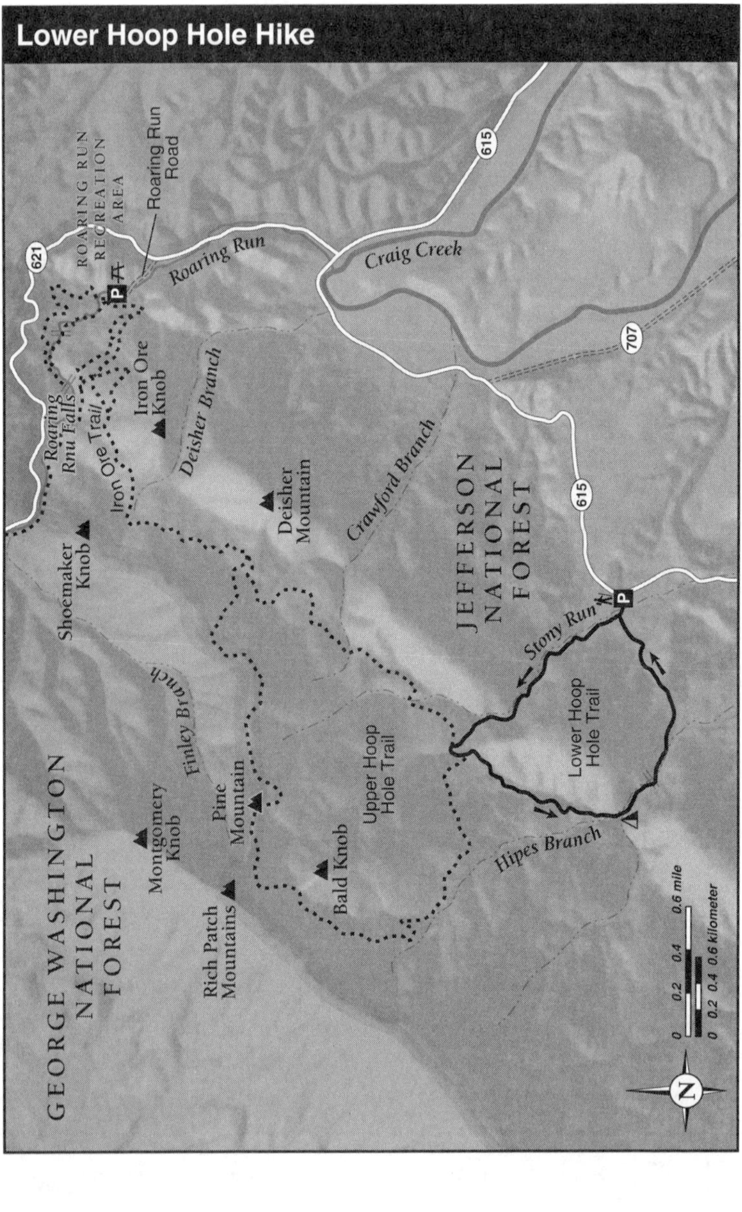
Lower Hoop Hole Hike
621
ROARING RUN RECREATION AREA
Roaring Run Road
615
Roaring Run
Craig Creek
707
Roaring Run Falls
Iron Ore Trail
Iron Ore Trail
Iron Ore Knob
Deisher Branch
Deisher Mountain
Crawford Branch
JEFFERSON NATIONAL FOREST
615
Shoemaker Knob
Stony Run
Finley Branch
Lower Hoop Hole Trail
Upper Hoop Hole Trail
Pine Mountain
Montgomery Knob
Bald Knob
Hipes Branch
GEORGE WASHINGTON NATIONAL FOREST
Rich Patch Mountains
0 0.2 0.4 0.6 mile
0 0.2 0.4 0.6 kilometer
N

fast and furious in the nadir of the canyon. Massive pale boulders—tattooed in lichens and moss—impress. Big, trouty pools far outstrip the size of the stream. Make your ninth crossing by 0.9 mile. You are on the left bank. Rise above Stony Run before returning to make another crossing at 1.1 miles. From here, leave the stream and reach a trail intersection at 1.2 miles. To your right the Upper Hoop Hole Trail leads right 1.7 miles to the Iron Ore Trail and another 2.5 miles to Roaring Run Recreation Area.

Our hike leads left, still on the Lower Hoop Hole Trail. Dip to cross Stony Run an 11th and final time. Meet the other leg of the Upper Hoop Hole Trail in a gap at 1.4 miles. Stay left on the Lower Hoop Hole Trail, aiming southwest in pine–oak–laurel woods mixed with black gum and sourwood trees. Enter a quiet, widening cove where a tributary of Hipes Branch trickles under patches of rhododendron. This perched valley evokes the gentle side of the mountains, contrasting with the crashing Stony Run gorge.

At 1.9 miles, pass some metal relics of mankind, then turn into a rhododendron thicket where several streams gather. Find a campsite on the right just before crossing Hipes Branch at 2.1 miles. Deep pools form between noisy rapids. At 2.2 miles, hop over to the left bank. Ahead, a short, rough trail leads right to a pool deeper than

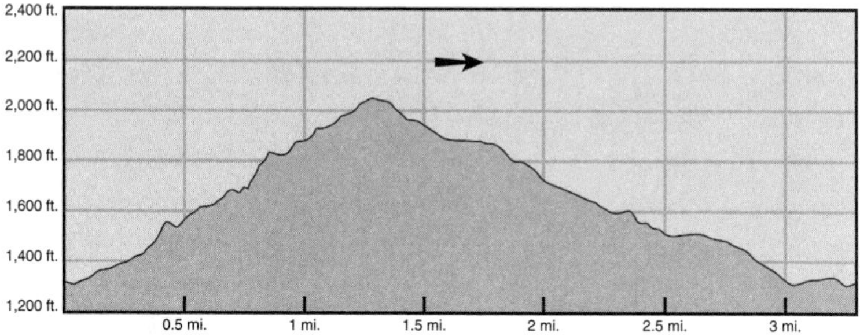

a grown man's height, just below an 8-foot cascade spilling over a mossy lip. The size of the pools relative to the size of the streams continues to amaze.

Keep cutting through Hipes Branch gorge, and look for big rock walls. Step over to the right bank at 2.3 miles. Skirt under a high bluff amid rhododendron, and make your final crossing at 2.4 miles; you are on the left bank. From here, Hipes Branch follows gravity's orders, eventually to feed Craig Creek, while the Lower Hoop Hole Trail peels away from Hipes Branch after emerging from the heart of the canyon, then turns northeast. Trailside vegetation becomes dominated again by pines and oaks on a gentle slope. Galax lines the path. The trailbed is sandy in spots.

The walking is easy as you descend through former farmland, now a tree-covered flat. Reach the other end of the Lower Hoop Hole Trail, then backtrack, completing the circuit at 3.3 miles.

Nearby Attractions

The **Roaring Run Recreation Area** is nearby. There, you can visit Roaring Run Furnace, a stone edifice from the 1830s that once fashioned iron; hike to Roaring Run Falls and return via the Roaring Run gorge; enjoy a fine picnic area; and fish for trout.

Directions

From Exit 150B on I-81, take US 220 North 8 miles to Fincastle and continue on US 220 for 12 more miles to VA 615 (Craig Creek Road) near Eagle Rock. Turn left on VA 615 and follow it 8 miles, then turn right into the Hoop Hole trailhead. (*Note:* You will pass the signed right turn toward Roaring Run Recreation Area 2.5 miles before you reach the trailhead.)

14 Craig Creek Loop Trail

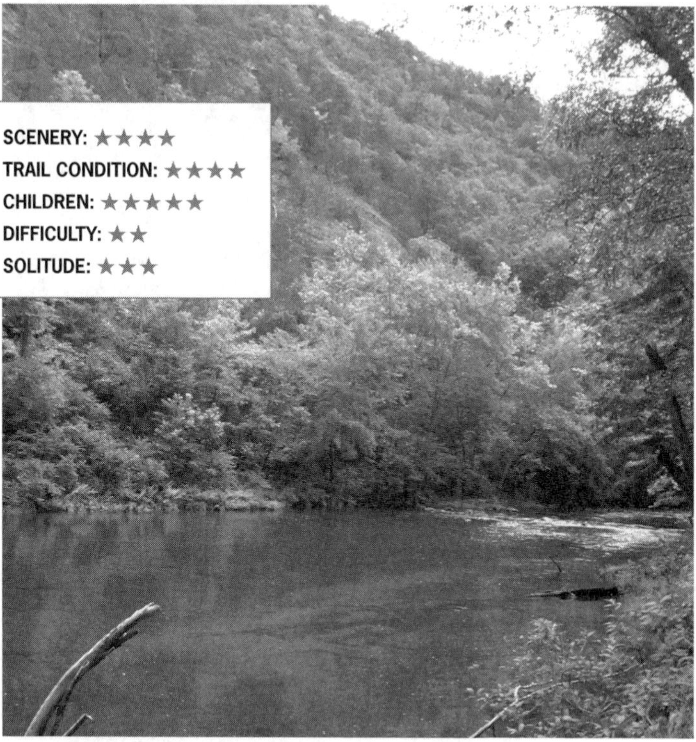

SCENERY: ★★★★
TRAIL CONDITION: ★★★★
CHILDREN: ★★★★★
DIFFICULTY: ★★
SOLITUDE: ★★★

CRAIG CREEK FLOWS CLEAR BENEATH PATTERSON MOUNTAIN.

GPS TRAILHEAD COORDINATES: N37° 36.800' W79° 57.383'

DISTANCE & CONFIGURATION: 1.9-mile loop

HIKING TIME: 1 hour

OUTSTANDING FEATURES: Mountain views, creek views, picnicking, swimming, fishing

ELEVATION: 1,095 feet at trailhead, 1,230 feet at high point

ACCESS: No fees or permits required

MAPS: National Geographic #788, *Covington/Alleghany Highlands;* USGS *Oriskany*

FACILITIES: Restrooms, picnic area at trailhead

WHEELCHAIR ACCESS: None

INFO: George Washington & Jefferson National Forests, Eastern Divide Ranger District, 110 Southpark Drive, Blacksburg, VA 24060; 540-552-4641, www.fs.usda.gov/gwj

Craig Creek Loop Trail

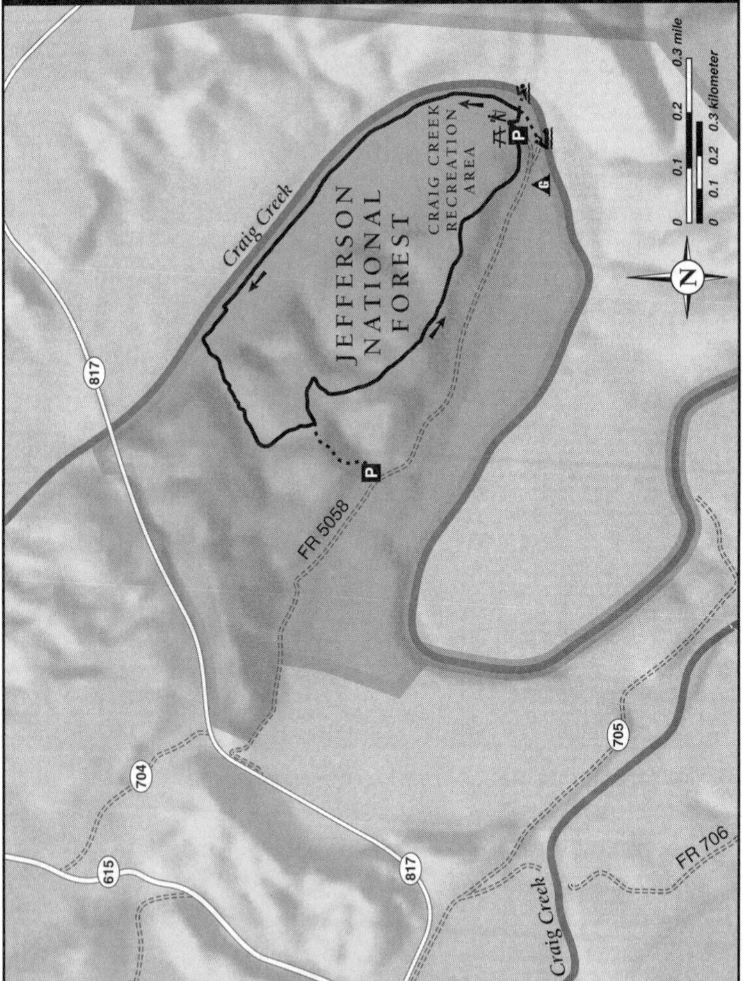

In Brief

This hike makes a circuit along lower Craig Creek as it bends in the shadow of the mountains. It's set at a fine national forest recreation area, so you can pair this fun family hike with water sports such as fishing, swimming, kayaking, or tubing. Also, enjoy the view from the picnic area, located at the trailhead.

Route Details

The Craig Creek Valley, located in the mountains west of Roanoke, is one of the most scenic watersheds in the Old Dominion. Flowing from southwest to northeast, Craig Creek originates just north of Blacksburg in Montgomery County, hemmed in by Sinking Creek Mountain to the north and Brush Mountain to the south. This clear trickle drains a mix of farms dotting bottomlands as well as wooded ridges of the Jefferson National Forest. Craig Creek enters Craig County and flows through the town of New Castle, where it leaves Sinking Creek Mountain behind. The valley widens and Craig Creek begins curving in huge arcs, with fertile bottomlands lying between these bends. The lowermost part of the stream flows through Botetourt County in the shadow of the Rich Patch Mountains and Patterson Mountain, finally meeting the James River at Eagle Rock, Virginia.

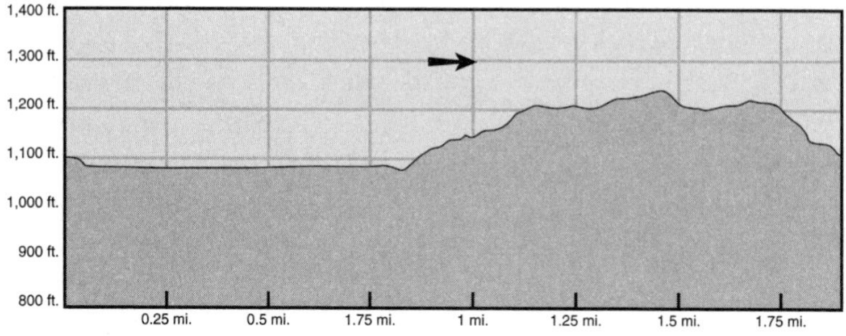

This normally clear stream is renowned for its smallmouth bass fishing, as well as paddling opportunities on its lower reaches. The paddling presents Class I–II rapids, perfect for family recreational floats or anglers plying the stream.

Part of the lowermost stream of Craig Creek is held by the Jefferson National Forest. Here, in a huge bend beneath pine and evergreen bluffs of Patterson Mountain, lies the Craig Creek Recreation Area, where visitors can not only paddle, float, swim, or fish Craig Creek but also picnic—and hike. A fun little circuit hike starts at the picnic area and makes the locale a worthy addition to this guide.

The trailhead offers great views. A small meadow beside the picnic area reveals a gorgeous panorama of the Rich Patch Mountains rising 2,500 feet over Craig Creek. So if you are feeling lazy, then have a picnic, enjoy this view, and call it good. However, if you want to see more—and there is more—take the Craig Creek Loop Trail heading east from the picnic area parking lot. A singletrack path makes a quick downhill switchback then descends to a grassy picnic area bordered with trees. Here, a trail leads right to the canoe access. There is another signed national forest canoe access upstream on VA 615 a little west of Oriskany. Another trail leads straight to a fine swimming hole, the deepest parts of which are over your head. This is also where anglers can be found.

At 0.1 mile, the Craig Creek Loop Trail heads left and parallels Craig Creek downstream under a canopy of ironwood, pawpaw, and tulip trees. The path follows an old farm road and makes for easy walking. User-created water accesses split right from the path. To your left a mix of forest and field becomes more forest every day. Gape across the water at the massive rock bluff pocked with cedars rising high above Craig Creek, part of Patterson Mountain. Chattering shoals divide lazy pools, and gravel bars are exposed in summer. Herons regally pose as they wait to strike minnows.

At 0.7 mile, the old road you've been following leaves right to a former ford. It is a good, shallow place for a road to cross, but these days it's just an informal river access. The Craig Creek Loop Trail briefly turns away from the water, only to follow it again. At 0.8 mile, the path abruptly turns left and crosses a small meadow that may be overgrown in summer. Stick with the plastic diamond blazes, and enter a shockingly steep-sided hollow cut by a small rill—a complete contrast to the wide streamside woods of Craig Creek. Hug the streambed.

At 1.1 miles, the Craig Creek Loop Trail cuts left, up a side drainage of the stream you've been following. Climb into woods of pine, mountain laurel, maple, and black gum. Reach a trail intersection at 1.2 miles, where a spur trail goes right to an alternate parking area and trailhead. We cut left, staying on the main loop. The rest of the hike is an easy walk through pines and oaks. Make sure to make a hard right turn at a power line you near, then pass under it at 1.4 miles. Patterson Mountain forms a backdrop through the trees. Drift down to an open meadow and reach the trailhead and picnic area at 1.9 miles, completing the circuit hike.

Nearby Attractions

The **Roaring Run Recreation Area** is just a few miles away off VA 615. There, you can visit Roaring Run Furnace, a stone edifice from the 1830s that once fashioned iron; hike to Roaring Run Falls and return via the Roaring Run gorge; enjoy a fine picnic area; and fish for trout. The **Hoop Hole National Recreation Trail** system is a few miles east on VA 615 and offers still more hiking opportunities.

Directions

From Exit 141 on I-81 just south of Roanoke, take VA 419 North 0.3 mile, then turn right on VA 311 North and follow it 19 miles to New Castle. From the intersection of VA 311, VA 42, and VA 615 in downtown New Castle, take VA 615 (Craig Creek Road) 11.9 miles to Oriskany. Turn right on VA 817/Old Rail Road and follow it 0.5 mile, then turn right onto the signed gravel road, Forest Road 5058, leading to Craig Creek Recreation Area. Dead-end at the picnic area after 1.3 miles. Join the Craig Creek Loop Trail here.

15 Fenwick Mines Walk

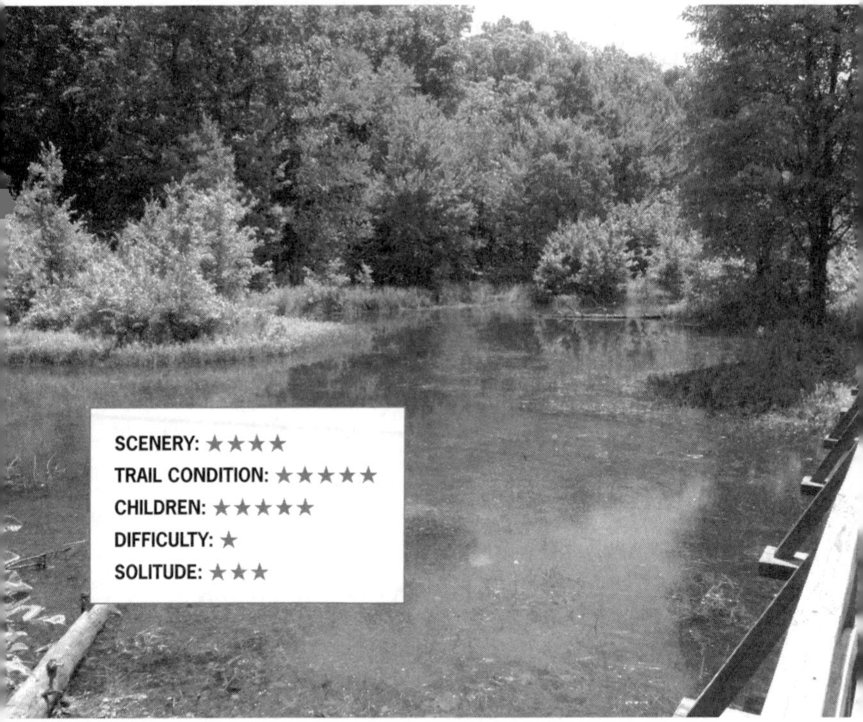

SCENERY: ★★★★
TRAIL CONDITION: ★★★★★
CHILDREN: ★★★★★
DIFFICULTY: ★
SOLITUDE: ★★★

WALK AMONG MOUNTAIN WETLANDS ON THIS HIKE.

GPS TRAILHEAD COORDINATES: N37° 34.104' W80° 3.339'

DISTANCE & CONFIGURATION: 1.9-mile double out-and-back

HIKING TIME: 1 hour

OUTSTANDING FEATURES: Pond, wetlands, waterfall, mining history

ELEVATION: 1,370 feet at trailhead, 1,410 feet at high point

ACCESS: No fees or permits required

MAPS: National Geographic #788, *Covington/Alleghany Highlands;* USGS *New Castle*

FACILITIES: Picnic shelter, vault restrooms, picnic area

WHEELCHAIR ACCESS: Yes, for entire trail

INFO: George Washington & Jefferson National Forests, Eastern Divide Ranger District, 110 Southpark Drive, Blacksburg, VA 24060; 540-552-464, www.fs.usda.gov/gwj

In Brief

This is an easy walk, fun for all ages. It explores the natural and cultural history of what was once a mining community. Today, a pair of all-access trails visit a pond, wetlands, and remnants of Fenwick. You will also wander down Mill Creek Valley to a surprisingly scenic waterfall.

Route Details

Back in the late 1800s, iron ore was discovered in the lower Craig Creek Valley, northeast of New Castle around Mill Creek, a tributary of Craig Creek. And by 1890, the Low Moor Iron Company established an iron ore mine and town named Fenwick. *Fen* is another word for "wetland," and the stretch of Mill Creek where the mine and community was located is a wetland to this day. Back then Fenwick boasted more than 300 residents and was even larger than New Castle, the seat of Craig County.

In addition to the mine and its facilities, such as a generating plant, ore-processing center, and loading dock, there stood a commissary, a hospital, a school, two churches, and even a playhouse. The residents were also served with a company clubhouse, and the company provided housing for their employees—black, white, and recently arrived Italian immigrants—all of whom lived in segregated sections of the town. Families rented individual dwellings while single men stayed in boardinghouses. Like many mining towns of the time, employees were paid in scrip, which could be used at the commissary. Monthly rent and other expenses were deducted from the scrip. However, it could be exchanged for dollars, and the Italian immigrants wanted dollars. It was said their goal was to save $1,000 and then return to their home country, where they could live well.

Today, no one lives in Fenwick, and there is surprisingly little evidence of the once bustling town and mine that thrived for 36 years. The most obvious trace is the stained upper segment of Mill Creek, where exposed iron ore gives the water a reddish tint. In addition to that, visitors can also see spoil piles of rock, the concrete abutments

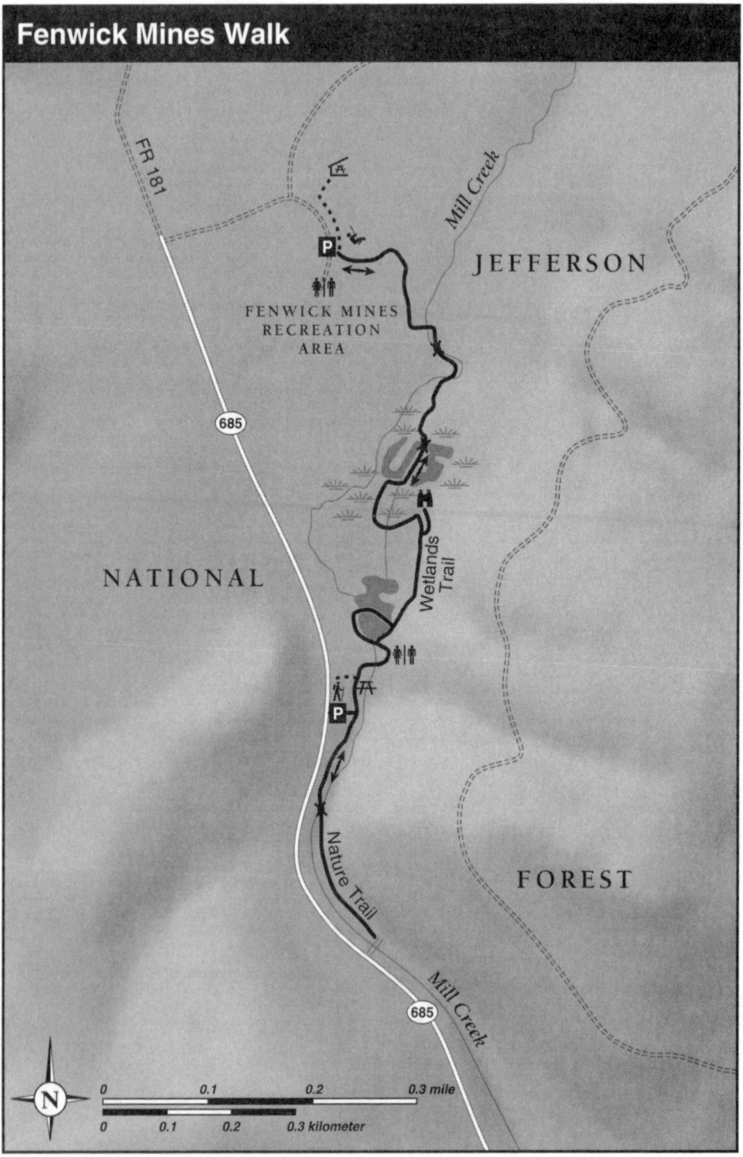
Fenwick Mines Walk
FR 181
Mill Creek
JEFFERSON
FENWICK MINES
RECREATION
AREA
685
NATIONAL
Wetlands
Trail
Nature Trail
FOREST
685
Mill Creek
N
0
0.1
0.2
0.3 mile
0
0.1
0.2
0.3 kilometer

of a bridge, and a few perennial flowers that rise from old homesites. The land is now owned by the US Forest Service and is a recreation area where we can explore the former mining community and the wildlife-rich wetlands.

Even the rail line linking Fenwick to the rest of the world has been completely dismantled. A branch of the Chesapeake and Ohio Railroad once ran through the Craig Creek Valley, with a spur track to the Fenwick mines. After the mines closed, the mine spur was abandoned. The Craig Creek Valley train ran less and less until it too was abandoned in 1958 and the tracks removed three years later.

Our visit to Fenwick mines leaves the VA 685 trailhead and heads left on the all-access Wetlands Trail. Walk just a few feet, passing through a picnic area and another trailhead access. Shortly cross Mill Creek on a footbridge. Notice the reddish tint from mining days. Pass some restrooms, then come to a fishing pond at 0.1 mile. Circle the auburn-colored little body of water, and then continue toward the Mill Creek wetlands. A hill rises to your right. Note the irregular spoil piles to your left. The terrain simply looks unnatural, and it is. At 0.3 mile, walk up the short distance to the overlook. If the overlook has been recently cleared, you can peer down on the Mill Creek wetlands below.

Beyond the overlook, a boardwalk and bridge take you through the wetlands, and benches are scattered along the trailside. Look for

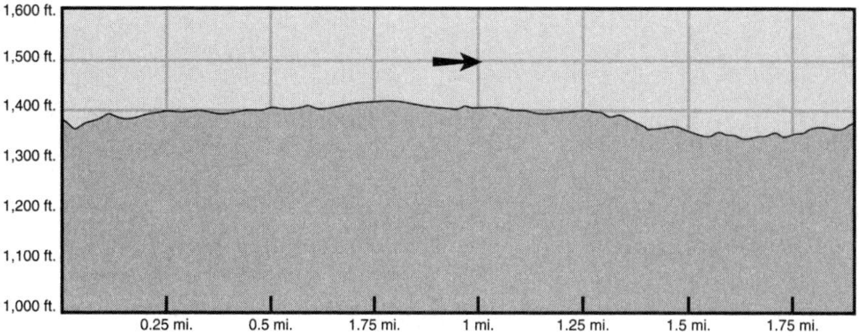

evidence of beavers. The level track spans Mill Creek on a bridge at 0.6 mile. Wander through flatwoods, then reach the Fenwick alternate parking and picnic area at 0.7 mile. A short spur path continues to the Fenwick picnic shelter.

From here, backtrack to the main trailhead, reaching it at 1.4 miles. This time take the Nature Trail downstream along Mill Creek. This is also a wheelchair-accessible trail. Walk the margin in woods, with VA 685 to your right and Mill Creek to your left, before soon bridging Mill Creek. After a quarter-mile, the trail ends at an observation deck overlooking a waterfall on Mill Creek. The spiller tumbles about 15 feet over stairstep ledges into a surprisingly large and deep pool bordered by a stone amphitheater, parts of which overhang the stream below. A gravel bar borders the waterfall pool. User-created trails lead to the top and bottom of the cataract. After you view the fall, it's just a quarter-mile back to the trailhead.

Nearby Attractions

The Pines Campground, a national forest facility, offers tent-camping sites in the cool of the Barbours Creek valley. The campground is open April–November and is accessible to other nearby paths in the national forest, such as Hipes Branch Trail and Potts Cove Trail.

Directions

From Exit 141 on I-81 just south of Roanoke, take VA 419 North 0.3 mile, then turn right on VA 311 North and follow it 19 miles to New Castle. From the intersection of VA 311, VA 42, and VA 615 in downtown New Castle, take VA 615 (Craig Creek Road) 5.1 miles to a four-way intersection. Turn left on Peaceful Valley Road (VA 611) and follow it 0.1 mile. Turn right on VA 685 and follow it 1.1 miles to the parking area on your right.

16 Sulphur Ridge Circuit

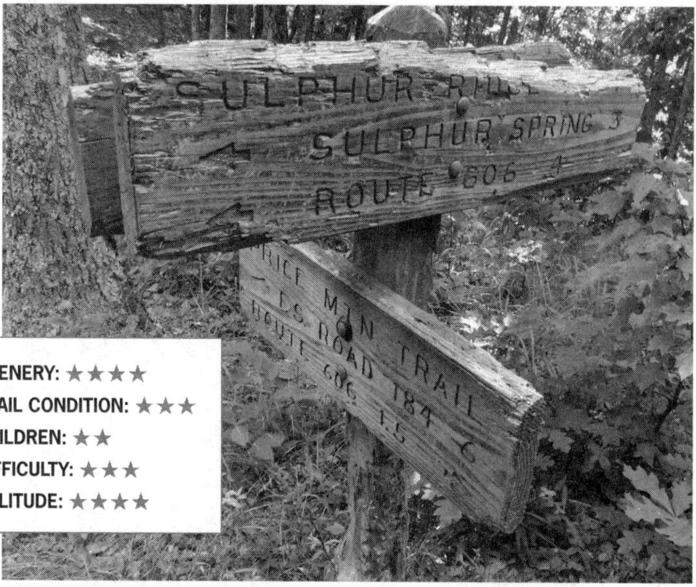

SCENERY: ★★★★
TRAIL CONDITION: ★★★
CHILDREN: ★★
DIFFICULTY: ★★★
SOLITUDE: ★★★★

BEARS USE THIS SIGN AS A TERRITORY-MARKING POST, GIVING IT A RUSTIC ASPECT.

GPS TRAILHEAD COORDINATES: N37° 32.655' W79° 58.099'

DISTANCE & CONFIGURATION: 4.7-mile loop

HIKING TIME: 2.5 hours

OUTSTANDING FEATURES: Solitude, vistas

ELEVATION: 1,970 feet at trailhead, 2,640 feet at high point, 1,390 feet at low point

ACCESS: No fees or permits required

MAPS: National Geographic #788, *Covington/Alleghany Highlands;* USGS *Oriskany*

FACILITIES: None

WHEELCHAIR ACCESS: None

INFO: George Washington & Jefferson National Forests, Eastern Divide Ranger District, 110 Southpark Drive, Blacksburg, VA 24060; 540-552-4641, www.fs.usda.gov/gwj

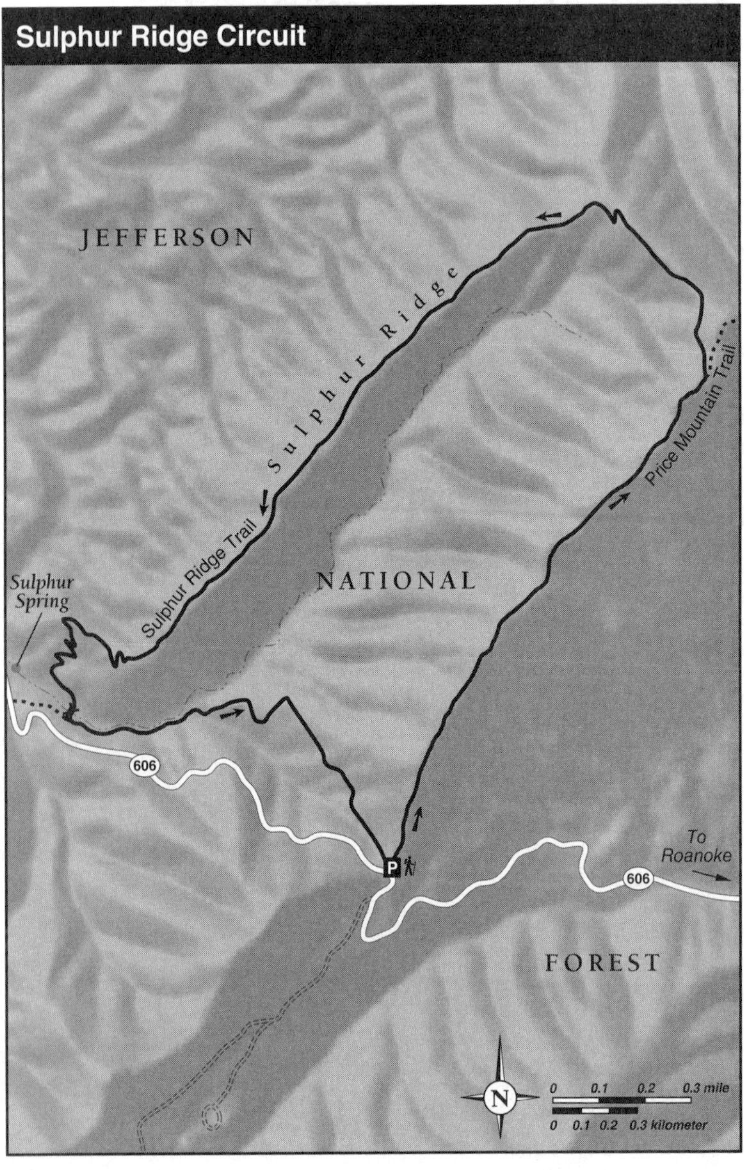
Sulphur Ridge Circuit
JEFFERSON
NATIONAL
FOREST
Sulphur Ridge
Sulphur Ridge Trail
Price Mountain Trail
Sulphur Spring
606
606
To Roanoke
0 0.1 0.2 0.3 mile
0 0.1 0.2 0.3 kilometer
N

In Brief

This is an often overlooked loop hike. Starting at a gap on Price Mountain, the circuit rises steeply on Price Mountain then runs the ridge, offering easterly views before joining piney Sulphur Ridge. Soak in scattered vistas of adjacent ridges and valleys before making a dive to an unnamed stream. Cross this stream, and then pick up an old wagon track turned trail, climbing back to the gap on Price Mountain.

Route Details

You will immediately discover that this hike has a few ups and downs. The first half-mile climbs 500 feet, nearly double the average gradient of national forest mountain trails. Nevertheless, do not let that dissuade you, since your legs and lungs will be fresh. Besides, we all need a challenge, don't we? You probably won't notice the scenery that first half-mile, but this loop provides eye-pleasing landscapes both near and far, whether you are traipsing underneath chestnut oaks interspersed with lichen-covered rocks or wandering pine needle–covered paths partly shaded by evergreens. Of course, there is a little aquatic action, too, at the lowest point of the hike, where you crisscross a stream before your final ascent.

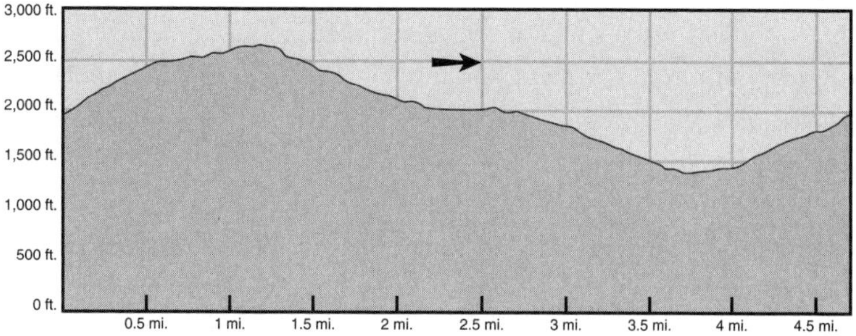

Start the circuit on the Price Mountain Trail. March east and upward in rocky woods flush with sassafras. Sassafras trees are easy to identify: Their leaves have three basic shapes: oval, three-lobed, and mitten-shaped. Mature trees have reddish-brown, deeply furrowed bark. Mostly an understory plant in the forest, these trees are known for their aromatic scent. Scratch the bark away from a twig, and the sweet smell is unmistakable. American Indians used sassafras for medicinal purposes, and pioneers and even people today make tea from boiling the roots. Birds eat the berries, and the wood, which shrinks when dried, is used for fence posts and hand tools. Sassafras trees can be found all over the Old Dominion and the South, though they do range to lower Michigan and even into Massachusetts.

Straddle the nose of the ridge, ever upward—no messing around with switchbacks here. Upturned rock slabs rise from the ground floor. Wintertime views open into the Catawba Creek Valley and points east. The last part of the ascent has a few nearly level spots. Reach a gap at 0.6 mile. *Whew!* What a climb.

Undulate still upward on the narrow ridge of Price Mountain. Make a short but solid pull at 1.0 mile. At 1.3 miles, reach a trail junction. Here, the Price Mountain Trail keeps straight 6 more miles. But this hike heads left, joining the Sulphur Ridge Trail. Angle left on the slope of Price Mountain to soon join a rib ridge. The singletrack footpath drops quickly amid scattered craggy pines and black gum. Views open of the Craig Creek Valley below and Bald Mountain beyond. At 1.7 miles, make a pair of switchbacks. At 1.8 miles, the Sulphur Ridge Trail turns northwest, picking up Sulphur Ridge. Roll under pines, oaks, and hickories, with more down than up. The trailbed can be faint in places; keep an eye peeled for blazes. Also, look for Price Mountain, now rising to your left. You are circling a hollow. Undulate along slender Sulphur Ridge, making a final uptick at 3.1 miles. Then drop toward the hollow below on a declivitous slope eased by switchbacks aplenty. You come near but not to Sulphur Spring, instead dropping to the unnamed creek coursing through the hollow below.

Reach a footbridge and the hike's low point of 1,390 feet at 3.7 miles. Cross the bridge and reach a campsite. VA 606 is above you. A rough road leads right to VA 606, but this loop heads left to shortly make a bridgeless crossing of the stream you just crossed. Note the small waterfall just below this second crossing. The ledge drop will be more impressive during higher flows. The trail now overlays on an old track leading up to the gap and trailhead; this route likely preceded the current route of VA 606. Cross the small stream three more times; you are now on the right bank. At 4.1 miles, leave the streambed and begin truly ascending in piney woods. You are aiming for the gap. This final assault makes another 500-foot climb, but it's spread over a mile, making it much easier than the hike's initial climb. At 4.7 miles, reach the gap on Price Mountain and the trailhead, completing the circuit.

Nearby Attractions

Fenwick Mines Recreation Area (see previous hike) offers a wheelchair-accessible, historic walk through a former mining community, through wetlands, and along Mill Creek to a waterfall. It also features fine picnicking facilities, including a shelter.

Directions

From Exit 150B on I-81, take US 220 North 8 miles to Fincastle and VA 606. Turn left on VA 606 and drive 6.8 miles to the Botetourt–Craig County line and trailhead in a gap on Price Mountain. Parking is on the right just before the county line sign.

17 Lick Branch Loop

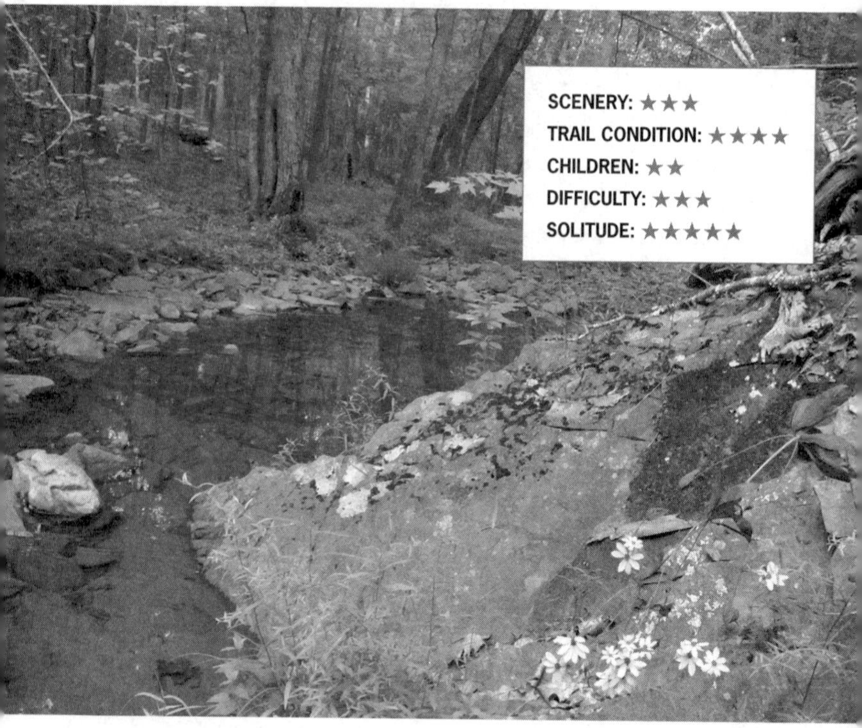

SCENERY: ★★★

TRAIL CONDITION: ★★★★

CHILDREN: ★★

DIFFICULTY: ★★★

SOLITUDE: ★★★★★

LICK BRANCH CAN BE MORE ROCK THAN WATER FOR MUCH OF THE YEAR.

GPS TRAILHEAD COORDINATES: N37° 29.501' W80° 4.569'

DISTANCE & CONFIGURATION: 6.3-mile out-and-back

HIKING TIME: 3.5 hours

OUTSTANDING FEATURES: Solitude, remote valley, seasonal waterfalls

ELEVATION: 1,340 feet at trailhead, 2,080 feet at high point

ACCESS: No fees or permits required

MAPS: National Geographic #788, *Covington/Alleghany Highlands;* USGS *Catawba*

FACILITIES: None

WHEELCHAIR ACCESS: None

INFO: George Washington & Jefferson National Forests, Eastern Divide Ranger District, 110 Southpark Drive, Blacksburg, VA 24060; 540-552-4641, www.fs.usda.gov/gwj

In Brief

This circuit hike is long on solitude. The woodsy walk leads up a slender hollow then climbs Lick Mountain before dropping to Lick Branch. Descend narrow Lick Branch valley, making seemingly innumerable crossings of the oft-dry upper creek, then delve deep into the lower perennial segment, crossing more. Pass a couple of wet-weather waterfalls. Leave the stream at an alternate trailhead, and return to the trailhead via a gravel forest road.

Route Details

This is a low-elevation mountain hike, good for when the high country is excessively cold yet you want to be in the mountains. It is good for solitude as well, as the circuit is off the beaten path and doesn't have any specific highlights, rather a constant level of beauty expected in the Appalachian Mountains of the Old Dominion. However, this is not a recommended hike after heavy rains. The hollows that you will be heading up and down require more than several bridgeless crossings, and the hiking could be tough if the streams are up. A good way to gauge the level of Lick Creek and the other unnamed tributary along which you hike is checking the unnamed tributary at the Ferrier Trail trailhead. Just before reaching the official parking area, Forest Road 5026 crosses the unnamed tributary you will be hiking up. If this stream is flowing boldly, then expect to have wet-footed stream fords on it and Lick Creek. An upside is you will also see a couple of small waterfalls. Conversely, if this streambed is dry then you will be crossing mostly rocky streambeds. Expect more flow on the streams in winter and spring, and dry conditions in summer and fall, except after heavy thunderstorms.

A trail sign and map mark the beginning of the Ferrier Trail. With any luck, the pole gate at the trail's beginning will be restored upon your arrival. Leave FR 5026 and enter the hollow of an unnamed branch, a tributary of Craig Creek flowing off Lick Mountain. The path is marked with paint blazes and plastic diamonds as it enters pine–oak

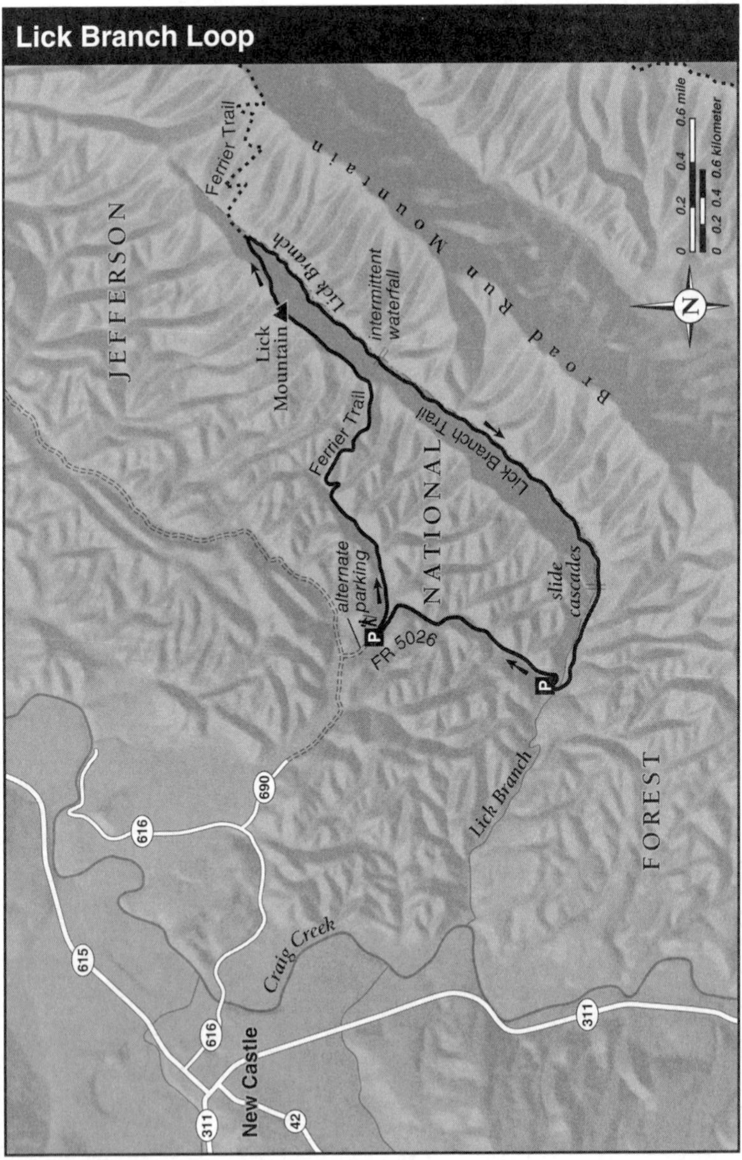
Lick Branch Loop
Ferrier Trail
Broad Run Mountain
JEFFERSON
NATIONAL
FOREST
Lick Branch
intermittent waterfall
Lick Mountain
Lick Branch Trail
Ferrier Trail
alternate parking
slide cascades
FR 5026
P
P
Lick Branch
Craig Creek
690
616
615
616
311
311
42
New Castle
0 0.2 0.4 0.6 mile
0 0.2 0.4 0.6 kilometer
N

woods. Pass near an old wildlife clearing to the right of the trail, and bisect a wildlife clearing at 0.3 mile. Cross more tributaries, likely to be just stony stream bottoms.

White oaks are prevalent here. Interestingly, oaks are technically part of the beech family. White oaks grow throughout the state of Virginia and most of the eastern United States, from Texas north to Minnesota, then east to Maine and south to Florida. The high-quality white oak wood has been prized by Americans for generations. Among other uses, it once was made into barrel staves, bringing about the "barrel oak." Wildlife may love white oaks more than man does: Woodpeckers and turkeys are among the birds that enjoy the nuts; raccoons and chipmunks also savor the nutrient-packed treat; and deer both eat the acorns and graze on the tender twigs.

Cross the waterway of the hollow several times in succession, then turn right up a rib ridge at 0.8 mile, amid scads of blueberries topped with pines. Ascend east to reach the crest of Lick Mountain at 1.4 miles. Turn northeast, rolling over knobs on a singletrack path. Gain views of the Rich Patch Mountains across the Craig Creek Valley and even parts of the town of New Castle. At 2.0 miles, slip right off Lick Mountain into Lick Branch.

Reach a trail intersection at 2.3 miles. Turn right on the Lick Branch Trail, as the Ferrier Trail continues onward to meet the North

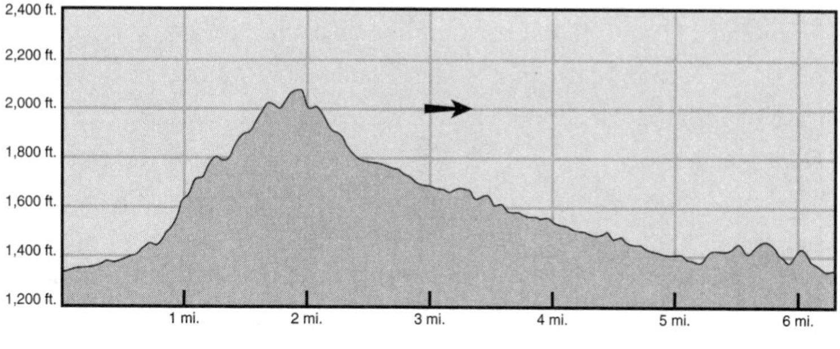

Mountain Trail. We delve into the upper reaches of Lick Branch, hemmed in by the parallel ridges of Lick Mountain and Broad Run Mountain. Ahead lie crossing after crossing of Lick Branch. It's fun making your way across the rock cobbles and picking up the path again—and again—in addition to stepping over side hollow streams on your downhill adventure.

At 3.2 miles, cross Lick Branch just above a 12-foot wet-weather waterfall. Continue down the bluff-bordered vale. By 4.5 miles, the valley has widened and Lick Branch flows perennially. The stream and trail curve northwest. At 4.7 miles, look for a slide cascade angling about 10 feet over a rock slab. Come under a power line at 4.9 miles. Ahead, enter a pine grove, and quickly descend right to cross Lick Branch a final time to emerge at the end of FR 5026 and an alternate parking area at 5.2 miles. From here, trace the gravel forest road over a low ridge, returning to the trailhead at 6.3 miles

Nearby Attractions

Fenwick Mines Recreation Area (see Hike 15, page 100) features a wheelchair-accessible, historic walk to a former mining community, through wetlands, and along Mill Creek to a waterfall. It also features fine picnicking facilities, including a shelter.

Directions

From Exit 141 on I-81 just south of Roanoke, take VA 419 North 0.3 mile, then turn right on VA 311 North and follow it 19 miles to New Castle. From the intersection of VA 311, VA 42, and VA 615 in downtown New Castle, take VA 615, (Craig Creek Road) 0.1 mile to turn right on VA 616 (Court Street). Follow VA 616 for 1.2 miles, then turn right on VA 690. Follow 690 0.3 mile; then it turns gravel. At 0.9 mile, split right on FR 5026. Follow FR 5026 just a short distance to a ford an unnamed stream. You can park before the ford, but the official parking area is just after the ford.

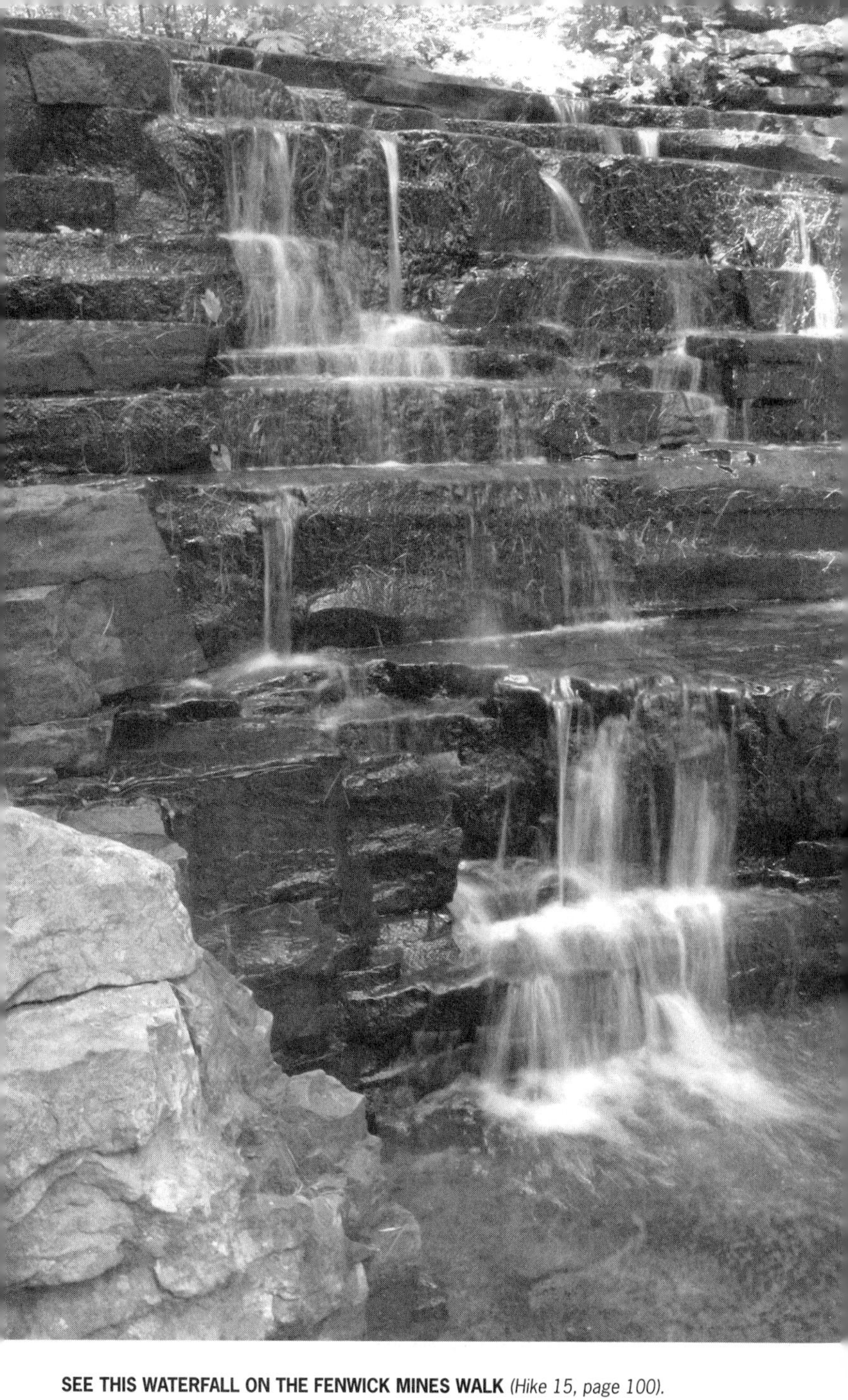

SEE THIS WATERFALL ON THE FENWICK MINES WALK *(Hike 15, page 100).*

Catawba

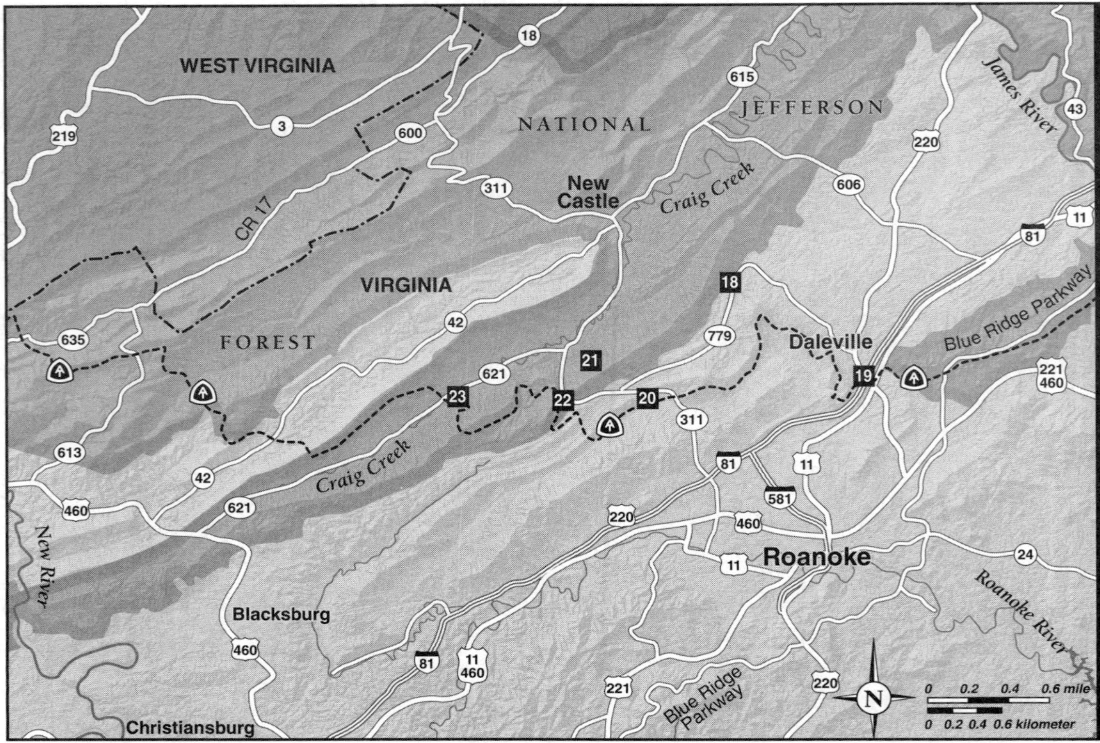
WEST VIRGINIA
NATIONAL
JEFFERSON
VIRGINIA
FOREST
New Castle
Daleville
Roanoke
Blacksburg
Christiansburg
James River
Craig Creek
Craig Creek
New River
Roanoke River
Blue Ridge Parkway
Blue Ridge Parkway
CR 17
18
19
20
21
22
23
N
0 0.2 0.4 0.6 mile
0 0.2 0.4 0.6 kilometer

Catawba

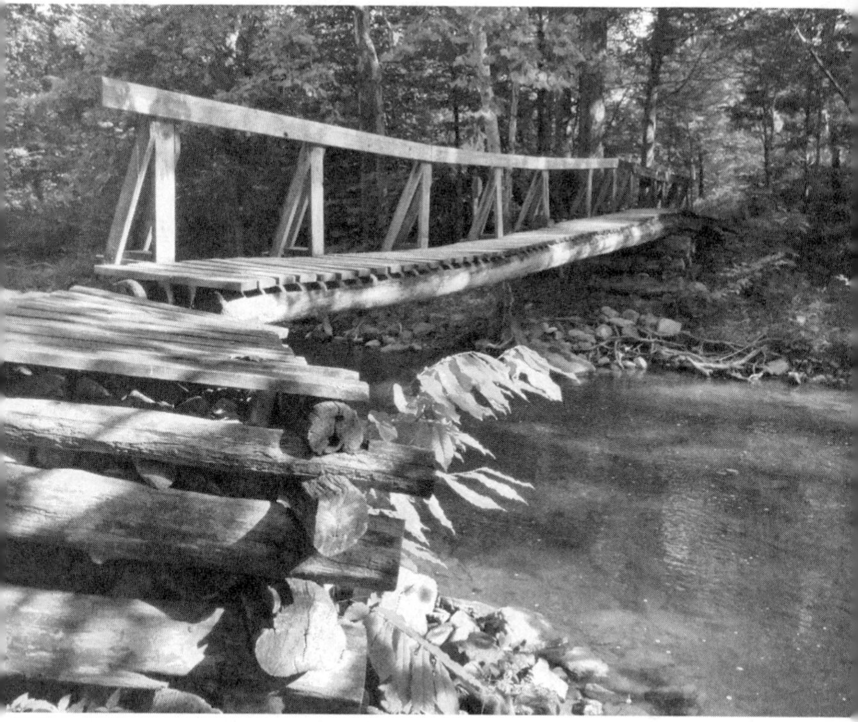

CROSS THIS HIKER BRIDGE OVER CATAWBA CREEK EN ROUTE TO THE TINKER CLIFFS. *(See next page.)*

18 Tinker Cliffs

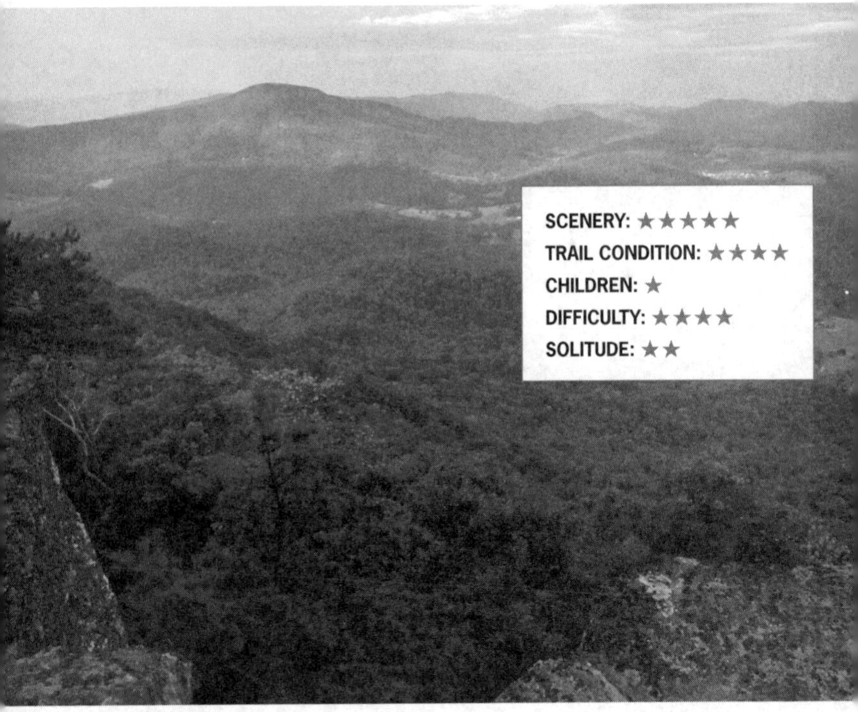

SCENERY: ★★★★★
TRAIL CONDITION: ★★★★
CHILDREN: ★
DIFFICULTY: ★★★★
SOLITUDE: ★★

THE CATAWBA CREEK VALLEY AND A HOST OF MOUNTAINS STRETCH OUT BELOW THE TINKER CLIFFS.

GPS TRAILHEAD COORDINATES: N37° 27.451' W80° 1.037'

DISTANCE & CONFIGURATION: 7.2-mile out-and-back

HIKING TIME: 4 hours

OUTSTANDING FEATURES: Multiple views from multiple locations, streams

ELEVATION: 1,480 feet at trailhead, 1,330 at low point, 2,900 feet at high point

ACCESS: No fees or permits required

MAPS: National Geographic #788, *Covington/Alleghany Highlands;* USGS *Catawba, Daleville*

FACILITIES: None

WHEELCHAIR ACCESS: None

INFO: George Washington & Jefferson National Forests, Eastern Divide Ranger District, 110 Southpark Drive, Blacksburg, VA 24060; 540-552-4641, www.fs.usda.gov/gwj

In Brief

Tinker Cliffs features some of the finest panoramas in Western Virginia. And the hike—with a 1,500-foot climb—has other rewards, too, such as two streams and views of Tinker Cliffs en route. A well-constructed trail with multiple switchbacks eases the ascent to one of the Roanoke Valley's iconic destinations.

Route Details

The route to the fabulous Tinker Cliffs uses the Andy Layne Trail, named for an outdoors enthusiast of the first degree. After leading an interesting life that included a stint in World War II and helping to develop trails, Layne returned to his native Roanoke Valley to take care of his aging mother and there embarked on yet another career: member extraordinaire of the Roanoke Appalachian Trail Club. He was one of the core members of the organization and not only was involved in everything but also encouraged others, whether they were meeting, leading hikes, or doing trail maintenance.

Layne personally managed what is now known as the Andy Layne Trail for more than a decade. Back then, however, it was the Appalachian Trail, before the AT was rerouted off North Mountain and onto Catawba Mountain. Luckily for us, this route to Tinker Cliffs remains. Today we have a well-constructed direct path to Scorched Earth Gap and the current route of the AT on the deservedly renamed Andy Layne Trail. And from Scorched Earth Gap—one of the all-time greatest Appalachian mountain names—it's less than a mile on the AT to the series of spectacular views that can be had from Tinker Cliffs.

Leave the trailhead parking area on the Andy Layne Trail. You are on land donated by nearby Roanoke Cement Company. Other portions along the trail are owned by the business, but they allow passage. Pass an informative kiosk, then rise through hardwoods. Angle downhill through a cedar forest, and cross a stile, entering grazing land. Reach sycamore-bordered Little Catawba Creek and a footbridge at 0.5 mile. Cross the creek and enter an open meadow.

Tinker Cliffs

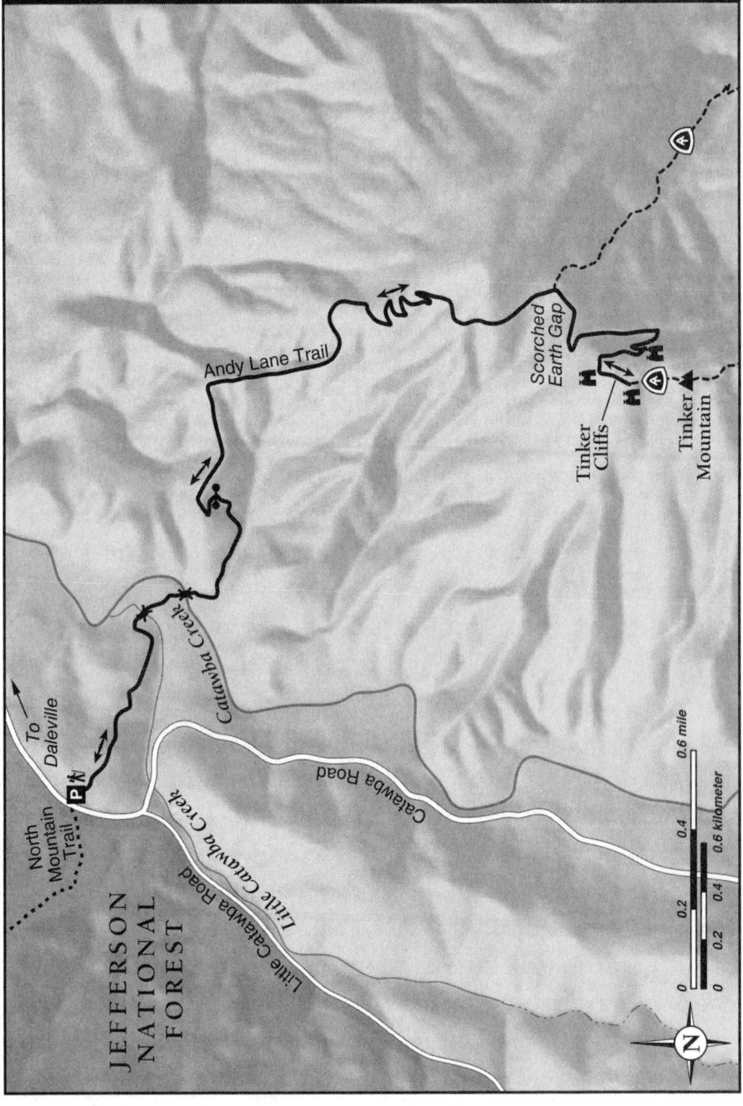

Make sure to look up toward Tinker Cliffs as you cross the meadow. Pass through a second stile and enter a riparian buffer area, where purple coneflowers and black-eyed Susans grow among replanted trees. Bridge Catawba Creek at 0.7 mile, just upstream of a sheer bluff that forces a turn in Catawba Creek.

You are near your low point. Let the climbing begin. And it does as you turn into a hollow and begin ascending in woods. Keep working uphill, and come to a gate at 1.1 miles. The Andy Layne Trail joins an old roadbed, then joins a rib ridge of Tinker Mountain, rising above you. The walking is easy among cedar, redbud, and locust.

At 1.5 miles, the path turns south, aiming for the crest of Tinker Mountain. Drop to a gap at 1.6 miles, and then make up for the decline with a short, very steep stretch. Wood water bars provide steps and discourage erosion. At 2.0 miles, you are on the steep upper slope of Tinker Mountain. However, a series of switchbacks makes the trail gradient manageable. By 2.4 miles, the Andy Layne Trail circles around the northwest side of the mountain.

Pull into Scorched Earth Gap, and meet the AT at 2.8 miles. To your left (north), it's 0.6 mile to the Lamberts Meadow trail shelter. Our hike goes right (south) toward Tinker Cliffs. But first you may want to grab a seat at the sizable repose boulder in the gap. The trail climbs from the gap, makes a switchback at 3.0 miles, then miraculously levels

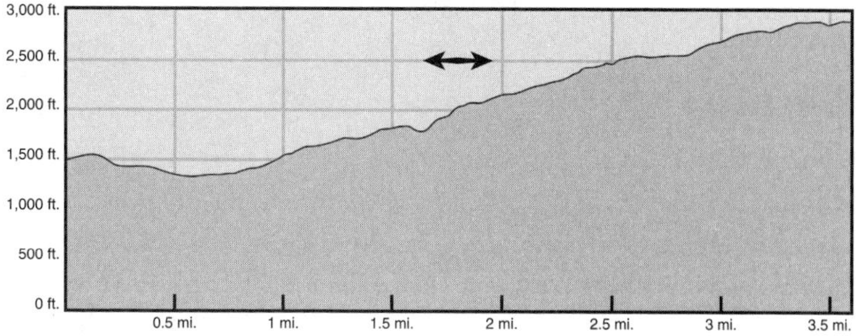

off on a shoulder of the mountain in viney hardwoods. That soon ends and you switchback up to the base of Tinker Cliffs.

The AT finds a break in the pale cliffline at 3.3 miles. Just ahead, a flat outcrop to the left of the trail allows a partial view to the east. Far better views lie ahead. Stay with the AT as it curves around the north end of the mountain. Stone slabs beckon a view. In other places, stacked outcrops—disconnected from the mountain—dare hikers to jump over deep crevasses to them. Don't do it; ahead are more-accessible panoramas. One opens at 3.5 miles. Here, you can look northwest to North Mountain, Broad Run Mountain, Caldwell Mountain, and the Catawba Creek Valley below.

Continuing onward, the rocky edge curves to the west side of Tinker Mountain. The views get better. The AT runs along the edge of open outcrops. They beckon you out to first-rate views. Mountains and valleys open to the west of the Catawba Creek Valley and waves of mountains, then southwest even to McAfee Knob. Tinker Cliffs, McAfee Knob, and the Dragons Tooth form the Roanoke Valley's Triple Crown. You can win your own triple crown using this guide, as hikes to all three destinations are detailed within.

Nearby Attractions

Along the way to this hike, you pass the trailhead leading to another fabled Roanoke-area hiking destination: **Hay Rock.** The Hay Rock and Beyond hike, also on the AT, is profiled next.

Directions

From Exit 150B on I-81 north of Roanoke, emerge from the off-ramp at US 11. Head south 0.2 mile on US 11 to a traffic light and US 220. Turn right, northbound for Daleville on Cloverdale Road. Drive north on US 220 for 1.5 miles, then turn left on Catawba Road at a traffic light. Follow Catawba Road 8.3 miles to the Andy Layne Trail parking area on your left.

19 Hay Rock and Beyond

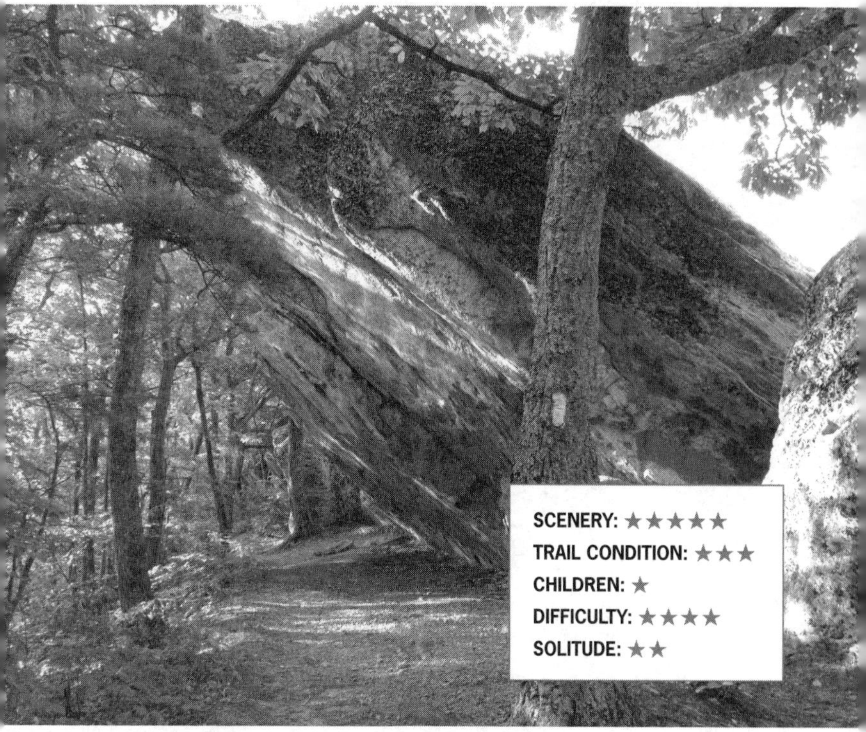

SCENERY: ★★★★★
TRAIL CONDITION: ★★★
CHILDREN: ★
DIFFICULTY: ★★★★
SOLITUDE: ★★

YOU CAN'T MISS ANGLED HAY ROCK, WHICH LIES DIRECTLY ON THE APPALACHIAN TRAIL.

GPS TRAILHEAD COORDINATES: N37° 23.471' W79° 54.392'

DISTANCE & CONFIGURATION: 9.2-mile out-and-back

HIKING TIME: 5 hours

OUTSTANDING FEATURES: Multiple panoramas, geological interest, Hay Rock

ELEVATION: 1,230 feet at trailhead, 1,980 feet at high point

ACCESS: No fees or permits required

MAPS: National Geographic #788, *Covington/Alleghany Highlands;* USGS *Daleville*

FACILITIES: None

WHEELCHAIR ACCESS: None

INFO: George Washington & Jefferson National Forests, Eastern Divide Ranger District, 110 Southpark Drive, Blacksburg, VA 24060; 540-552-4641; www.fs.usda.gov/gwj

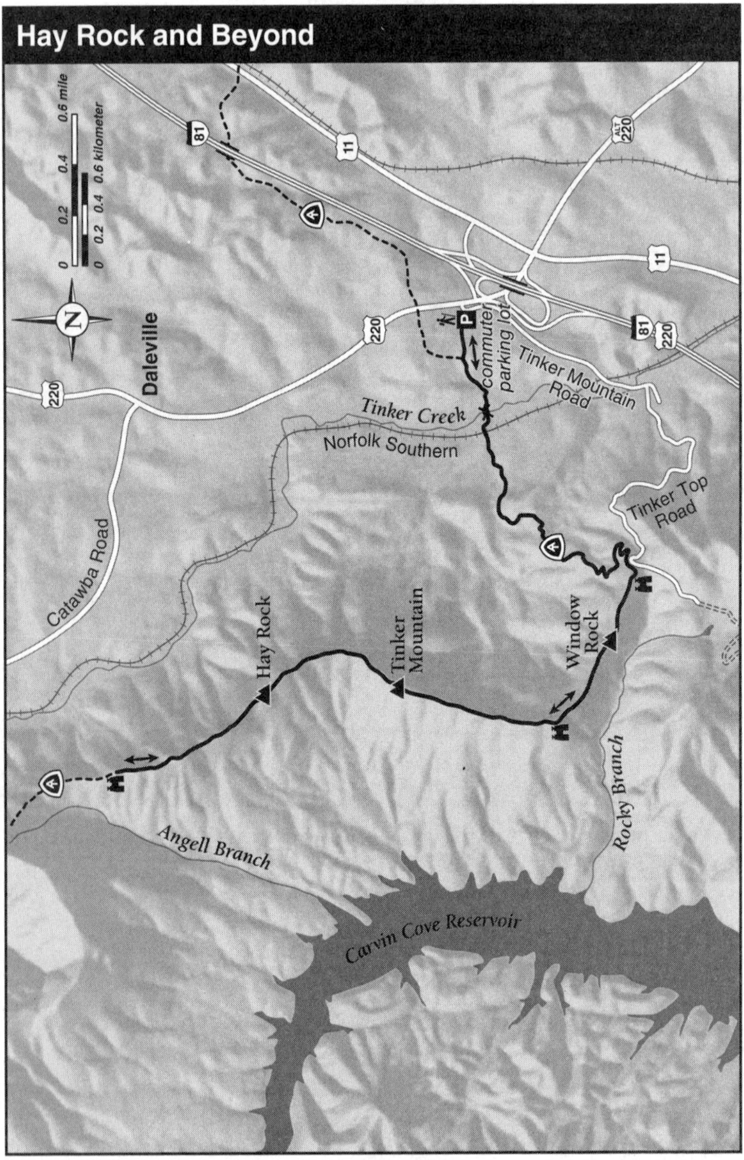
Hay Rock and Beyond
0 0.2 0.4 0.6 mile
0 0.2 0.4 0.6 kilometer
N
Daleville
81
11
ALT 220
220
commuter parking lot
P
Tinker Mountain Road
Tinker Creek
Norfolk Southern
Catawba Road
Tinker Top Road
Hay Rock
Tinker Mountain
Window Rock
Rocky Branch
Angell Branch
Carvin Cove Reservoir

In Brief

Reap multiple Appalachian Trail rewards while climbing Tinker Mountain. Rock outcrops, upthrusts, and geological underpinnings present views galore and massive, tilted Hay Rock. Continue the AT, viewing a long fortresslike wall, and finally reach a signed overlook where Carvins Cove Reservoir forms the centerpiece of an inspiring mountain panorama.

Route Details

This ultrascenic hike starts at a decidedly nonscenic location—a commuter parking lot off I-81. However, the parking is convenient, and you soon enter a world vastly different from the network of roads, bridges, and byways that take us to and through Western Virginia. From the commuter parking lot, look for a wide gravel track leaving west. Pass around an aluminum guardrail, joining the gravel track. Quickly enter scrubby woods and reach a trail kiosk outlining the local route of the AT.

Continue tracing a crumbly roadbed to meet and join the AT southbound at 0.2 mile. Keep west, still in brushy woods, before descending into a pine grove, then reach Tinker Creek. The AT uses an old road bridge to span Tinker Creek. There is a shaded campsite to the right of the trail beyond the former road bridge. Ahead, the

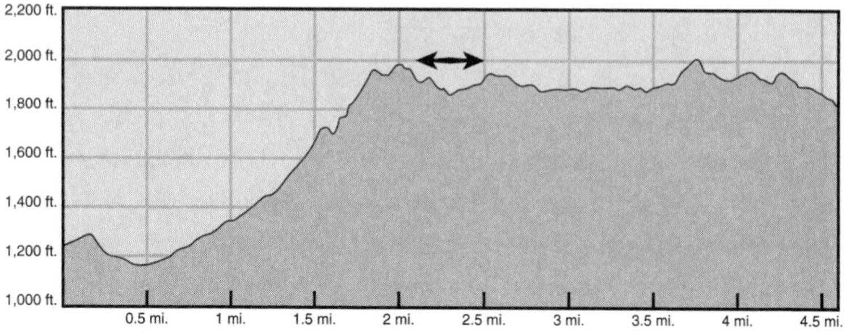

trail crosses railroad tracks—yet another part of the infrastructure. It then cuts across a gas-line clearing to bridge a smaller stream at 0.6 mile. It is fascinating to see how trail managers route the AT through areas like this, near interstates and populated areas.

Enter a rich hardwood flat at 0.8 mile, then cross a power-line clearing at 1.0 mile. Start climbing in earnest, which is what you've been expecting from this hike all along. At 1.5 miles, short, tight switchbacks compensate the increasing steepness of Tinker Mountain. Begin winding among boulder gardens, stone walls, and bluffs. At 1.6 miles, the AT curves around the point of the ridge, cloaked in stunted pines, laurel, and oaks. Limited views open between the trees, north toward Troutville and the Blue Ridge Parkway.

At 1.8 miles, the AT takes you directly under a power-line transmission tower and through a clearing. Here you can look primarily east toward the Glade Creek valley. Beyond the power line, join the crest of Tinker Mountain, traversing a pine needle–carpeted track brightened with pale rock outcrops. The path is rocky as it tightropes a narrow ridge, dropping sharply on both sides. At 2.1 miles, look for Window Rock, a natural arch resembling a small window in a boulder, to the left of the trail. (The arch is too small for an adult to pass through.) Ahead, the valley of Angell Branch opens below, allowing the first of numerous views of Carvins Cove Reservoir, which lies at 1,170 feet, 700 feet below Tinker Mountain. Sand, pines, and pale tan and gray outcrops characterize the ridge here. More views continue ahead, on a line of cliffs overlooking Carvins Cove.

At 2.5 miles, an unobstructed outcrop and high point to the left of the trail delivers a westerly prospect across the reservoir, over I-81 and the Roanoke Valley. The balance of Tinker Mountain, Catawba Mountain, and a host of ridges stretches onward. Wow! Keep southbound on the AT, though the trail at this point is traveling north. The path becomes extremely rocky, slowing travel and forcing you to watch your every step. The good news is that elevation changes are minimal from here on out.

At 2.6 miles, pass under another transmission-tower clearing, opening more views. Continue among boulders, uptilted rocks, and stony trailbed. Trees and brush find their place where the soil allows. At 3 miles, the rockiness of the path eases, with breaks of unobstructed trailbed between stonier segments. At 3.6 miles, the AT makes a "Fat Man's Squeeze" between chest-high boulders. Keep north along Tinker Mountain, the crest dropping off both east and west. Climb over a little knob, then descend along the ridgetop, coming to Hay Rock at 3.9 miles. The upthrust rock rises to the left of the AT and overhangs the path, forming a shelter of sorts. Little trails run among the boulders here. Hay Rock itself is challenging to climb. Most visitors admire it from the ground, rather than scale its extremely slanted heights.

Hay Rock is a fine destination in and of itself, but there are more geological wonders and views beyond. So onward we go. Quickly come along another upthrust rock, and then saddle alongside a rock wall, the "Great Wall of Tinker Mountain." The barricade stretches along the path and eventually gives way, and you meander stony track. Emerge at a power-line clearing at 4.6 miles. Here, a short signed spur trail leads left to a bouldery view. Below, Angell Branch flows to meet Carvins Cove Reservoir, itself encircled by ridges. Brushy Mountain rises ahead, while the Roanoke Valley stretches in the distance, backed by still more mountains. Tinker Mountain curves west to meet Catawba Mountain.

Nearby Attractions

Carvins Cove Reservoir has not only a boat-accessible lake but also a vast network of trails, albeit dominated by mountain bikers.

Directions

From Exit 150B on I-81 North of Roanoke, emerge from the off-ramp at US 11. Head south 0.2 mile on US 11 to a traffic light and US 220. Turn right (northbound) for Daleville on US 220/Cloverdale Road. Drive north on US 220/Cloverdale under the interstate; then, at 0.2 mile, turn left on Tinker Mountain Road and immediately reach the commuter parking lot.

20 McAfee Knob

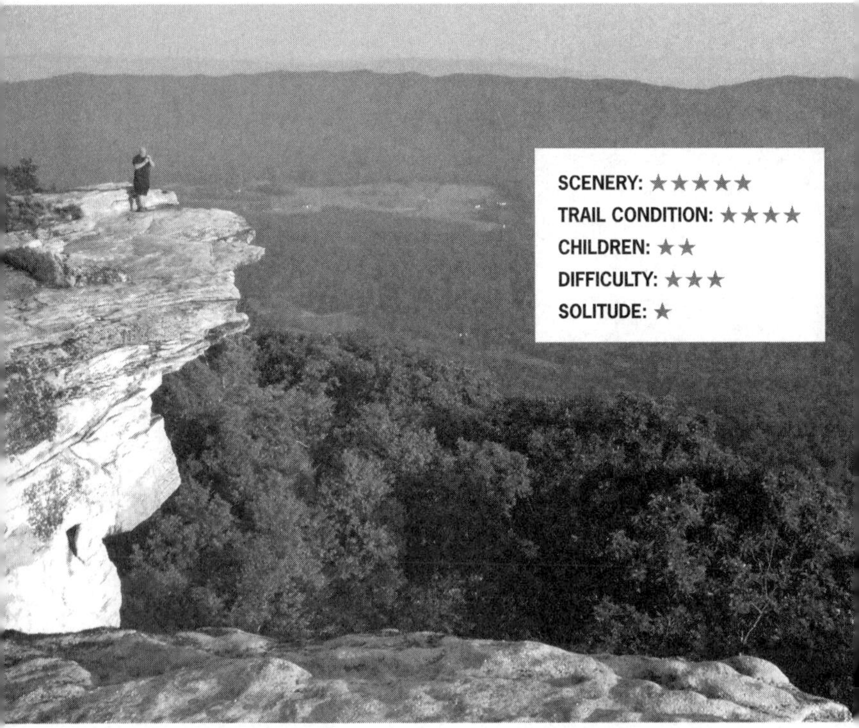

SCENERY: ★★★★★
TRAIL CONDITION: ★★★★
CHILDREN: ★★
DIFFICULTY: ★★★
SOLITUDE: ★

McAFEE KNOB IS PERHAPS THE MOST PHOTOGRAPHED OVERLOOK ON THE ENTIRE APPALACHIAN TRAIL.

GPS TRAILHEAD COORDINATES: N37° 22.812' W80° 5.360'

DISTANCE & CONFIGURATION: 7.8-mile out-and-back

HIKING TIME: 4.5 hours

OUTSTANDING FEATURES: Views from the most photographed trailside vista in Virginia

ELEVATION: 1,950 feet at trailhead, 3,150 feet at high point

ACCESS: No fees or permits required

MAPS: National Geographic #788, *Covington/Alleghany Highlands;* USGS *Catawba*

FACILITIES: None

WHEELCHAIR ACCESS: None

INFO: George Washington National Forest, Eastern Divide Ranger District, 110 Southpark Drive, Blacksburg, VA 24060; 540-552-4641, www.fs.usda.gov/gwj

In Brief

Take a hike to the outcrop of McAfee Knob, arguably the icon of the Appalachian Trail in Virginia. Start at busy VA 311 and trace the AT northbound along Catawba Mountain. The moderate hike skirts past two trail shelters then works up the slope of McAfee Knob. Emerge onto a long brow of overhanging rock, where a mass of mountainlands extends to the horizon. A fire road offers an alternate return route.

Route Details

This trek is a rite of passage for Roanoke and New River Valley hikers. Not only is McAfee Knob great for snapping pictures of hikers standing atop its overhang, but the views from the outcrop are far-reaching. At the same time, expect no solitude. The first part of the adventure is crossing VA 311 from the trailhead parking lot. It is a semiblind curve, and you just have to listen for approaching cars and then go. Join the AT northbound. Quickly pass under a brushy power-line crossing. By 0.1 mile, you have crested Catawba Mountain. Ascend via wood and earth steps. The Catawba Creek Valley falls away to your left, backed by North Mountain. Views also open right (east) toward the Roanoke Valley.

At 0.3 mile, reach a trail intersection and informational kiosk. Here, the AT leaves right, and a short path splits left then reaches the fire road running the length of Catawba Mountain. Stay with the AT, briefly stopping at the southerly overlook near the kiosk. Now, the AT resumes its easterly tack running beneath the mountain crest. Pass over and near open rock slabs and stony segments. Bridges rise above some of the slabs, and they are especially appreciated when the slabs are wet or icy. At 1 mile, pass just above the Johns Spring trail shelter. The wooden structure is set in a small cove. Not only do AT thru-hikers use this shelter, but it's also popular with local backpackers. Campers are asked to stay only at shelters and designated camping areas along Catawba Mountain to concentrate the heavy use here.

McAfee Knob

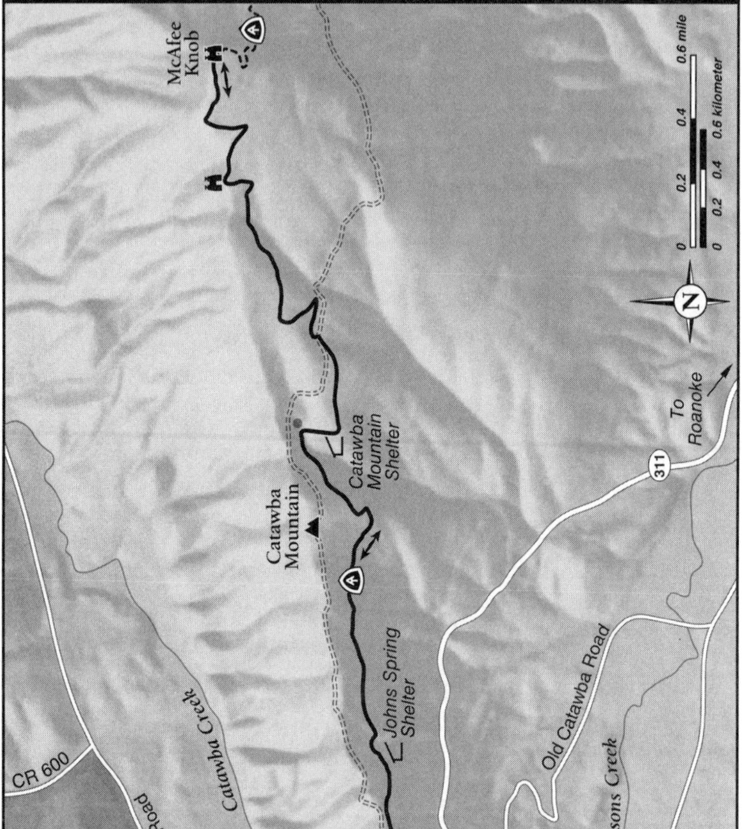
McAfee Knob
Catawba Mountain
Catawba Mountain Shelter
Johns Spring Shelter
311
To Roanoke
Old Catawba Road
Masons Creek
Catawba Creek
Catawba Creek Road
CR 600
JEFFERSON NATIONAL FOREST
0 0.2 0.4 0.6 mile
0 0.2 0.4 0.6 kilometer
N

Climb from the shelter to enter oak, pine, gum, and sassafras. Pass by more rock slabs and bridges traversing them. At 2.1 miles, the AT curves just below a box spring that can run dry by late summer/early fall. Just ahead, pass the spur to the Catawba Mountain shelter. This three-sided wooden refuge is set in a small cove as well. The AT passes some designated campsites, turns uphill, and then begins the first real climb of the day. You have gained only 250 feet in elevation thus far. By 2.6 miles, you have gained another 200 feet and reach the fire road, which can be used as a return route to the trailhead. You cut off a half-mile of distance on a more foot-friendly track, but the fire road isn't the AT.

Onward to McAfee Knob, staying with the AT and still climbing. At 3.1 miles, bisect a power-line clearing. The uptick continues as the AT parallels the clearing. This is a good area to see wildlife around dusk or dawn. By 3.4 miles, you have crested Catawba Mountain. Views once again open to the north. Walk along the rock brow, and keep climbing to reach what seems like a trail intersection at 3.6 miles. The only way to go is left, however, as the trail leading right is closed. Begin curving around the south side of McAfee Knob. Pass an agglomeration of giant squared-off boulders in silent repose. Hikers have created side trails, passing among these geological giants. The AT turns

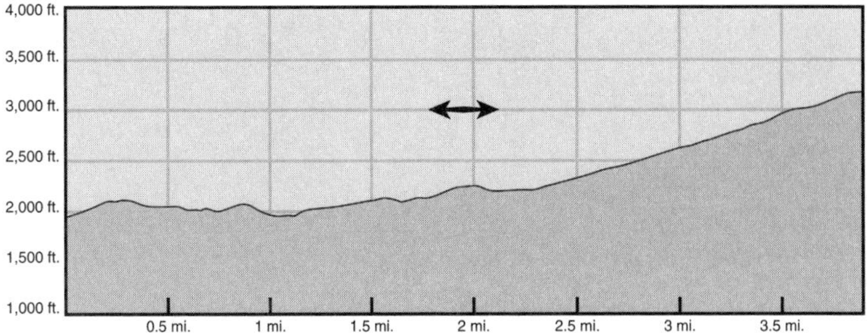

around the boulders in its quest for McAfee Knob then passes through brushy, wind-stunted woodland. At 3.9 miles, the AT takes you to the western edge of McAfee Knob. Take the short spur left to the stony edge of the mountain. Here you see the overhanging rock outcrop so often seen in photos. The area is truly picturesque—a large upthrust outcrop overlooking the Catawba Creek Valley and a host of ridges and valleys to the north and west. If you continue along the outcrop rim, it curves around to the right enough to allow northeasterly views of the Roanoke Valley. This is a popular spot, and you will likely share it with others. No camping is allowed directly on the knob, but nearby camping areas on both sides allows backpackers to view the sunset from the outcrop, then return to their campsites. Sunrise, sunset, midday—it doesn't matter; what matters is getting to McAfee Knob. It is one of the jewels in the crown of the AT in the South.

Nearby Attractions

The hike to **Dragons Tooth** (page 138)—with its 360-degree views—is just 4.6 miles farther down VA 311.

Directions

From Exit 141 on I-81 just south of Roanoke, take VA 419 North 0.3 mile; turn right on VA 311 North and follow it 5 miles. As you approach the gap in Catawba Mountain, look for the road-crossing sign with the yellow hiker; turn left into the large parking area for McAfee Knob.

21 North Mountain Loop

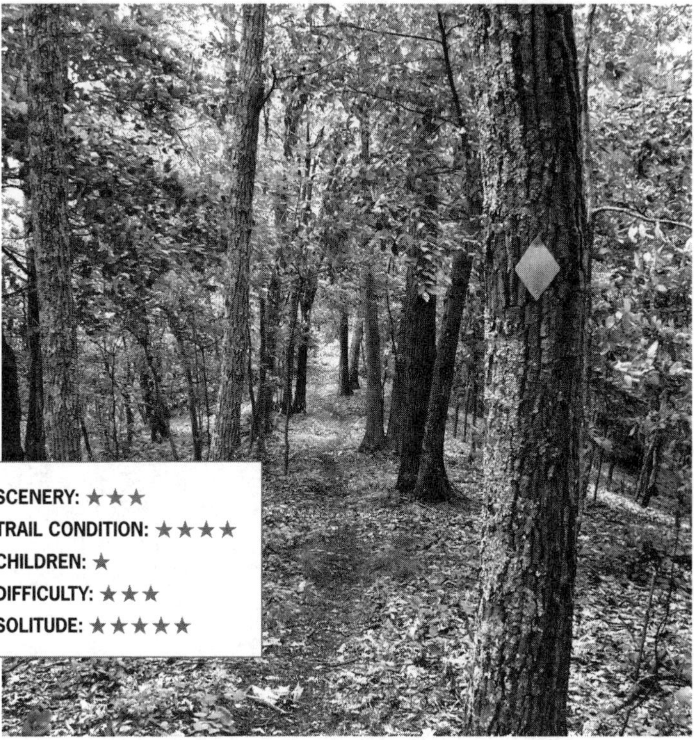

SCENERY: ★★★
TRAIL CONDITION: ★★★★
CHILDREN: ★
DIFFICULTY: ★★★
SOLITUDE: ★★★★★

NORTH MOUNTAIN OFFERS SOLITUDE ON ITS SINGLETRACK TRAIL.

GPS TRAILHEAD COORDINATES: N37° 24.306' W80° 8.086'

DISTANCE & CONFIGURATION: 6.3-mile loop

HIKING TIME: 3.5 hours

OUTSTANDING FEATURES: Solitude, partial views, challenge

ELEVATION: 1,730 feet at trailhead, 2,880 feet at high point

ACCESS: No fees or permits required

MAPS: National Geographic #788, *Covington/Alleghany Highlands;* USGS *Looney, Catawba*

FACILITIES: None

WHEELCHAIR ACCESS: None

INFO: George Washington & Jefferson National Forests, Eastern Divide Ranger District, 110 Southpark Drive, Blacksburg, VA 24060; 540-552-4641, www.fs.usda.gov/gwj

North Mountain Loop

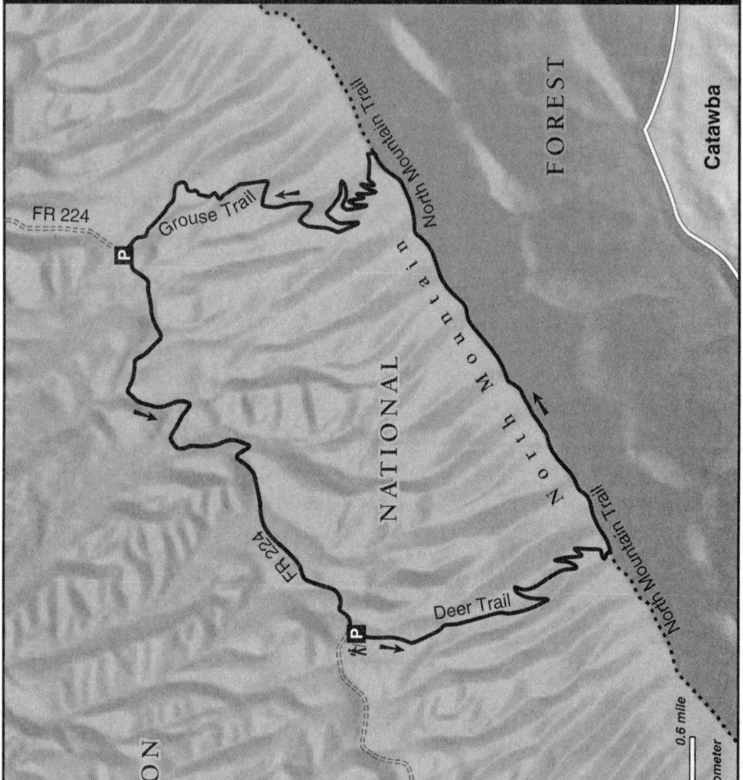

In Brief

This forgotten loop on North Mountain is overshadowed by the nearby Dragons Tooth and McAfee Knob hikes, but solitude lovers will revel in the challenging circuit. Take the Deer Trail steeply to the crest of North Mountain. Roll the rocky crest of the ridge, peering down on adjacent ridges and valleys. The Grouse Trail leads you off North Mountain. The final part of the hike uses a remote forest road to complete the loop.

Route Details

This loop hike is very near Roanoke to be so filled with solitude. North Mountain rises to form the boundary between Roanoke and Craig Counties. Part of the Jefferson National Forest, North Mountain begins at nearby McAfee Gap, near where the famed Dragons Tooth hike starts. In fact, North Mountain is also known as the Dragon's Back. The northeast-running ridge forms a rampart between Craig Creek and Catawba Creek. A monolith of rocks, trees, and solitude, North Mountain is left mostly to the deer, bear, and grouse that bolt when the infrequent hiker or mountain biker darkens the ridgecrest. Just west of North Mountain, throngs are tackling the worthwhile Dragons Tooth, and the next ridge south—Catawba Mountain—hosts a parade of trail trekkers aiming for venerable McAfee Knob.

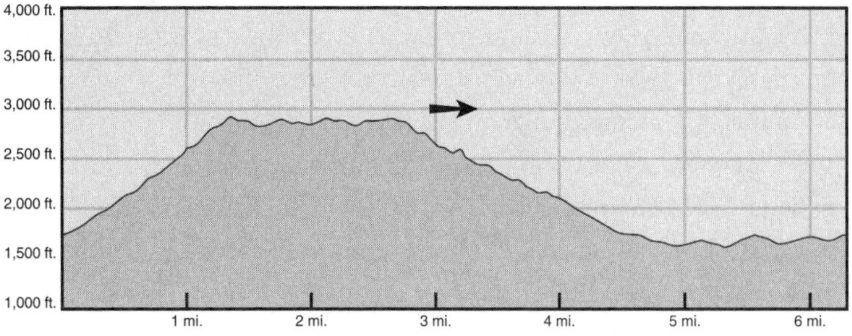

However, North Mountain has no such outcrops attracting hikers. Nor does the Appalachian Trail tread over its heights, though the AT ran atop North Mountain from 1978 to 1987. Instead, North Mountain languishes in solitude where smaller rock protrusions and breaks between the trees provide partial views that don't hold the lure of nearby destinations. Though North Mountain Trail runs more than 13 miles along its crest from McAfee Gap to Broad Run Creek, it lacks the glamour of the AT.

Thus, this hike is left to solitude and wildlife seekers. Begin the trek by leaving Forest Road 224 on the Deer Trail. A trailside kiosk displays an area map. The Deer Trail gently rises north, a slender natural-surface track rambling under oaks, black gum, and sassafras. The ascent steepens, eventually to climb 1,100 feet just in the next 1.3 miles. That is another reason hikers avoid North Mountain. However, fear not, as the trail is well graded and uses switchbacks to make the very steep upper slope of North Mountain doable.

At 0.3 mile, sidle alongside a hollow dropping off to your right. Partial views of Brush Mountain and Sinking Creek Mountain open to the west, through breaks in the bedraggled evergreens. Craig Creek Valley stretches below in alternating forests and fields. At your feet, blueberries rise to your thighs, offering succulent fruit in summertime. At 0.6 mile, the Deer Trail comes near the streambed of the hollow you have been paralleling, then turns away to join a rib ridge of North Mountain, cloaked in wind-stunted oaks and pines. Switchbacks come more frequently the higher you climb. Partial views continue. At 1.2 miles, big boulders crowd the trail; then you reach the crest of North Mountain and a trail intersection. Congratulations! You just climbed 1,100 feet.

Catch your breath, for the rest of the hike is just a walk in the national forest. To your right, the North Mountain Trail heads 2.2 miles to US 311 near the Dragons Tooth trailhead. We head left (northeast) on the North Mountain Trail. Roll along the crest of the mountain, enjoying partial views north and south, and excellent vistas in leafless winter. In most places, the trail rides the crest of North Mountain, but elsewhere "hogbacks" or upturned rock outcrops make treading atop the ridge too difficult. Then the path drops over to the mountainside a bit on sloped but manageable, less-boulder-strewn terrain.

The path remains mostly level atop North Mountain, varying less than 100 feet in elevation, averaging around 2,850 feet. Hickories and oaks rise where rock isn't, growing more robustly than the scraggly side-slope pines. Pass a Forest Service survey marker at 1.7 miles. Crisscross the crest, occasionally passing big boulders.

Meet the Grouse Trail at 2.7 miles. The North Mountain Trail continues northeast. Head left on the Grouse Trail, dropping off the crest and working down the north slope of North Mountain. Switchbacks commence, and along these you can peer north to see the east end of Sinking Creek Mountain and the town of New Castle in the distance. At 3.2 miles, curve into a hollow, walking directly underneath a huge northern red oak tree. Turn away from the hollow, back in the pines.

From here on out, the trail angles down the mountain, crossing small streambeds divided by modest pine–oak ridges. By 4.2 miles, the Grouse Trail has become gentler. Emerge onto FR 224 at 4.5 miles. Head left and commence walking the gravel doubletrack forest road as it undulates southwest. Cross small hills dividing streams flowing off North Mountain. The walking is easy and the traffic is light. At 6.3 miles, you're back at the Deer Trail parking area, completing the hike.

Nearby Attractions

The hike to **Dragons Tooth** (next page)—with its 360-degree views—is on US 311, just before you reach the final turn to this hike.

Directions

From Exit 141 on I-81 just south of Roanoke, take VA 419 North 0.3 mile; then turn right on VA 311 North and follow it 12.8 miles to turn right and uphill on gravel Wildlife Road (FR 224). (If you reach the left turn for VA 621, you've gone 0.5 mile too far.) Turn right on gravel FR 224—an SUV is recommended—and continue 1.7 miles to reach the parking area on your left and the Deer Trail on your right.

22 Dragons Tooth

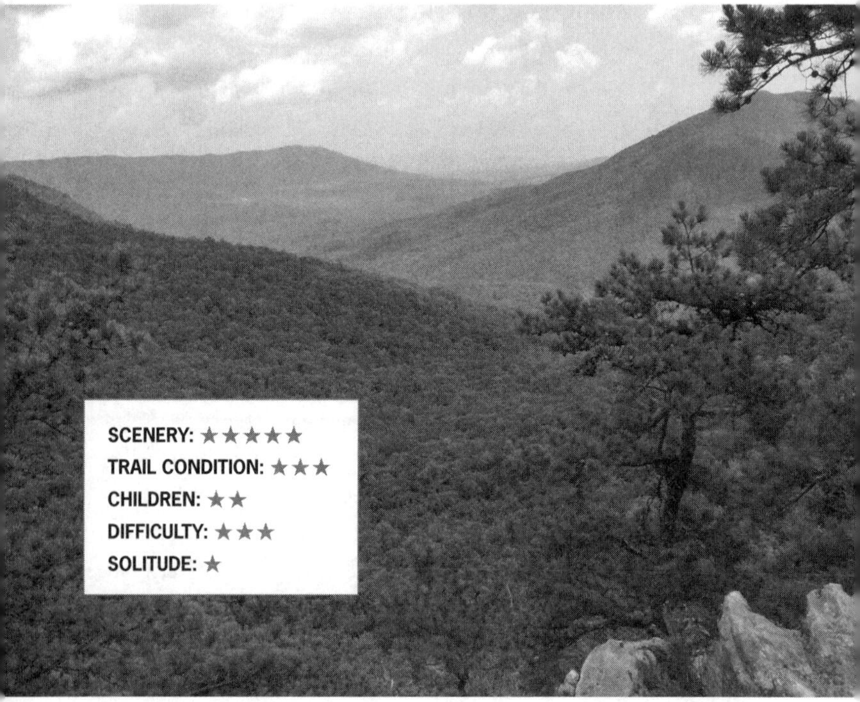

SCENERY: ★★★★★
TRAIL CONDITION: ★★★
CHILDREN: ★★
DIFFICULTY: ★★★
SOLITUDE: ★

DESPITE THE DIABOLICAL NAME, THE VIEW FROM DEVILS CHAIR IS HEAVENLY.

GPS TRAILHEAD COORDINATES: N37° 22.716' W80° 9.370'

DISTANCE & CONFIGURATION: 4.9-mile loop

HIKING TIME: 3 hours

OUTSTANDING FEATURES: Panoramas from Dragons Tooth and Devils Chair, rock scrambling

ELEVATION: 1,800 feet at trailhead, 3,020 feet at high point

ACCESS: No fees or permits required

MAPS: National Geographic #787, *Blacksburg/New River Valley;* USGS *Glenvar*

FACILITIES: Restroom at trailhead

WHEELCHAIR ACCESS: None

INFO: George Washington National Forest, Eastern Divide Ranger District, 110 Southpark Drive, Blacksburg, VA 24060; 540-552-4641, www.fs.usda.gov/gwj

In Brief

This deservedly popular circuit hike travels up Cove Mountain to a vertical stone slab providing 360-degree panoramas. Along the way, you will ascend a small stream valley, then meet the Appalachian Trail. From there, the AT traverses boulder fields and upturned rock slabs that require some scrambling. Climb the Dragons Tooth, then return via the AT, passing more views, including Devils Chair.

Route Details

This is a fun, popular, yet challenging hike to a geological formation that is fascinating to see while providing a vista from its tip. Be apprised that part of the hike, a part that is on the AT, does require a modicum of rock scrambling using hands and feet. That being said, the hike is done by thousands every year. And it certainly shows off the Roanoke River Valley in a spectacular setting.

Start out on the Dragons Tooth Trail. The singletrack path quickly leads away from the large parking area into the valley of a tributary of McAfee Run. Small bridges pass smaller tributaries. After a quarter-mile, you reach a trail intersection and the loop portion of the hike. Stay right with the Dragons Tooth Trail. Begin crisscrossing the stream of the valley you are ascending. The small watercourse can go nearly dry in summer, but stepping-stones will aid your passage when the stream is higher. Rise into classic pine, oak, and hickory woods with a smattering of sassafras. Occasional switchbacks ease the ascent. Wander through quiet coves of tulip trees, then reach Lost Spectacles Gap and the AT at 1.4 miles. Turn right, southbound on the AT. Begin a benign climb toward the crest of Cove Mountain.

Then things change. A sign accurately warns you of extremely rocky trail ahead. However, it is not simply rocks in the trail but big boulders, naked rock slabs, and upturned formations that challenge the hiker. Stone steps help in places. Pines and black gum trees find their place in the thin soil among lichen-covered boulders. At 2.0 miles, the trail becomes normal again for a minute; then you renew

Dragons Tooth

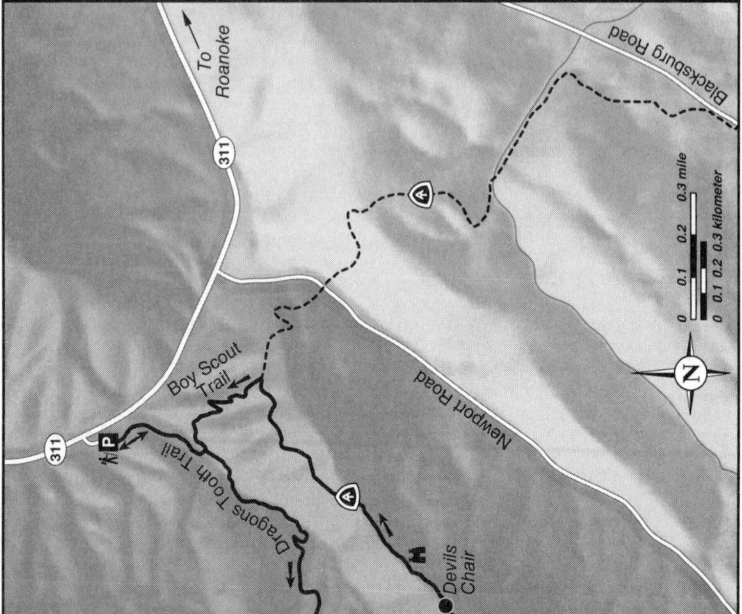

your close relationship with the geology of Cove Mountain. The pathway begins angling up a sloped rocky slab and opens onto your first great view of the Catawba Creek Valley below and Fort Lewis Mountain to the southeast. Beyond the view, you will be using all fours. Two spots have iron rungs placed into the rock for improved hand and foot placement. Exciting!

At 2.2 miles, leave the AT left, joining the ridgetop spur to the Dragons Tooth. The blue-blazed spur curves right around some upturned rocks in a preview of what you are about to reach. Break the 3,000-foot barrier. At 2.4 miles, come to the Dragons Tooth, an upturned rock that does have a fangish look to it. (There are other, lesser "teeth" as well.) Views can be had from its base, but far better ones await atop the tooth. Walk around the far side of the pillar, then scramble to its narrow apex. It is a little scary up there but worth the 360-degree visions of the ridges and valleys near and far. Sinking Creek Mountain stands to the northwest, and marks the Virginia–West Virginia boundary. Craig Creek Valley stretches into the distance. Myriad southwest-to-northeast-running parallel ridges and valley proffer a panorama of the first order.

Be careful descending the narrow Dragons Tooth, especially when it is wet or other hikers are on it. Once on terra firma, backtrack

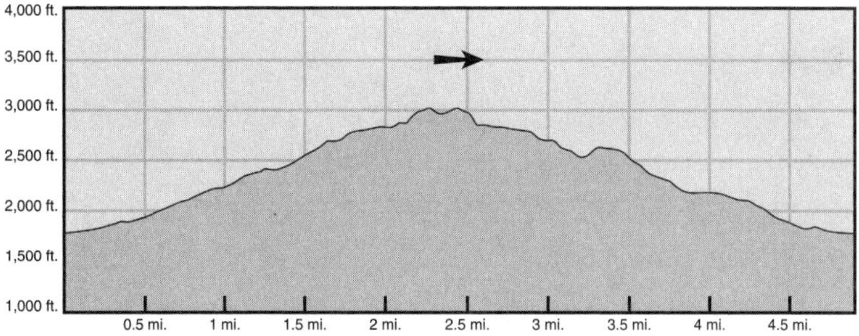

on the spur, then backtrack on the AT, now northbound. Descending the rock slabs and stone steps is harder than climbing them, in a way. Return to Lost Spectacles Gap at 3.2 miles. Continue northbound on the AT, now covering new terrain. Switchback uphill through laurel, galax, and oak. Regain the ridgecrest among squat pines, blueberry, and mountain laurel. Pass an outcrop and a southerly view at 3.4 miles. Ahead, keep an eye peeled for a short spur trail leaving left to a squarish rock with a north-facing perch. This is Devils Chair. Beyond McAfee Run below, the linear ridge of North Mountain stands tall and proud. Resume the AT as it makes a rocky downgrade over a slender ridgeline. At 3.7 miles, reach another southerly view. You have descended quite a bit, and Catawba Creek Valley is much closer.

A continual downgrade leads you to the Boy Scout Trail at 4.3 miles. Leave the AT for a foot-friendly, pine needle–carpeted path. The Boy Scout Trail switchbacks downhill in thickening woods. Come along a little drainage, then, at 4.6 miles, return to the Dragons Tooth Trail. From here, it is a simple backtrack to the trailhead, completing the hike.

Nearby Attractions

The hike to the famed **McAfee Knob** (page 128), another AT icon, is just 4.6 miles away on VA 311 toward Roanoke. In addition, the **North Mountain Loop** (see previous hike), offering solitude aplenty, is even closer, off Forest Road 224.

Directions

From Exit 141 on I-81 just south of Roanoke, take VA 419 North 0.3 mile. Turn right on VA 311 North and follow it 9.6 miles; turn left into the signed parking area for the Dragons Tooth.

23 Audie Murphy Monument

SCENERY: ★★★★
TRAIL CONDITION: ★★★★
CHILDREN: ★★
DIFFICULTY: ★★★
SOLITUDE: ★

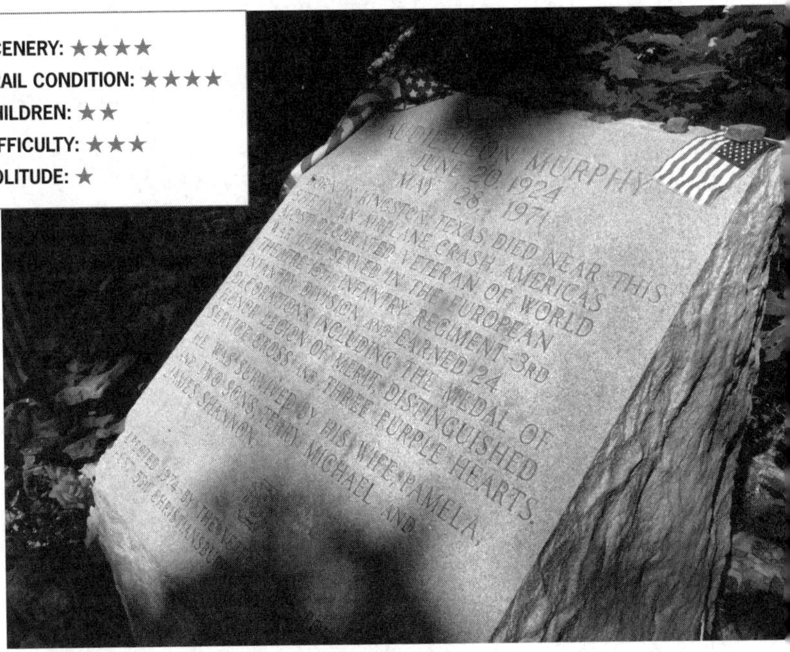

A CLOSE-UP LOOK AT THE AUDIE MURPHY MONUMENT

GPS TRAILHEAD COORDINATES: N37° 22.754' W80° 15.010'

DISTANCE & CONFIGURATION: 7.6-mile out-and-back

HIKING TIME: 4.5 hours

OUTSTANDING FEATURES: Monument to World War II hero, view

ELEVATION: 1,540 feet at trailhead, 3,080 feet at high point

ACCESS: No fees or permits required

MAPS: National Geographic #788, *Covington/Alleghany Highlands;* USGS *Craig Springs, Looney, Glenvar*

FACILITIES: None

WHEELCHAIR ACCESS: None

INFO: George Washington & Jefferson National Forests, Eastern Divide Ranger District, 110 Southpark Drive, Blacksburg, VA 24060; 540-552-4641, www.fs.usda.gov/gwj

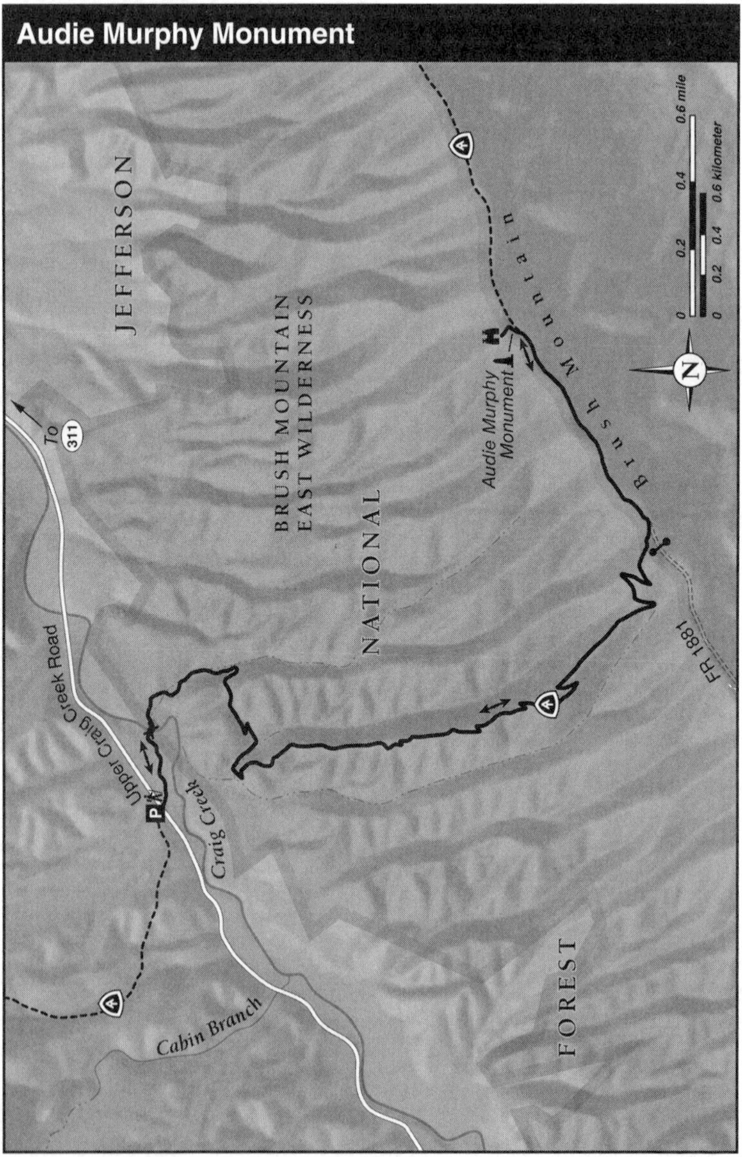
Audie Murphy Monument
JEFFERSON
BRUSH MOUNTAIN
EAST WILDERNESS
NATIONAL
FOREST
Brush Mountain
Audie Murphy Monument
To 311
Upper Craig Creek Road
Craig Creek
Cabin Branch
FR 1881
N
0 0.2 0.4 0.6 mile
0 0.2 0.4 0.6 kilometer

In Brief

This Appalachian Trail hike takes you from bucolic Craig Creek into the Brush Mountain East Wilderness, where you climb Brush Mountain on piney ridges. Once atop Brush, the AT picks up an old roadbed and leads you to a spur trail and the Audie Murphy Monument, commemorating the most decorated American soldier of World War II. A stellar view awaits of the Craig Creek Valley just beyond the monument. Though the hike is never steep, it does gain 1,500 feet from bottom to top.

Route Details

The story of Audie Murphy is an American classic. Known as a movie actor to millions, the way he came into such a position is amazing. Born to poor Texas sharecroppers, his mother passed away as World War II loomed. Times were tough, so Murphy fibbed about his age and joined the Army to help support his siblings. His days of hunting squirrels for food paid off, and Murphy's expert marksmanship, bravery, and leadership stood out. He earned 33 awards and decorations, including the Medal of Honor, the highest military award for bravery that can be given to any individual in the United States. Murphy started out as a private then rose to 2nd Lieutenant while fighting

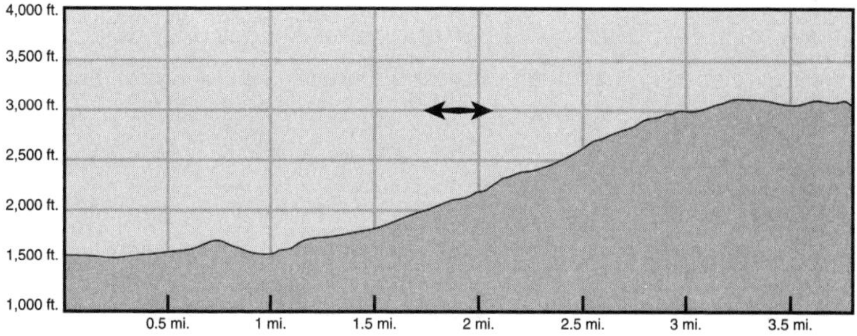

nine major campaigns in Europe. He was wounded three times in his three years of active service.

At the close of World War II, his valor put Murphy on the cover of *Life* magazine. Actor James Cagney saw the photo of Murphy and invited him to Hollywood. Murphy's acting career started slowly, but by 1949 he had starred in his first movie. That same year, his autobiography, *To Hell and Back,* was released and became a best seller. In 1955, *To Hell and Back* was made into a movie starring Murphy as himself and remained Universal Studios' most successful release for two decades. Murphy ended up taking part in 44 films while also engaging in the racehorse business. On May 28, 1971, Murphy was killed when a small private plane he was on crashed into Brush Mountain, near the monument site.

The hike to the monument has the added benefit of traversing the Brush Mountain East Wilderness. Leave Craig Creek Road, heading northbound on the AT, even though the trail is currently traveling south. Walk through the wooded flat of Craig Creek. Immediately bridge a stream flowing through nearby Lee Hollow, then bisect a power-line clearing. Enter Brush Mountain East Wilderness and come to normally clear and alluring Craig Creek at 0.2 mile. Here, climb steps to a raised span built to withstand occasional floods that sweep this flat and cross Craig Creek. A small swimming hole is located just below the bridge. Ahead you will enter more floodplain, likely exhibiting the effects of high water such as brush pushed against the upstream side of trees, small gravel bars, and dry stream braids. Quickly bridge a tributary flowing off Brush Mountain. The AT then enters the white pine–filled hollow of this unnamed stream. Ahead, more bridges cross the tributary, which will likely be dry in summer and fall.

At 0.7 mile, the AT rises to a gap then surprisingly descends to cross the stream of the next hollow over at 0.9 mile. And you were prepared for a relentless climb. Well, here is where it begins. Turn south, beginning the assault on Brush Mountain. Join a piney ridge with an understory of blueberries, ripe for the picking from mid-June to mid-July. Chestnut oaks find their place. While you climb, glimpses of Brush Mountain loom ahead, while behind you, the rampart of Sinking Creek Mountain stretches across the horizon. At 1.3 miles, the AT briefly levels off then resumes the uptick. Enjoy another level area at 1.9 miles.

You have been working up the nose of a ridge, but at 2.1 miles the AT angles right and switchbacks to mitigate a steep segment of the ridge. Pine needles carpet the trailbed. Breaks between the evergreens allow limited vistas. However, these same gaps in the trees allow summer afternoon sun to bake the hiker. I recommend doing this trek in the morning during the warm season.

At 2.3 miles, regain the nose of the ridge and pass a little campsite. Continue ascending, placing your feet between tree roots and crumbly shale. At 2.6 miles, leave the ridge nose again to make a big switchback. Make yet another switchback at 2.8 miles. Leave the Brush Mountain East Wilderness at 3.1 miles to reach the crest of Brush Mountain and a welcome resting bench. The AT heads left on an old

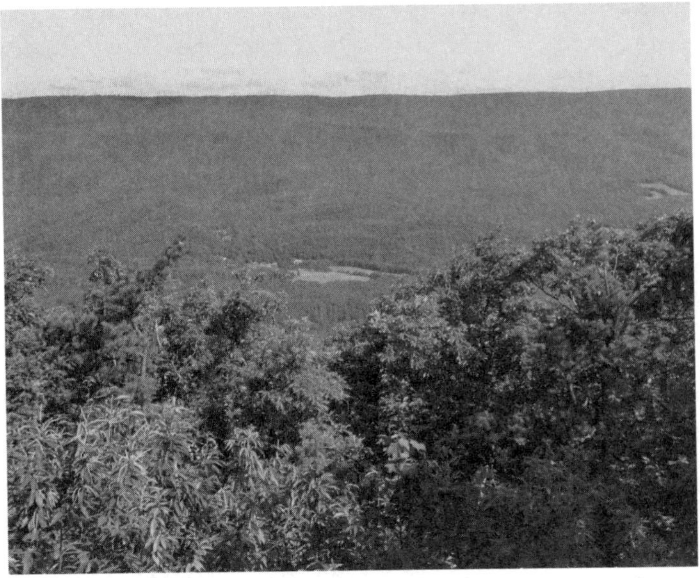

SINKING CREEK MOUNTAIN FORMS A RAMPART ACROSS THE CRAIG CREEK VALLEY.

closed forest road while the monument access from Forest Road 1881 leaves right. Follow the AT, tracing Brush Mountain northeast. Climb a little more, topping out at 3.3 miles. From here the hiking is easy and glorious. Cruise the ridgecrest on a singletrack path overlaying the old forest road.

Pass an old wildlife pond at 3.7 miles, then just ahead you reach a flat and the spur to the Audie Murphy Monument. Split left and make the short climb to the inscribed granite tribute to a bona fide World War II hero. Others have added pebbles to the spot as well as other personalized tributes. After admiring the monument, follow a singletrack path down to an open rock outcrop and a view. From here, hikers can scan across the Craig Creek Valley to the wooded wall forming Sinking Creek Mountain, along with a few outcrops over there. The panorama is a fitting complement to the monument dedicated to Audie Murphy.

Nearby Attractions

From this trailhead, the AT heads south past the Niday trail shelter up to Sinking Creek Mountain.

Directions

From Exit 141 on I-81 just south of Roanoke, take VA 419 North 0.3 mile; turn right on VA 311 North and follow it 13.3 miles to turn left on Upper Craig Creek Road (VA 621). Follow VA 621 for 6.4 miles to the AT crossing at Craig Creek Road. Parking is on the right as you approach the crossing.

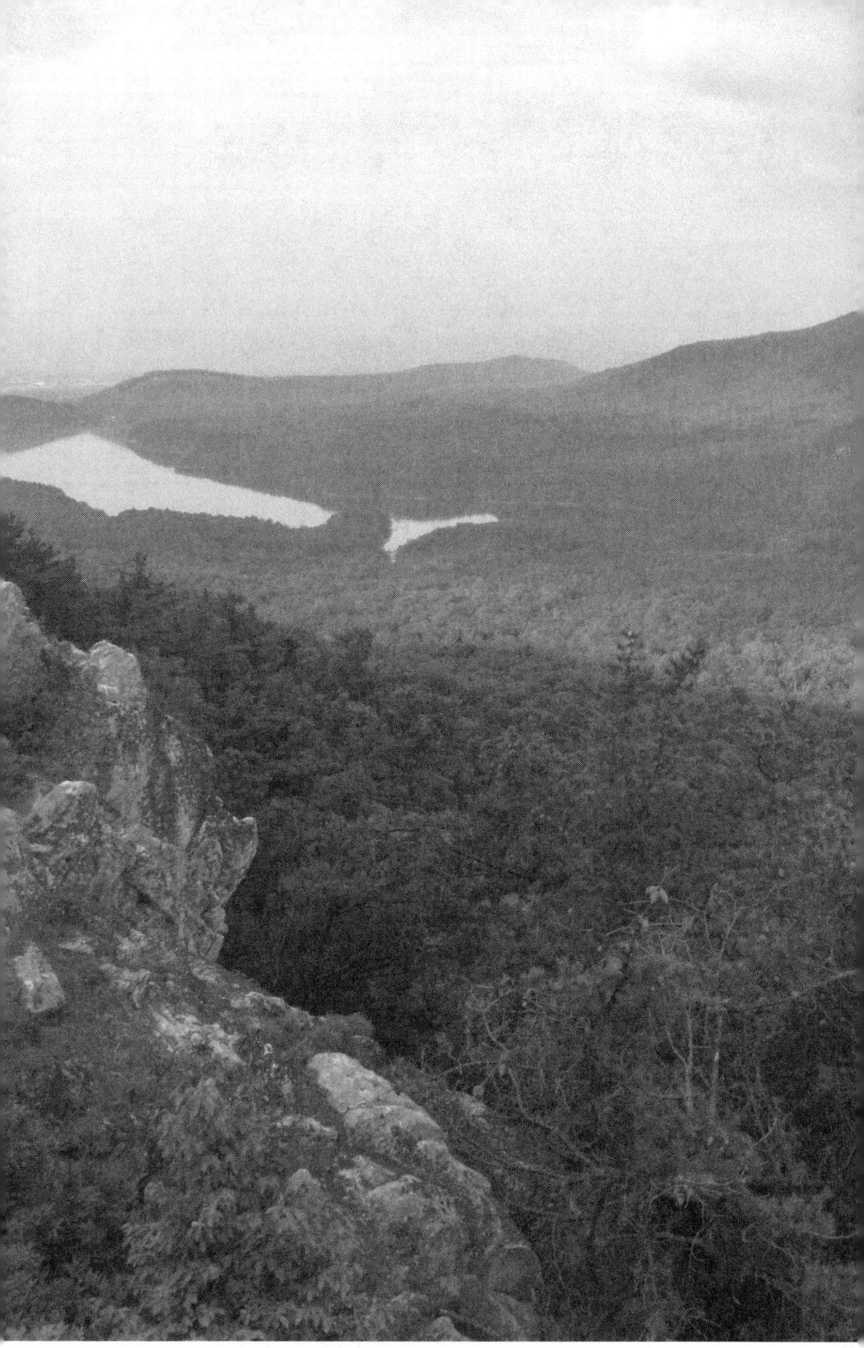

VIRGINIA HIGHLANDS RISE IN THE DISTANCE FROM AN OVERLOOK ON HIKE 19, HAY ROCK AND BEYOND. *(See page 123.)*

Peaks of Otter

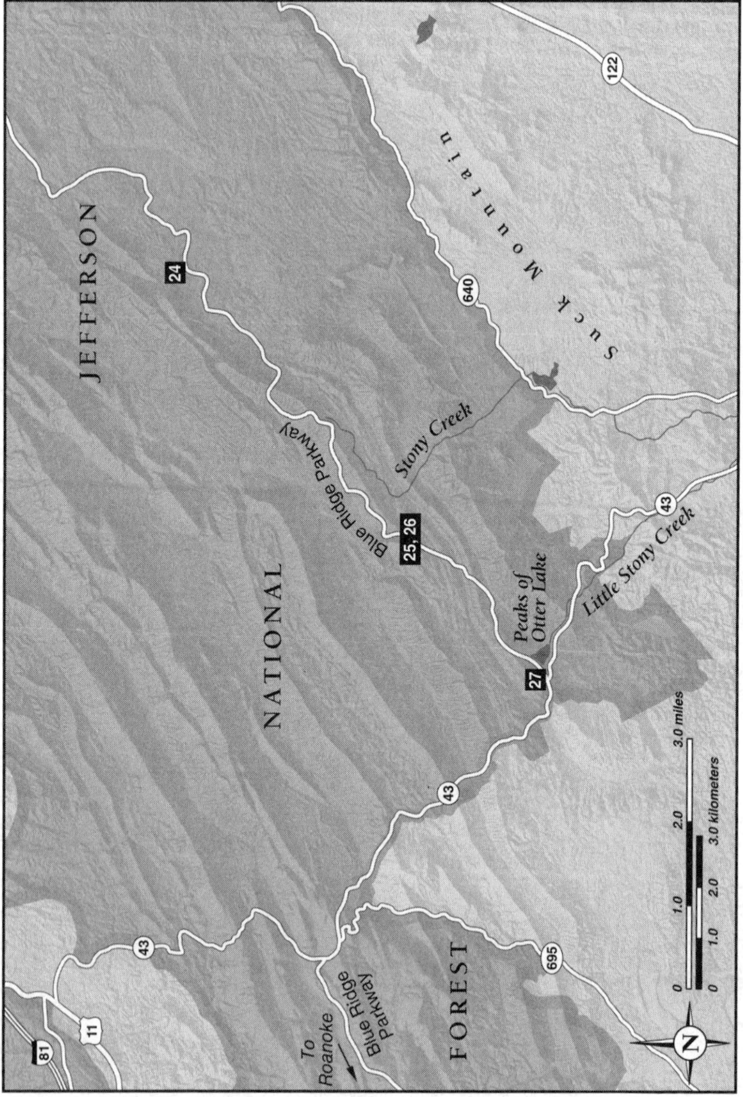

Peaks of Otter

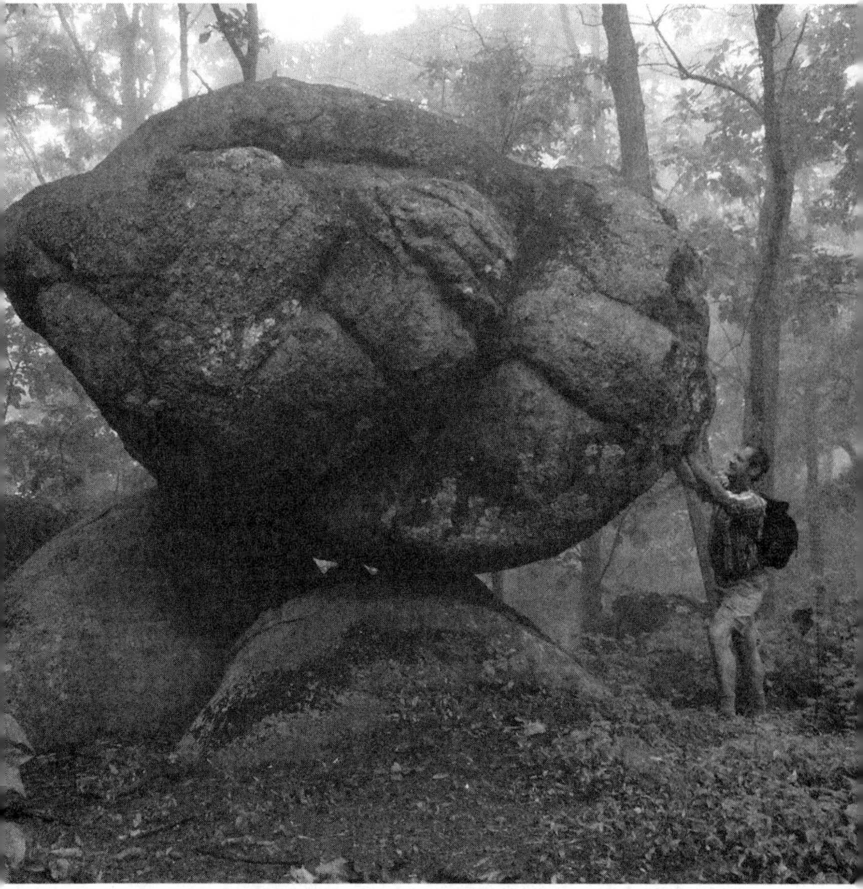

THE AUTHOR FEIGNS AN ATTEMPT TO PUSH OVER A PRECARIOUS TRAILSIDE ROCK ON THE JOHNSON FARM HIKE. *(See Hike 27, page 167.)*

24 Apple Orchard Falls Loop

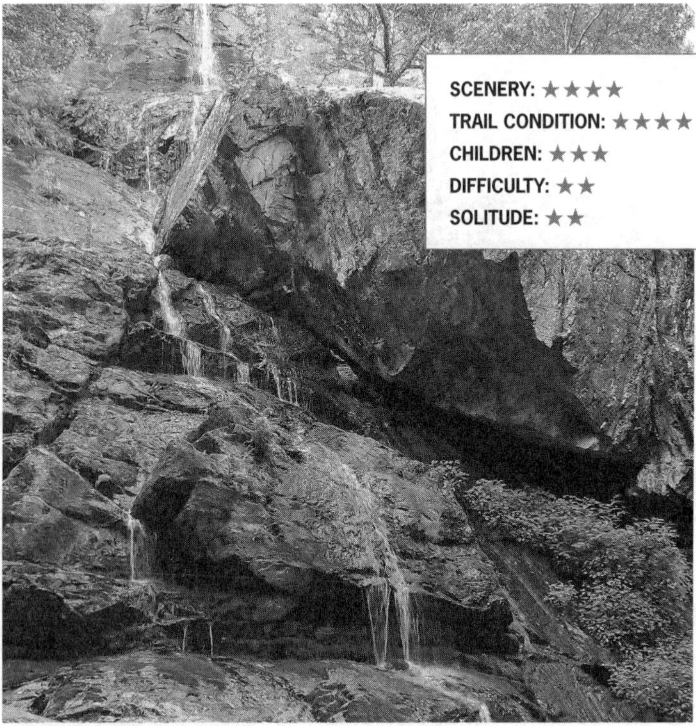

SCENERY: ★★★★
TRAIL CONDITION: ★★★★
CHILDREN: ★★★
DIFFICULTY: ★★
SOLITUDE: ★★

ITS HARD TO CAPTURE ALL 150 FEET OF APPLE ORCHARD FALLS IN JUST ONE PHOTO.

GPS TRAILHEAD COORDINATES: N37° 30.466' W79° 31.448'

DISTANCE & CONFIGURATION: 5.1-mile loop

HIKING TIME: 3 hours

OUTSTANDING FEATURES: Apple Orchard Falls, view

ELEVATION: 3,450 feet at trailhead, 2,420 feet at low point

ACCESS: No fees or permits required

MAPS: National Geographic #789, *Lexington/Blue Ridge Mountains;* USGS *Arnold Valley*

FACILITIES: None

WHEELCHAIR ACCESS: First 200 feet

INFO: George Washington National Forest, Glenwood-Pedlar Ranger District, 27 Ranger Lane, Natural Bridge Station, VA 24579; 540-291-2188, www.fs.usda.gov/gwj

In Brief

Leave the Blue Ridge Parkway at Sunset Fields, and descend Apple Orchard Mountain to tall and varied Apple Orchard Falls. From there, loop via the Cornelius Creek Trail to meet the Appalachian Trail. A high-country ramble on the slope of Apple Orchard Mountain leads you back to the parkway.

Route Details

You may not want to leave your starting point on the Blue Ridge Parkway. Sunset Fields Overlook provides a western vista from atop lofty Apple Orchard Mountain, so named for the rounded-off, weathered oaks that grow atop it, resembling ranks of apple trees. Nevertheless, the AT is calling, and so is high Apple Orchard Falls, tumbling in its wide-ranging fashion, a menagerie of cascades in one location.

The first part of the Apple Orchard Falls Trail is asphalt and all access, leading across the small roadside meadow. From there, join a singletrack natural-surface path descending into rich hardwoods. Circle around an upland cove. At 0.2 mile, intersect the AT. This will be your return route. For now, stay straight with the Apple Orchard Falls Trail, as it begins a headlong descent along a fast-gathering, unnamed tributary of North Creek, making small cascades along the way. At 0.6 mile, spot some old rock walls from a hardscrabble farm. Life must have been tough up here, with cold winters; thin, sloped soils chock-full of rocks; and extreme isolation. At 0.8 mile, come to Apple Orchard Falls Road, closed to vehicles. Keep straight, still descending on the Apple Orchard Falls Trail. Step over a trickling branch contributing its waters to Apple Orchard Falls, then rejoin the main creek, which has now picked up steam and volume as it dashes between boulders. At 1.0 mile, squeeze through a boulder garden, a stone portal of sorts, then cross the main creek on a hiker bridge, near a campsite and small ledge waterfall.

The valley opens beyond the bridge, and you make a wide switchback. Work down an amazing number of wooden stairs, daring

Apple Orchard Falls Loop

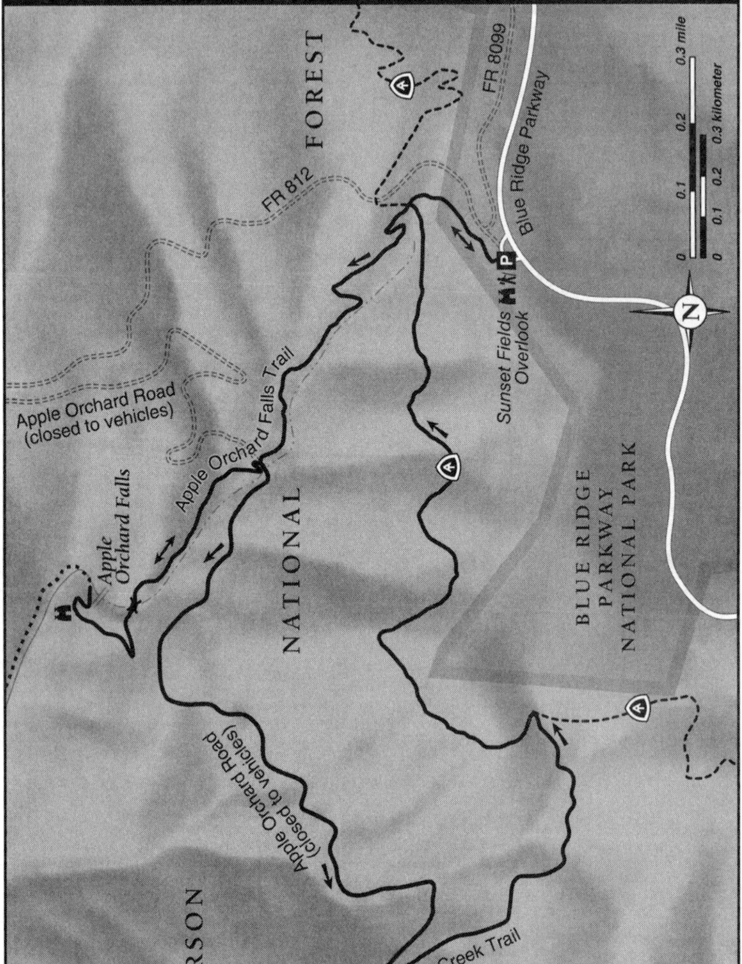

for Apple Orchard Falls. Pass a big boulder and cleared overlook at 1.2 miles. Here, you can gaze west into ridges and hills toward the James River Valley. Look for the bolts of a bench once connected to the boulder. Continue negotiating wooden steps through rhododendron and mountain laurel. At 1.3 miles, reach a bridge crossing the base of Apple Orchard Falls. The span makes for an ideal viewing platform. Look up—from here you can see the cataract spill over an open ledge, then slide down an angled chute. From there the foam encounters a huge mid-cataract boulder, where water disperses into multiple spills, then filters into a rock jumble as it passes underneath the bridge. There is a little bit of everything in this waterfall.

Beyond here, the Apple Orchard Falls Trail continues down to North Creek, but we backtrack away from the falls, returning to Apple Orchard Road at 2.0 miles. Turn right, westbound, on the former forest road turned trail. The roadbed is still grassy, but trees are closing in these days. The walking is easy on the north slope of Apple Orchard Mountain. At 2.7 miles, turn into a stream valley. Ahead, step over this unnamed branch, then rise to meet the Cornelius Creek Trail at 3.1 miles. Head left, joining a ridgeline clad in galax, laurel, and oaks. Climb, and then dip to a gap and small campsite at 3.4 miles. Ahead, recross the aforementioned branch, then rise to meet the AT at 3.6 miles. From here, head left, northbound on the

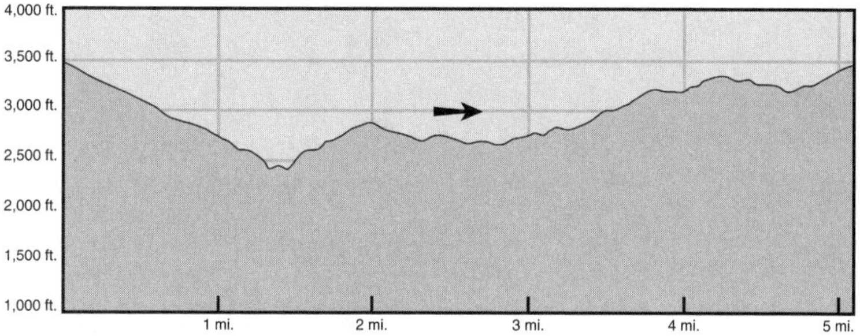

AT. The master path of the East wanders in and out of rich coves of Apple Orchard Mountain, where sturdy, gray-trunked tulip trees fashion a regal mantle. Stinging nettle borders the path in late summer. The trail undulates but little, making for easy walking. Bisect a mossy boulder garden at 4.3 miles. At 4.9 miles, the AT returns you to the Apple Orchard Falls Trail. From here, it is a simple backtrack to the trailhead. If it's late afternoon, consider lingering at the Sunset Fields Overlook to watch Sol sink below the mantle of Old Dominion ridges fading into the distance.

Nearby Attractions

This part of the Blue Ridge Parkway makes for an alluring drive as it travels from the lowest part of the parkway in Virginia at the James River to the highest stretch of Old Dominion Parkway atop Apple Orchard Mountain.

Directions

From Exit 167 on I-81, northeast of Roanoke, take US 11 South 1.2 miles to the town of Buchanan. Turn left on VA 43 East. Follow it to reach the Blue Ridge Parkway after 4.7 miles. Turn left and follow the Blue Ridge Parkway to Sunset Fields Overlook at milepost 78.4. The trailhead is in the middle of the parking area.

25 Fallingwater Cascades

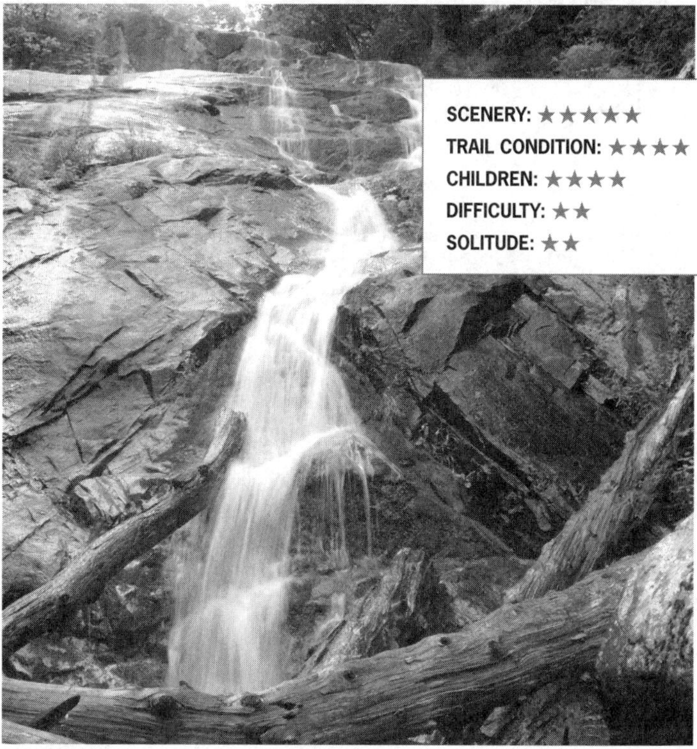

SCENERY: ★★★★★
TRAIL CONDITION: ★★★★
CHILDREN: ★★★★
DIFFICULTY: ★★
SOLITUDE: ★★

FALLINGWATER CASCADES TUMBLES MORE THAN 100 FEET FROM TOP TO BOTTOM.

GPS TRAILHEAD COORDINATES: N37° 28.128' W79° 34.827'

DISTANCE & CONFIGURATION: 1.5-mile loop

HIKING TIME: 1 hour

OUTSTANDING FEATURES: Fallingwater Cascades, old-growth trees, views

ELEVATION: 2,500 feet at trailhead, 2,140 feet at low point

ACCESS: No fees or permits required

MAPS: National Geographic #789, *Lexington/Blue Ridge Mountains;* USGS *Peaks of Otter*

FACILITIES: None

WHEELCHAIR ACCESS: None

INFO: Blue Ridge Parkway, 199 Hemphill Knob Road, Asheville, NC 28803; 828-298-0398; nps.gov/blri

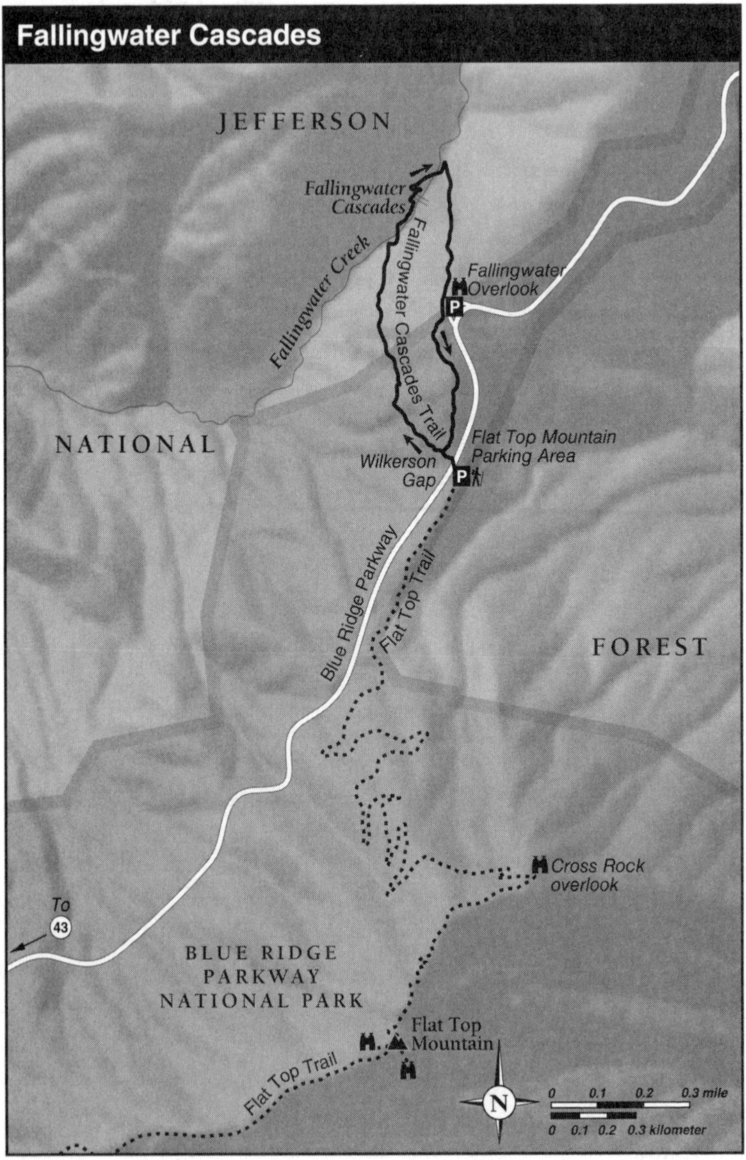
Fallingwater Cascades
JEFFERSON
NATIONAL
FOREST
Fallingwater Cascades
Fallingwater Creek
Fallingwater Cascades Trail
Fallingwater Overlook
Flat Top Mountain Parking Area
Wilkerson Gap
Blue Ridge Parkway
Flat Top Trail
Cross Rock overlook
To
43
BLUE RIDGE PARKWAY NATIONAL PARK
Flat Top Mountain
Flat Top Trail
N
0 0.1 0.2 0.3 mile
0 0.1 0.2 0.3 kilometer

In Brief

This relatively short hike makes a loop to view one of the prettiest waterfalls around, near the Peaks of Otter Recreation Area along the Blue Ridge Parkway. Hike downhill into the geologically rich canyon of Fallingwater Creek, where boulders and woods lend a rugged aspect. Reach Fallingwater Cascades, a scenic waterfall; then climb out of the canyon, soaking in views of mountains down the stream valley before returning to the trailhead.

Route Details

This hike delivers looks at Fallingwater Cascades from multiple viewpoints. You see it from below at a distance, from its base, beside the cataract, and from above it. These varied perspectives deliver an added appreciation of the 100-plus-foot sloping, slipping stream and allow you to see the entirety of Fallingwater Cascades.

The 1.6-mile loop down to the falls is pretty easy, doable by children and older hikers, though parts of the pathway are boulder strewn and irregular. Leave Wilkerson Gap and the Flat Top parking area on the Fallingwater Cascades Trail, a designated national recreation trail built in 1982. Walk down from the west side of the Blue Ridge Parkway on a singletrack natural-surface path. Immediately

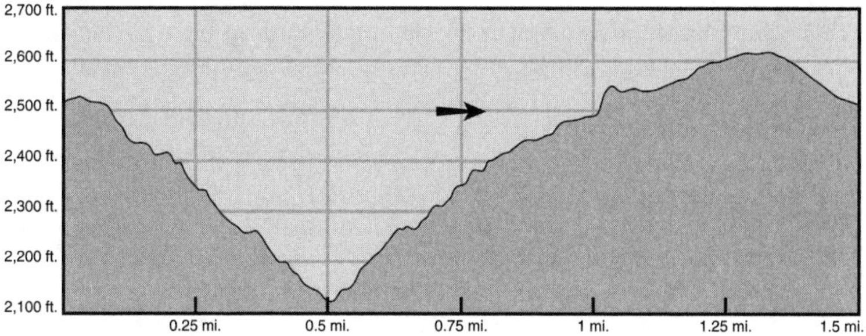

enter an impressive grove of old-growth tulip trees. These towering giants somehow escaped the logger's ax. Quickly reach the loop portion of the hike. Keep straight here, drifting into the steep-sided Fallingwater Creek valley. This stream originates on the slopes of Chestnut Mountain and Floyd Mountain, cutting a chasm to meet its mother stream, Jennings Creek, which then flows on to feed the James River. Pines and rocks border the path. At 0.2 mile, curve around an evergreen-cloaked rib ridge. Pass through a stony talus slope, representative of this rugged canyon that at times seems more stone than soil.

At 0.5 mile, come to Fallingwater Creek and a contemplation bench. There has been a bridge here in the past, and there may be one in the future, but be prepared to rock-hop the watercourse. Here is the catch-22 of waterfall hiking: If the falls are vigorous, then crossing the stream might be challenging. If such is the case, just take off your shoes and make a short wade. However, if the stream is low, the crossing will be an easy rock-hop, but the falls will be less bold. Just hope the bridge has been rebuilt when you come here. Periodic floods have washed it out in the past.

In the depths of the gorge, moving water intersperses huge boulders and rock walls. Vegetation finds its place where soil and slope allow. Ascend along Fallingwater Creek after crossing it, passing lesser falls. The terrain is rugged and steep, and the canyon hems you in. Stone steps, wood steps, and rock walls aid your passage through this otherwise decidedly non-trail-friendly terrain. At 0.6 mile, reach an intersection. Keep straight, soon finding the base of 100-foot Fallingwater Cascades. It spills over a naked rock face into a shallow pool at your feet. The lowermost part of the waterfall is visible from here, as the uppermost fall is too sloped to view in its entirety. The open rock face gets lots of light, even when summer's growth is at its thickest. Repose boulders and photo opportunities are numerous.

Backtrack to continue the loop, climbing to another spur path that leads to the top of the falls, skirting along a stone wall. Use caution here, as slippery slabs of stone are numerous. The open rock face of the falls allows you to look downstream beyond the spreading valley toward the Peaks of Otter.

Continue up the geologically fascinating vale. Look back in this area at a host of mountains through the window formed by the valley of Fallingwater Creek. The sharp top of Sharp Top is easily discernible. Harkening Hill is visible, too. The wild terrain makes civilization seem far away. Bridge Fallingwater Creek at 0.8 mile. Rock slabs below the wooden footbridge make ideal relaxation spots.

The trail then aims for the parkway in pine, oak, and mountain laurel woods. Pass the Fallingwater Overlook and alternative parkway parking at 1.2 miles. Continue uphill in woods, drifting over a knob to finish the loop. From there, turn left, reaching Wilkerson Gap and the Flat Top parking area at 1.5 miles.

Nearby Attractions

The **Peaks of Otter Recreation Area** features not only this trek but also other hikes, such as the 1.5-mile trip to Sharp Top, the peak of which can almost be reached by bus, with but 0.3 mile to the top, where 360-degree views await. In addition, Peaks of Otter has a lodge, campground, and picnic area, open in season.

Directions

From Exit 167 on I-81, northeast of Roanoke, take US 11 South 1.2 miles to the town of Buchanan. Turn left on VA 43 east. Follow it to reach the Blue Ridge Parkway after 4.7 miles. Turn left and follow the Blue Ridge Parkway northeast 7.5 miles to milepost 83.5, with Flat Top Overlook on your left, about 2.4 miles beyond the Peaks of Otter Visitor Center. The Fallingwater Cascades Trail starts across from the viewless Flat Top Overlook on the parkway, opposite the road from the Flat Top Trail, which also starts at this overlook.

26 Flat Top

SCENERY: ★★★★★
TRAIL CONDITION: ★★★★
CHILDREN: ★★
DIFFICULTY: ★★★
SOLITUDE: ★★★

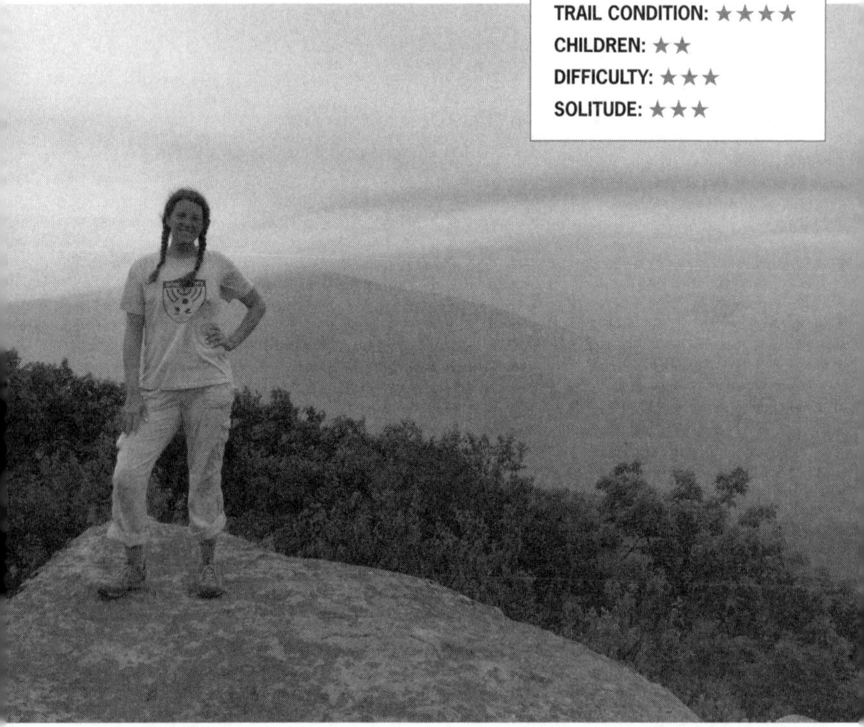

THIS HIKER STRIKES A HAPPY POSE AFTER HAVING CLIMBED 1,500 FEET TO THE CREST OF FLAT TOP MOUNTAIN.

GPS TRAILHEAD COORDINATES: N37° 22.754' W80° 15.010'

DISTANCE & CONFIGURATION: 5.6-mile out-and-back

HIKING TIME: 3.5 hours

OUTSTANDING FEATURES: Views from Cross Rock, Flat Top

ELEVATION: 2,500 feet at trailhead, 4,001 feet at high point

ACCESS: No fees or permits required

MAPS: National Geographic #789, *Lexington/Blue Ridge Mountains;* USGS *Peaks of Otter*

FACILITIES: None

WHEELCHAIR ACCESS: None

INFO: Blue Ridge Parkway, 199 Hemphill Knob Road, Asheville, NC 28803; 828-298-0398; nps.gov/blri

In Brief

A switchback-laden ascent takes you to the top of Flat Top Mountain, where views of the adjacent Peaks of Otter and beyond can be had on both sides. Along the way you will wind through attractive woods that open to Cross Rock and a warm-up vista. The 1,500-foot climb to the top of Flat Top is mitigated by first-rate trail construction and the aforementioned switchbacks.

Route Details

If you can, choose a clear, crisp day to make this trek. The views are marvelous. A crystalline fall day will reveal a cornucopia of color, while winter's bite will be on your nose and hands but allow views to stretch as far as the clarity of the sky allows. A post-front spring day will expose the greens of spring inexorably climbing from the James River 3,000 feet below.

Unfortunately, most hikers visit the Peaks of Otter area and its trails during summer, when views can be obscured by haze, fog, or rain. However, a summer visit beats no visit at all, and you might encounter a fine day. In summer, start early to beat the thunderstorms and heat. The well-marked and -maintained Flat Top Trail leaves from the parking area, southbound, roughly paralleling the parkway in rich hardwoods. The walking is easy at first. Reach a gap at 0.3 mile; then the climb really begins. However, the path is well graded and rarely steep, punctuated by several switchbacks. In fact, the Flat Top Trail is known for its switchbacks. Make the first of these 0.7 mile from the trailhead, in a dry, rocky pine forest. You are working up the northwest slope of Flat Top Mountain. Look for Turk's cap lily and columbine in summer. Make the second switchback at 0.9 mile and the third at 1.3 miles, in the middle of a boulder field. The trailbed becomes rockier as you rise. The Jennings Creek valley falls away far below.

More switchbacks come at 1.4, 1.6, 1.7, and 1.8 miles. You are climbing slowly but surely. Reach the first boulder garden. Here, car-sized stones are heaped upon one another like giant toy blocks. From

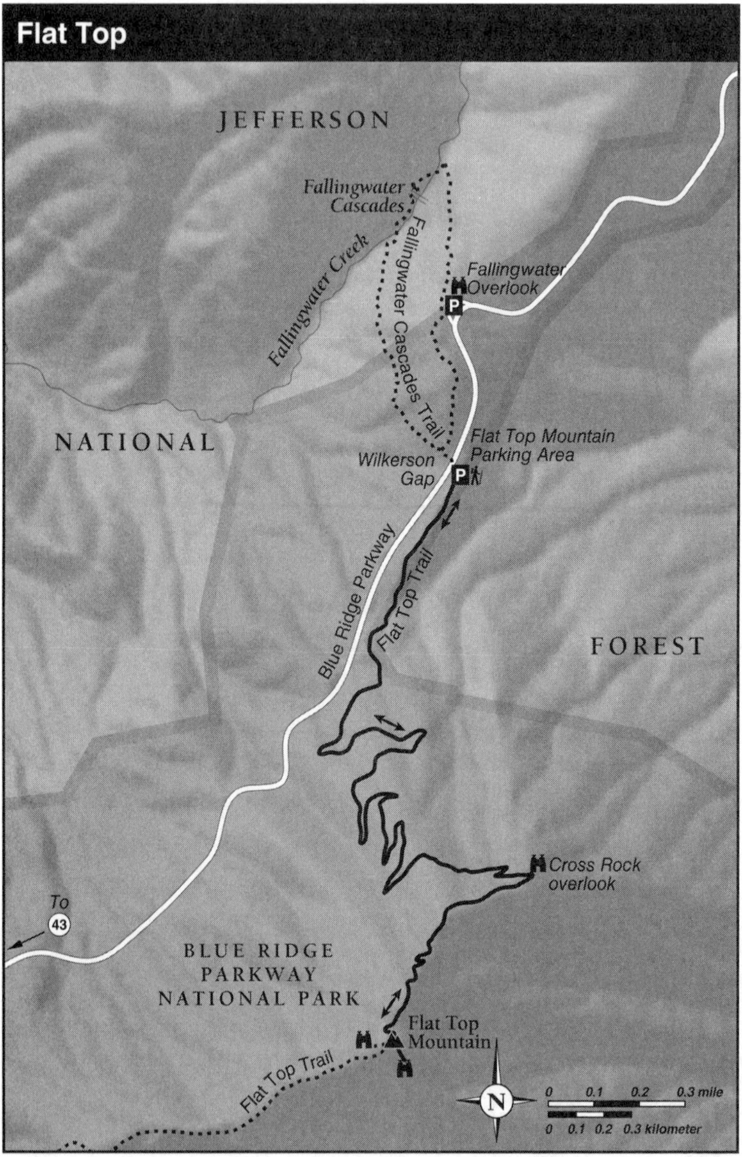
Flat Top
JEFFERSON
NATIONAL
FOREST
Fallingwater Cascades
Fallingwater Creek
Fallingwater Cascades Trail
Fallingwater Overlook
Flat Top Mountain Parking Area
Wilkerson Gap
Blue Ridge Parkway
Flat Top Trail
Cross Rock overlook
To
43
BLUE RIDGE PARKWAY NATIONAL PARK
Flat Top Mountain
Flat Top Trail
N
0 0.1 0.2 0.3 mile
0 0.1 0.2 0.3 kilometer

here on out, boulder gardens become a regular but fascinating element of the mountainscape. The Flat Top Trail often twists and turns among them, adding to a hiker's appreciation of both the trail and the terrain through which it travels.

At 2.1 miles, a very short spur trail leads up to the Cross Rocks, an open outcrop presenting views to the north and east, including the Blue Ridge Parkway, Headforemost Mountain, and east toward the Piedmont. From there, the Flat Top Trail shortly reaches the crest of its namesake mountain, then aims southwest along its spine. At 2.5 miles, the path begins winding through boulder gardens, still ascending for the summit of Flat Top. Look for yellow birch trees, which grow only at the higher elevations in these parts. They can be identified by yellowish-gold, peeling bark with horizontal stripes. The twigs and leaves, when crushed, have a slight wintergreen aroma. Primarily a tree of the north, ranging from Minnesota to Maine, it stretches south down the spine of the Appalachians of Virginia, existing in moist, cool, and high environments. It will often sprout on nutrient-rich rotting logs. Later, the yellow birch grows, and the nurse log rots completely away, leaving the yellow birch looking as if it grew up on its root "legs."

At 2.6 miles, a spur leads left to a decent view, but keep going. Drop to a gap, then work your way up through one more boulder garden

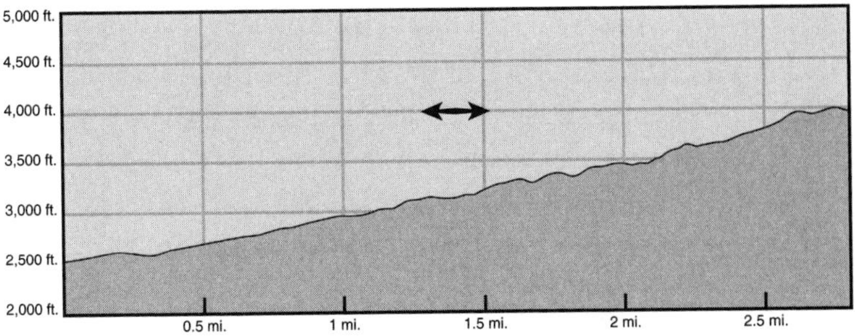

mixed with stone bluffs. Just before the summit, at 2.7 miles, a spur leads left to a wide outcrop and a sweeping panorama to the south. Below lie Bedford Lake and the Big Otter River valley—and Bedford itself. To your left the crest of the Blue Ridge stretches to the horizon. To the right, craggy Sharp Top stands out. This was worth every step.

Resume the Flat Top Trail to shortly reach the signed summit, elevation 4,001 feet. Just beyond the sign, a trail leads right to yet another outcrop, this one on the north side of the mountain. Here, the view extends across Jennings Creek to the James River Valley and beyond toward Purgatory Mountain. Two superlative panoramas from one mountain! The multiple views from the top of Flat Top provide ample recompense for the climb.

Nearby Attractions

The **Peaks of Otter Recreation Area** features not only this trek but also other hikes, such as the 1.5-mile trip to Sharp Top, the peak of which can almost be reached by bus, with but 0.3 mile to the top, where 360-degree views await. In addition, Peaks of Otter has a lodge, campground, and picnic area, open in season. The **Fallingwater Cascades Trail** (see previous hike) starts across the parkway from this hike.

Directions

From Exit 167 on I-81, northeast of Roanoke, take US 11 South 1.2 miles to the town of Buchanan. Turn left on VA 43 East. Follow it to reach the Blue Ridge Parkway after 4.7 miles. Turn left and follow the Blue Ridge Parkway northeast 7.5 miles to milepost 83.5, with Flat Top Overlook on your left, about 2.4 miles beyond the Peaks of Otter Visitor Center. The Flat Top Trail leaves from the southeast corner of the parking area.

27 Johnson Farm via Harkening Hill

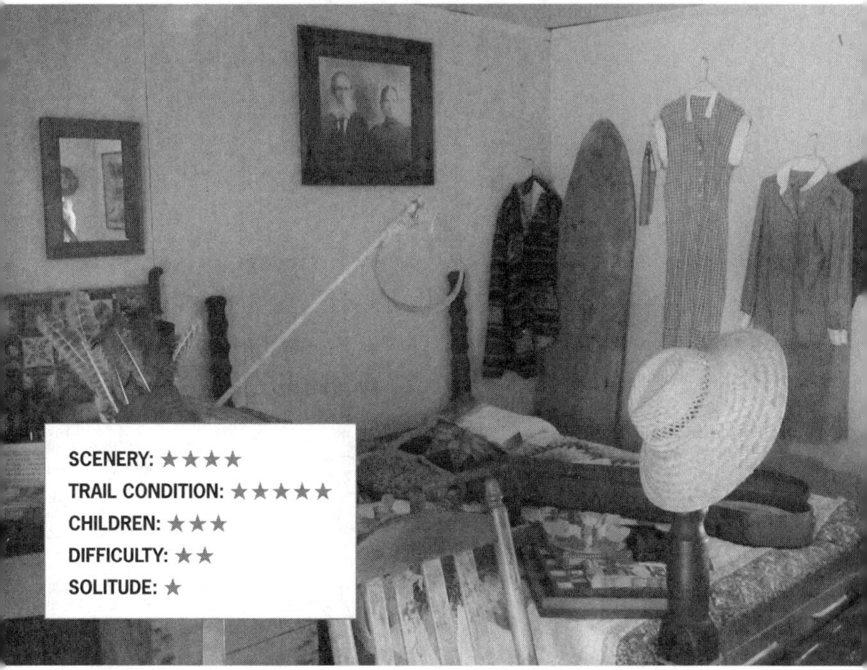

SCENERY: ★★★★
TRAIL CONDITION: ★★★★★
CHILDREN: ★★★
DIFFICULTY: ★★
SOLITUDE: ★

THE JOHNSON FARM REFLECTS 1930S-ERA APPALACHIAN VIRGINIA.

GPS TRAILHEAD COORDINATES: N37° 26.730' W79° 36.584'

DISTANCE & CONFIGURATION: 4.8-mile loop

HIKING TIME: 2.5 hours

OUTSTANDING FEATURES: Balance Rock, Johnson Farm, Abbott Lake, mountain views, geology

ELEVATION: 2,540 feet at trailhead, 3,364 feet at high point

ACCESS: No fees or permits required

MAPS: National Geographic #789, *Lexington/Blue Ridge Mountains;* USGS *Peaks of Otter*

FACILITIES: Visitor center, restrooms, gift shop in season

WHEELCHAIR ACCESS: Around Abbott Lake

INFO: Blue Ridge Parkway, 199 Hemphill Knob Road, Asheville, NC 28803; 828-298-0398; nps.gov/blri

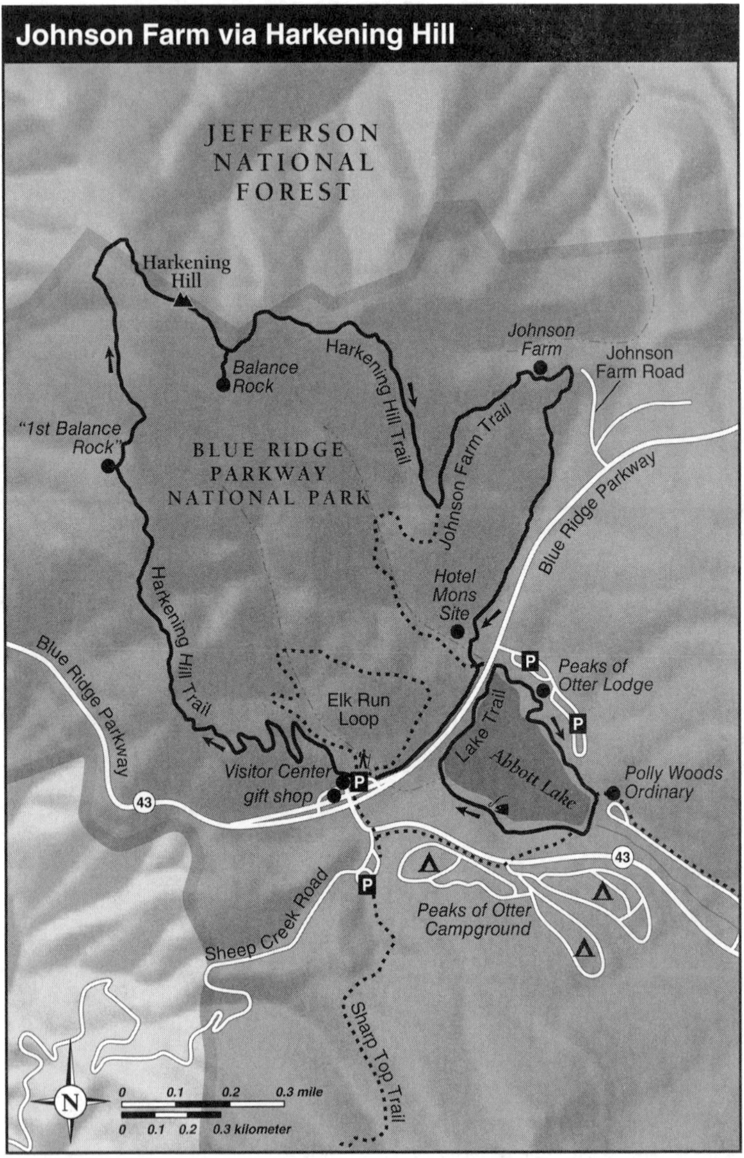
Johnson Farm via Harkening Hill
JEFFERSON NATIONAL FOREST
Harkening Hill
Balance Rock
Harkening Hill Trail
Johnson Farm
Johnson Farm Road
Johnson Farm Trail
"1st Balance Rock"
BLUE RIDGE PARKWAY NATIONAL PARK
Blue Ridge Parkway
Hotel Mons Site
Harkening Hill Trail
Blue Ridge Parkway
Peaks of Otter Lodge
Elk Run Loop
Lake Trail
Abbott Lake
Visitor Center
gift shop
Polly Woods Ordinary
43
43
Sheep Creek Road
Peaks of Otter Campground
Sharp Top Trail
N
0 0.1 0.2 0.3 mile
0 0.1 0.2 0.3 kilometer

In Brief

This hike at the Peaks of Otter area of the Blue Ridge Parkway offers three distinct pleasures. The Harkening Hill Trail takes you first to a geologically entrancing mount with partial views and Balance Rock, then on to historic Johnson Farm, a preserved home replicating local life in the 1930s. Finally, take an easy stroll around Abbott Lake, soaking in water-reflected vistas of the surrounding mountains.

Route Details

This is a fun and varied hike that explores multiple features of the Peaks of Otter area. You will scale one of these peaks—Harkening Hill—first. Leave the Peaks of Otter visitor center, passing through the breezeway separating it from the restrooms. Head left, cutting across an outdoor amphitheater. Join the well-marked and -maintained singletrack Harkening Hill Trail. Cruise beside a branch flowing off Harkening Hill before executing a series of gentle switchbacks. At 0.5 mile, join a north-running ridgeline clothed in hardwoods with a light understory. Note the old apple trees and locust trees, likely from when this hillside was part of a farm—the locusts were pioneers, taking over former grazing lands. Come along the first of

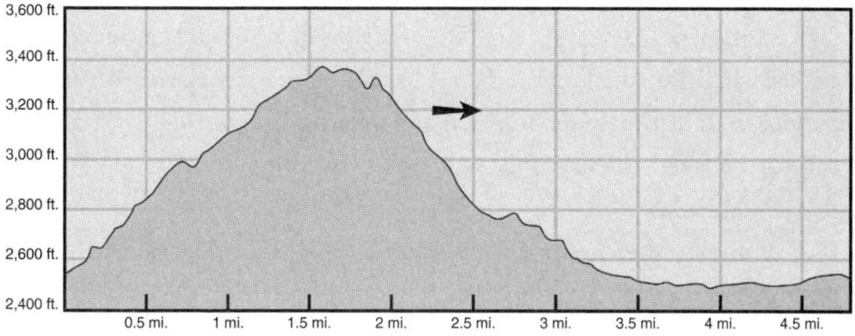

an increasing number of mounded boulders, piles of giant rocks that beckon kids young and old to climb them.

Stairstep to the crest of Harkening Hill. At 1.1 miles, pass a noteworthy stone pile, where a large boulder sits atop others; however, this is not *the* Balance Rock, just a balanced rock. At 1.5 miles, cut through a boulder garden and turn south, now on the crest of Harkening Hill. Reach the summit of Harkening Hill, elevation 3,364 feet. A boulder jumble near the trail provides limited views to the north of the James River Valley and adjacent mountains. Continue on the trail, descending, then turning right to Balance Rock at 1.8 miles. The spur descends a short distance to pass another false Balance Rock on the right, then reaches the bona fide Balance Rock just below. This 10-by-10-foot or so flat boulder stands on a small stone pedestal.

Rejoin the Harkening Hill Trail, descending through youngish forest to pass through a pair of fields at 2.1 miles. At 2.3 miles, briefly join then leave the road accessing the fields. At 2.5 miles, turn left at an intersection, joining the Johnson Farm Trail, reaching the clearing of Johnson Farm at 2.8 miles.

The site of Johnson Farm, occupied since the late 1750s, stands at 2,800 feet in a gap on the shoulder of Harkening Hill. Despite this farm's presence, the Peaks of Otter area became a tourist retreat for those beating the summer lowland heat and hiking the same places we visit today.

The Johnson clan purchased the farm in 1852, occupying the spot for nearly a century more. They worked at some of the prepark tourist facilities, such as the Hotel Mons, before the National Park Service bought the Johnson Farm and adjacent properties. The park service restored the farmhouse's look—including furnishings—to the 1930s era.

Initially, the dwelling was stripped to a bare log cabin that originally stood from the 1700s. Restoring the cabin to its 1930s appearance provides contrast with most other preserved pioneer cabins, which normally depict pre–Civil War periods. Living members of the Johnson family contributed items from the house and used their knowledge to restore the home to what we see today. In season, interpreters are stationed at the farm and can answer all sorts of questions you may have. Prepare to spend some time there.

Leave the home on the old Johnson Farm Road and soon split right from the road on a hiking path. Pass through fields, then come to the Hotel Mons site on your right at 3.5 miles. Ahead, cross a stream, then split left to pass under the Blue Ridge Parkway via tunnel to emerge near the Peaks of Otter Lodge. Turn left on the Lake Trail, now circling Abbott Lake, named for the Blue Ridge Parkway's chief architect. Flat Top and Sharp Top rise in the distance.

At 3.9 miles, a spur leads left to Polly Woods Ordinary, a replica of a rural boardinghouse that once stood where Abbott Lake is now. The Lake Trail spans Abbott Lake Dam, then curves west, passing a spur to Peaks of Otter Campground. At 4.2 miles, another spur leads right to a fishing pier with a stellar view. Continue cruising through woods and grassy area, returning to the tunnel under the parkway. From here, turn left (southwest) on the Johnson Farm Trail, returning to the Peaks of Otter visitor center and completing the loop at 4.8 miles.

Nearby Attractions

The Peaks of Otter Recreation Area features not only this trek but also other hikes, such as the 1.5-mile trip to Sharp Top, the top of which can almost be reached by bus, with but 0.3 mile to the top, where 360-degree views await. Also, Peaks of Otter has a lodge, campground, and picnic area, open in season.

Directions

From Exit 167 on I-81, northeast of Roanoke, take US 11 South 1.2 miles to the town of Buchanan. Turn left on VA 43 East. Follow it to reach the Blue Ridge Parkway after 4.7 miles. Turn left and follow the Blue Ridge Parkway northeast 5 miles to the Peaks of Otter Visitor Center, at milepost 85.9, on your left.

Roanoke and Smith Mountain Lake

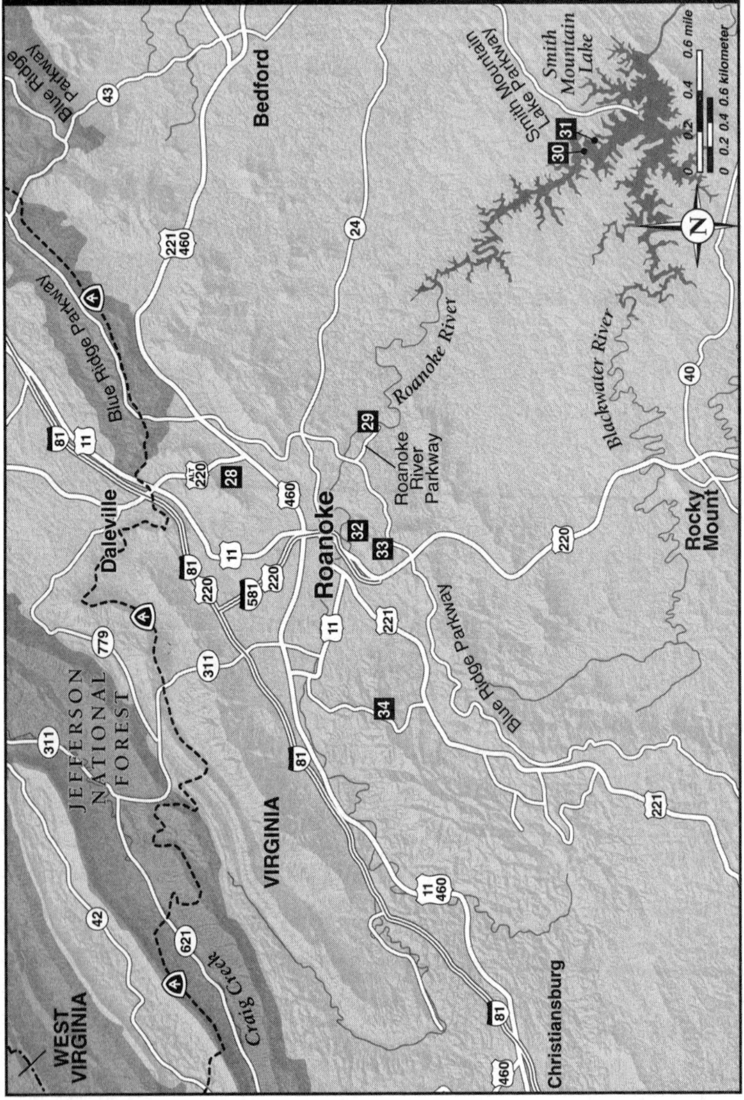

Roanoke and Smith Mountain Lake

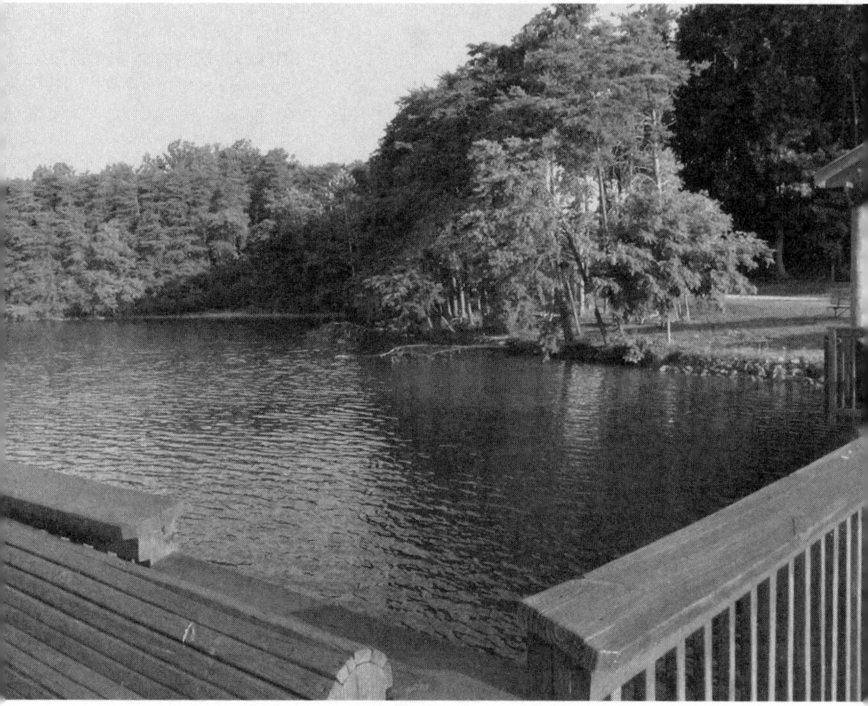

HIKERS CAN CATCH VIEWS FROM THIS TRAILSIDE FISHING PIER AT SMITH MOUNTAIN LAKE. *(See Hike 30, Lake View Walk, page 184.)*

28 Read Mountain Preserve

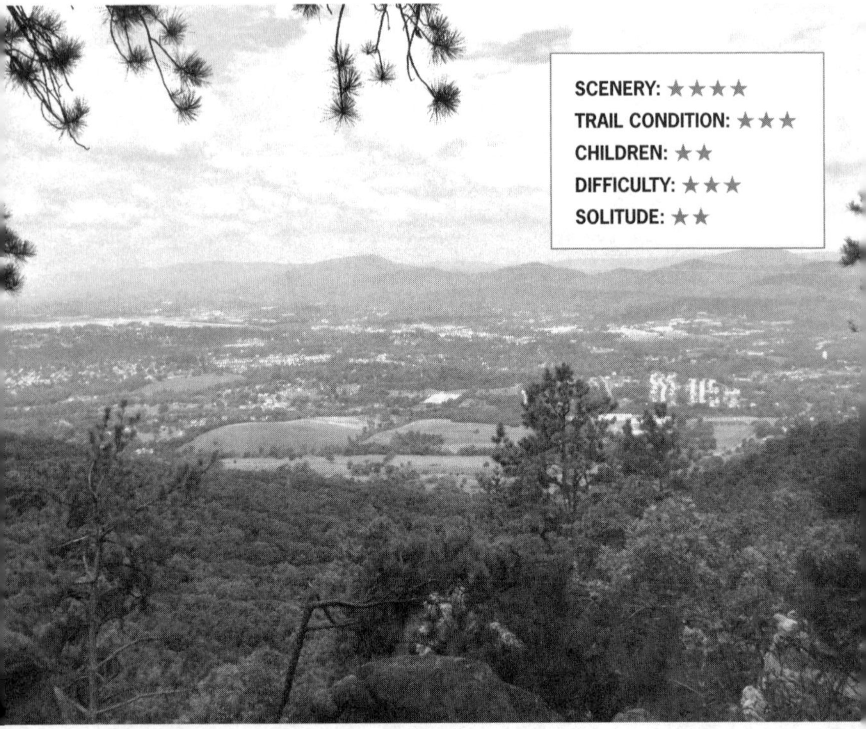

SCENERY: ★★★★
TRAIL CONDITION: ★★★
CHILDREN: ★★
DIFFICULTY: ★★★
SOLITUDE: ★★

READ MOUNTAIN PRESERVE PRESENTS MOUNTAIN AND VALLEY SCENERY FROM BUZZARD ROCK.

GPS TRAILHEAD COORDINATES: N37° 22.754' W80° 15.010'

DISTANCE & CONFIGURATION: 5.0-mile balloon loop

HIKING TIME: 3.5 hours

OUTSTANDING FEATURES: Views from Buzzard Rock and Devils Drop, geology

ELEVATION: 1,350 feet at trailhead, 2,270 feet at high point

ACCESS: No fees or permits required

MAPS: Read Mountain Preserve, USGS *Roanoke*

FACILITIES: Covered picnic table at trailhead

WHEELCHAIR ACCESS: None

INFO: Read Mountain Preserve, 6101 Crumpacker Drive, Bonsack, VA 24019; 540-387-6078, roanokecountyparks.com

In Brief

This hike explores the 258-acre preserve at Read Mountain, a wooded ridge rising northeast of downtown Roanoke. Climb along a hollow, then work your way up the rocky south slope, making view-filled Buzzard Rock. Travel the mountain crest, then complete your loop on the aptly named Rocky Way Trail, grabbing another stellar view from the Devils Drop.

Route Details

Read Mountain is one of those hiking destinations that, once you discover them, you can't help but return to time and again, season to season, while bragging that you were the first among your hiking compadres to go there. Sure, there are sexier destinations like McAfee Knob and higher destinations like Mountain Lake Wilderness, but Read Mountain Preserve, a Roanoke County park, holds its own—and it keeps getting better. It has been a recreation destination since the 1930s, when the Civilian Conservation Corps built trails atop Read Mountain. Ever since, folks have been going up there to hike and reap views. Fast-forward to our times, when the Read Mountain Alliance has worked with Roanoke County to expand and improve access, parking, and trails, resulting in this "must hike" for residents of Roanoke and the New River Valley.

The Buzzard Rock Trail leaves the parking area at a trailhead kiosk. Join a path heading east through an open field. Curve north, entering woods. Pass through a power-line clearing. You are climbing alongside a desiccated tributary of Glade Creek. At 0.3 mile, cross an old ore-car grade. Like many other mountains in the Roanoke Valley, Read Mountain was mined for iron ore a century back. Switchback away from the steep hollow you've been climbing alongside at 0.4 mile. Curve east, intersecting the Rocky Way Trail at 0.6 mile; it is your return route. For now, continue on the Buzzard Rock Trail, entering Iron Mine Hollow. Cross the branch of this hollow, and continue east in scrub pines and oaks that dominate the south slope of Read Mountain, along with sassafras and sourwood.

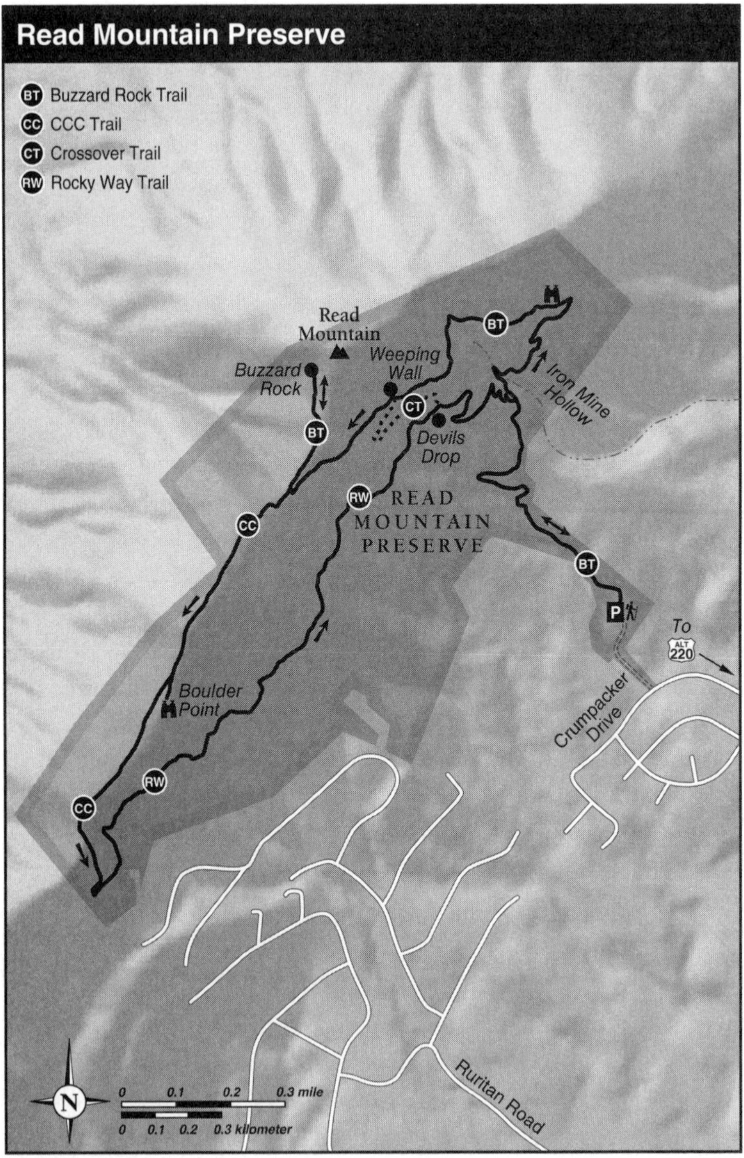
Read Mountain Preserve
BT Buzzard Rock Trail
CC CCC Trail
CT Crossover Trail
RW Rocky Way Trail
Read Mountain
Buzzard Rock
Weeping Wall
Devils Drop
Iron Mine Hollow
READ MOUNTAIN PRESERVE
Boulder Point
To ALT 220
Crumpacker Drive
Ruritan Road
N
0 0.1 0.2 0.3 mile
0 0.1 0.2 0.3 kilometer

Ignore old paths and user-created shortcuts. The Read Mountain Alliance is working hard to stabilize and expand the trail system here. Turn west at 0.9 mile, then pass a partial view to the south. Keep angling up the slope. Intersect the Crossover Trail at 1.3 miles. The short connector path switchbacks down a rocky slope, passing geological formations such as The Fortress and Jacob's Ladder before meeting the Rocky Way Trail near the Devils Drop. The abundance of rock formations on Read Mountain has inspired hikers to name these outcrops.

We continue with the Buzzard Rock Trail, still angling up the south slope of Read Mountain, passing the Weeping Wall, a stone bluff with a slow seep pouring over it. At 1.6 miles, come to a trail intersection atop the crest of Read Mountain. Head east, still on the Buzzard Rock Trail. At first, follow an old roadbed, then split left, coming alongside a mountainside bluff. Reach the open outcrop at 1.8 miles. Here, a stony drop-off opens a vista before you. I-81 crosses the landscape in the lowermost terrain. The Roanoke Airport is easy to spot, while Tinker Mountain and its fellow wooded ridges rise in rank all the way to West Virginia. No wonder this is the most popular destination at the preserve.

Backtrack from Buzzard Rock, then join the CCC Trail. It's an easy walk along the top of Read Mountain, not nearly as rocky as the

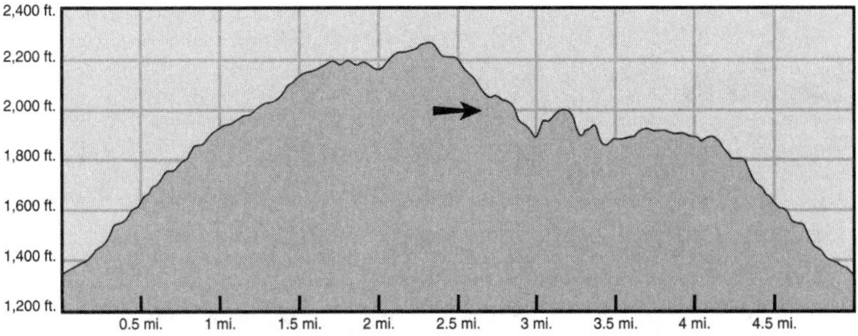

other preserve trails, and fairly level, too. At 2.2 miles, pass a posted private road dropping right down the mountain. Continue hiking the crest among stately oaks. At 2.4 miles, a short spur leads left to Boulder Point. Partial views extend south toward Roanoke. Beyond here, the CCC Trail mostly drops, cutting through a gap at 2.8 miles to meet the Rocky Way Trail near another closed access road at 3.0 miles.

Join the Rocky Way Trail easterly. This is a newer preserve path and is true to its name, especially at first. The singletrack trail picks its way around boulders, outcrops, and stony spots, all scenic areas just a little on the jagged side. Semi-open rock slabs afford partial views southeast. Stone steps make walking more manageable, but the going is slow. By 3.5 miles, the rocks ease and the scenery changes to viney, wooded coves. However, the rocks reappear, and at 4.1 miles you come to the fine view from the Devils Drop. Gaze toward Vinton, the Blue Ridge Parkway, and the Roanoke River as it cuts a swath east through the Piedmont.

Just ahead, pass the Crossover Trail and begin two long switchbacks, then meet the Buzzard Rock Trail at 4.4 miles. You have completed the loop. From here, backtrack to the trailhead, completing the hike.

Nearby Attractions

The hike on the Appalachian Trail up to **Hay Rock and Beyond** (see Hike 19, page 123) is just a few miles from here.

Directions

From Exit 151A on I-81 just north of Roanoke, take US 220 Alternate South 3.5 miles to turn right on Hillview Drive. Follow Hillview Drive into a neighborhood to a four-way stop, and keep straight where Hillview Road becomes Hunt Ridge Road. Continue 0.8 mile from US 220A, then turn right on Crumpacker Drive and follow it 0.2 mile. Turn right onto the signed road and narrow access to Read Mountain Preserve, between two houses. Follow the access road a short distance uphill to the trailhead.

29 Explore Park Hike

SCENERY: ★★★★
TRAIL CONDITION: ★★★★
CHILDREN: ★★★★
DIFFICULTY: ★★
SOLITUDE: ★★

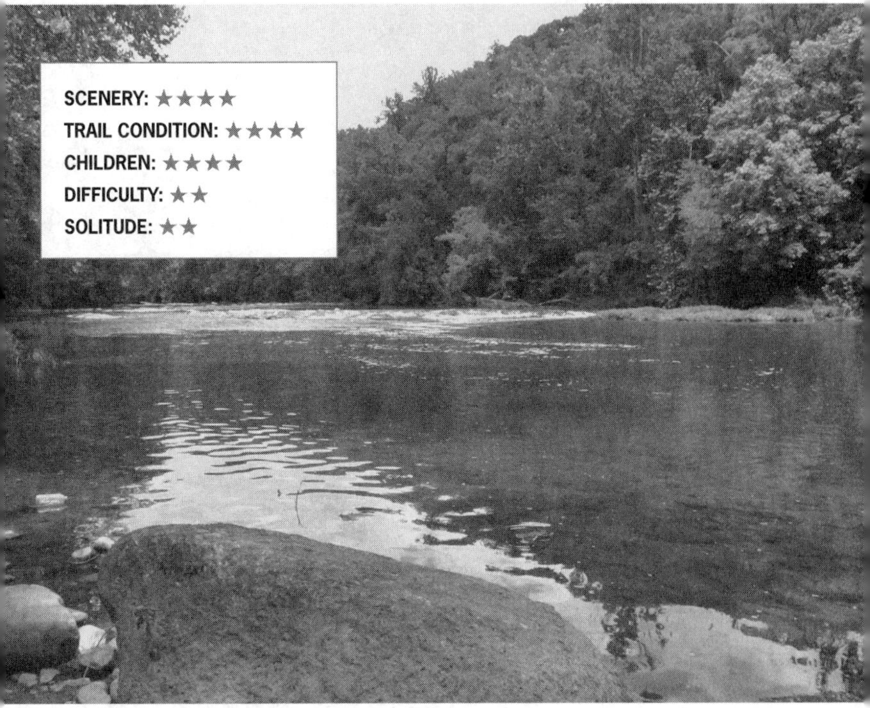

THE ROANOKE RIVER FLOWS THROUGH EXPLORE PARK.

GPS TRAILHEAD COORDINATES: N37° 14.238' W79° 50.760'

DISTANCE & CONFIGURATION: 3.0-mile loop

HIKING TIME: 1.5 hours

OUTSTANDING FEATURES: Historical buildings, Roanoke River

ELEVATION: 880 feet at trailhead, 990 feet at high point

ACCESS: No fees or permits required

MAPS: Explore Park, USGS *Hardy*

FACILITIES: Visitor center, restrooms, picnic area near trailhead

WHEELCHAIR ACCESS: None

INFO: Explore Park, 56 Roanoke River Parkway, Roanoke, VA 24014; 540-387-6078, explorepark.org

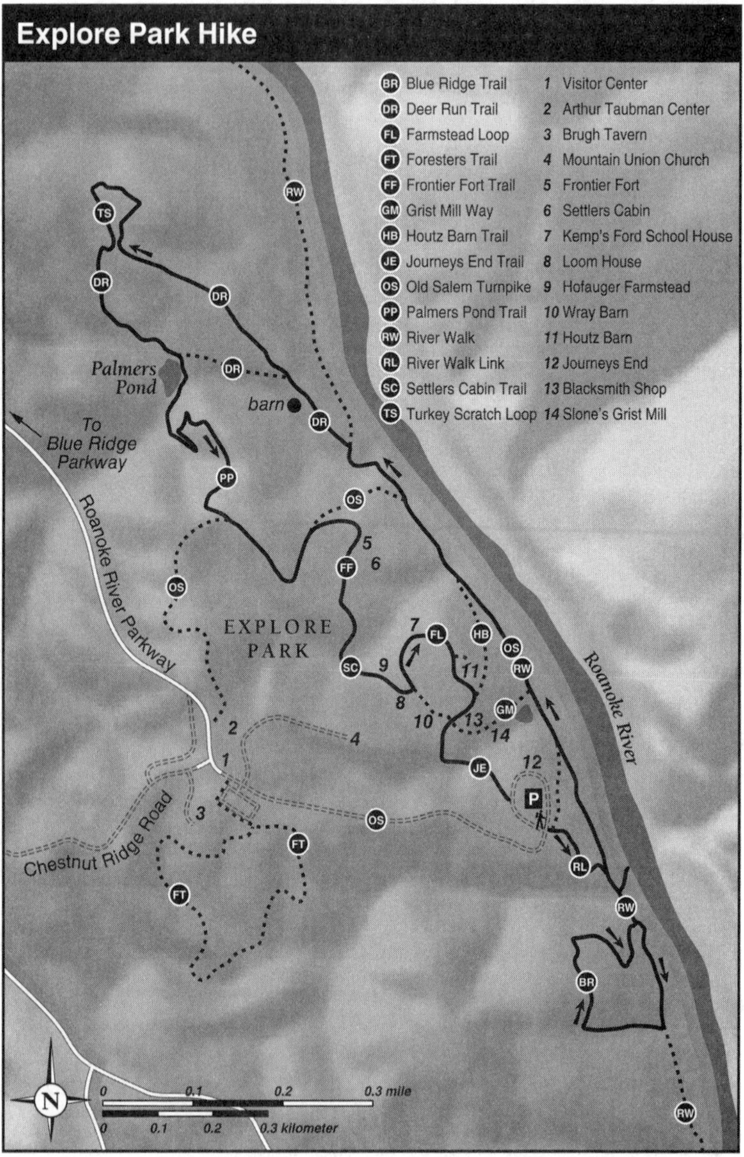
Explore Park Hike
BR Blue Ridge Trail
DR Deer Run Trail
FL Farmstead Loop
FT Foresters Trail
FF Frontier Fort Trail
GM Grist Mill Way
HB Houtz Barn Trail
JE Journeys End Trail
OS Old Salem Turnpike
PP Palmers Pond Trail
RW River Walk
RL River Walk Link
SC Settlers Cabin Trail
TS Turkey Scratch Loop
1 Visitor Center
2 Arthur Taubman Center
3 Brugh Tavern
4 Mountain Union Church
5 Frontier Fort
6 Settlers Cabin
7 Kemp's Ford School House
8 Loom House
9 Hofauger Farmstead
10 Wray Barn
11 Houtz Barn
12 Journeys End
13 Blacksmith Shop
14 Slone's Grist Mill
Palmers Pond
barn
To Blue Ridge Parkway
Roanoke River Parkway
EXPLORE PARK
Roanoke River
Chestnut Ridge Road
N
0 0.1 0.2 0.3 mile
0 0.1 0.2 0.3 kilometer

In Brief

This hike travels the hiker-only trails coursing through Explore Park. First, hike along a scenic portion of the Roanoke River with rocky rapids, pools, and beaches; then head for the hills, where you will wander through upland woods. Finally, make your way past the intriguing assemblage of historical buildings reflecting Virginia's past.

Route Details

Explore Park, located off the Blue Ridge Parkway, has never reached its potential and has often fallen short of expectations. Conceived in 1987, the 1,100-acre hilly tract along the Roanoke River was originally planned as an outdoorsy theme-park destination. It never got off the ground, and through the years, owners and investors have come and gone, spending some $60 million with little to show for it. Since 2014, however, Explore Park has been managed by Roanoke County and is on the rebound. Changes will continue to take place, yet the natural setting and trail infrastructure are in place. And if the trail system changes, it should be for the better.

This hike leaves Parking Lot D, Journeys End. Depart the east side of the parking area on the River Walk Link, a wide gravel

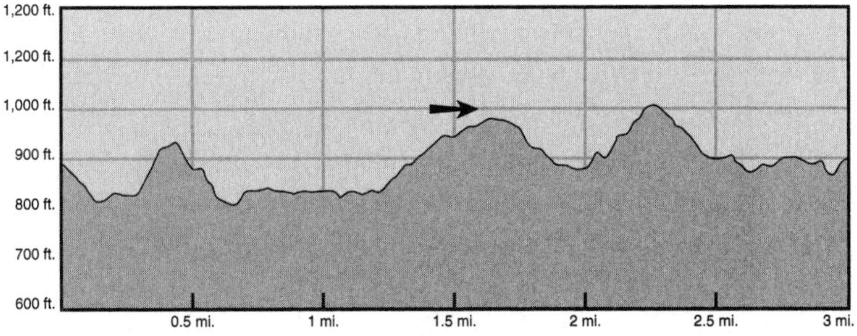

doubletrack. Descend to quickly reach the River Walk. Head right, following the energetic Roanoke River as it flows downstream. The trail is a wide, grassy doubletrack passing under hardwoods. Shortly, pass the north end of the Blue Ridge Trail. Keep going to turn right on the south end of the Blue Ridge Trail. Wind your way up a hill under oak, redbud, and pawpaw trees. Old washtubs and terraced land indicate previous habitation, despite the slope. Return to the River Walk at 0.6 mile. Backtrack toward Journeys End, now heading up the Roanoke River. Split right to visit a riverside beach and water access, used by anglers, swimmers, and sunbathers.

Beyond there, keep up the River Walk. Pass the intersections with Grist Mill Way and then Houtz Barn Trail. Those paths lead to the historical buildings assemblage; our hike will lead there later. For now, continue on the River Walk. More informal river accesses leave right for the water. At 1.1 miles, the Old Salem Turnpike leaves left—stay right with the River Walk, then meet the Deer Run Trail. Head left on the Deer Run Trail, climbing away from the water. Pass a barn still standing from the days when what is now Explore Park was farmland. As you continue, note the gullies created from poor farming practices in the past. Even at that, the forest has made a fine comeback.

Stay right at the loop portion of the Deer Run Trail. At 1.5 miles, split right on the Turkey Scratch Loop. It climbs to a pine- and oak-clad hill then curves back to rejoin the Deer Run Trail at 1.7 miles. Descend the Deer Run Trail to reach cattail-rich Palmers Pond at 1.9 miles. This former farm pond is now silting over to the point where it is more of a marshy wetland that an actual body of water. However, it is still rich in wildlife, especially turtles. Just ahead, turn right to cross the outflow and dam of Palmers Pond, joining the Palmers Pond Trail. This path works its way up a sharply sloped hillside using switchbacks. This is the steepest part of the hike.

Meet the Old Salem Turnpike ahead. Take the wide doubletrack trail left, descending back to the river and the historic area. At 2.4 miles, curve right to reach the old frontier fort. Note the wooden palisades around the buildings. Continue winding through the woods to pass the reconstructed settlers cabin. At 2.6 miles, come to the main grouping of historical structures, in a mix of woods and fields. These wooden wonders were moved here and placed together. Each has its own story. For example, the Kemps Ford schoolhouse was once situated in Franklin County, near a crossing of the Blackwater River. The one-room, fireplace-heated affair served the area in the 1800s. Esom Slone's gristmill was also located in Franklin County and operated until 1952 before being relocated here. It is undergoing a long restoration process. The Hofauger Farmstead, with its house and two original outbuildings, was once on Ogden Road in Roanoke County. It was built in 1837. Take your time exploring these pieces of the past. Roanoke County is working on the long-term future of the buildings. From here, it is but a short walk from near the Leininger Cabin to the parking area at Journeys End.

Nearby Attractions

Explore Park also features miles of mountain bike trails and a canoe/kayak launch to paddle the Roanoke River. Visitors can also fish and swim the Roanoke River from the park. Additionally, the Blue Ridge Parkway offers scenic driving and has a nearby 20-minute hike on the parkway, just north of Roanoke River Parkway and before the Blue Ridge Parkway crossing of the Roanoke River. The trail travels along cliffs above the Roanoke River.

Directions

From downtown Roanoke, take VA 24 East to the Blue Ridge Parkway and milepost 112. Head south on the Blue Ridge Parkway to milepost 115 and turn right on Roanoke River Parkway. Follow it 1.5 miles to the Blue Ridge Parkway Visitor Center. Turn left just beyond the visitor center and go 0.4 mile to Parking Lot D.

30 Lake View Walk

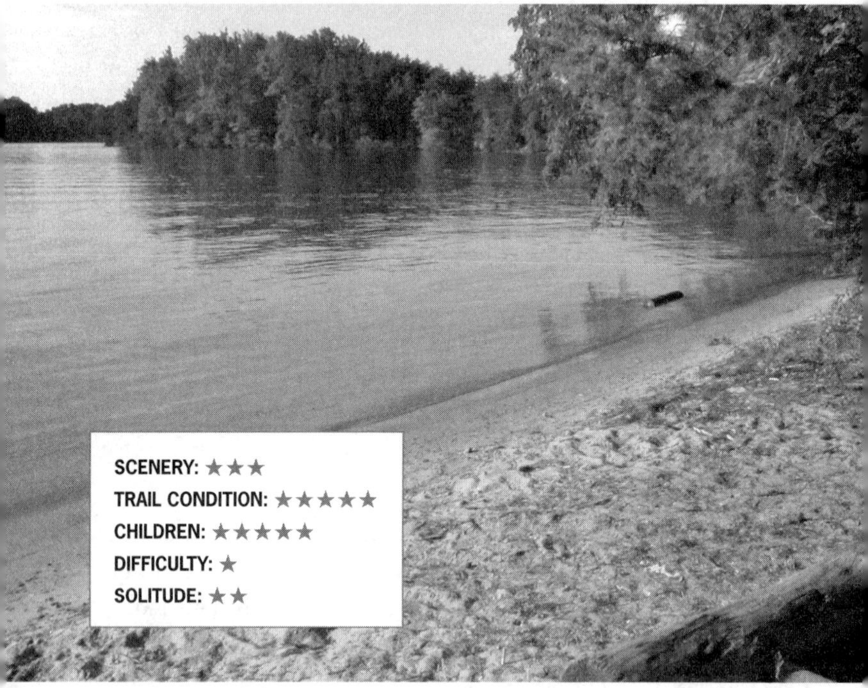

SCENERY: ★★★
TRAIL CONDITION: ★★★★★
CHILDREN: ★★★★★
DIFFICULTY: ★
SOLITUDE: ★★

PEERING INTO A SCENIC COVE FROM A SMALL BEACH ON SMITH MOUNTAIN LAKE

GPS TRAILHEAD COORDINATES: N37° 5.254' W79° 36.936'

DISTANCE & CONFIGURATION: 1.9-mile loop

HIKING TIME: 1 hour

OUTSTANDING FEATURES: Lake views, additional recreation opportunities

ELEVATION: 820 feet at trailhead, 795 feet at low point

ACCESS: No fees or permits required

MAPS: Smith Mountain Lake Community Park; USGS *Smith Mountain Dam*

FACILITIES: Swim beach, picnic area, restrooms, playground, fishing pier, picnic shelter

WHEELCHAIR ACCESS: First part of hike between trailhead and fishing pier

INFO: Smith Mountain Lake Community Park, 1480 Park Way Ave., Moneta, VA 24121; franklincountyva.gov/parks

In Brief

This is an excellent lowland watery destination for the entire family. Make a loop on a peninsula nearly encircled by water at Smith Mountain Lake. This Franklin County park not only features aquatic views on easy woodsy trails but also has a fishing pier, picnic area, and swim beach, allowing you to combine your outdoor activities.

Route Details

Smith Mountain Lake, a dammed impoundment of the Roanoke River southeast of the town of Roanoke, is known for its numerous peninsulas jutting into the water, forming near-islands that add to the 600 or so miles of shoreline. Franklin County's Smith Mountain Lake Community Park is situated on one of those peninsulas, on the Roanoke River arm of the tarn.

The trail system explores about every inch of the park's shoreline, allowing views in all directions. Start your hike on the pea gravel, all-access Picnic Point Trail, heading east toward the fishing pier. Scrub pines and oaks border the wide path. You can already see the lake ahead—and the fishing pier. It is an elaborate wooden structure, with built-in wooden benches and a roof covering part of it. Views open east of Smith Mountain Lake State Park's natural shoreline, as well as lakefront homes elsewhere. On land nearby stands a picnic shelter.

After watching the anglers and boaters and perhaps having a picnic, begin a counterclockwise loop around the park. Take the North Shore Trail, curving around the north side of the park. In the 1940s, you would have been on a hill overlooking the Roanoke River, but the Army Corps of Engineers came up with a plan to put 11 dams on the river to provide water storage, power generation, and recreation. However, Appalachian Power got wind of the plan and decided to beat the Army Corps of Engineers to the punch. The natural gap in Smith Mountain through which the Roanoke River flowed was an ideal location for a dam, and one was started in 1960. Property condemnation and purchases along the proposed lake were under way, as

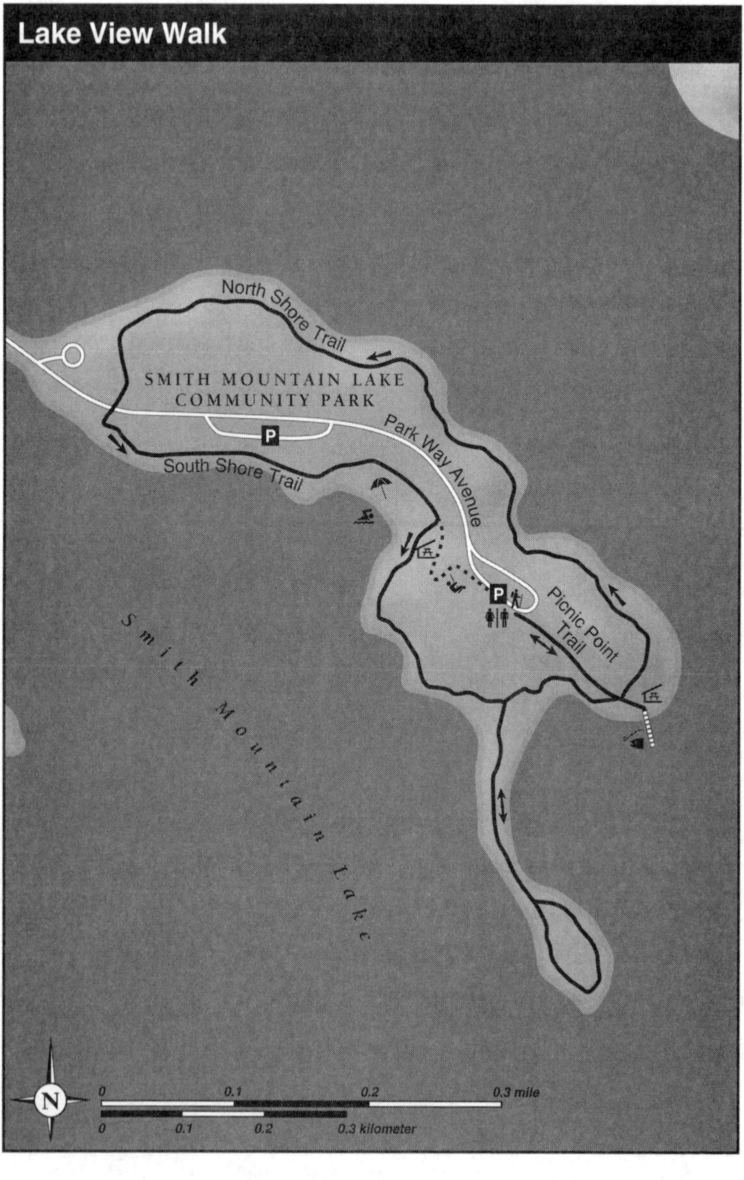
Lake View Walk
North Shore Trail
SMITH MOUNTAIN LAKE
COMMUNITY PARK
Park Way Avenue
South Shore Trail
P
P
Picnic Point
Trail
Smith Mountain Lake
N
0
0.1
0.2
0.3 mile
0
0.1
0.2
0.3 kilometer

was removal of structures that would eventually be inundated—and perhaps cause navigational hazards. Graves were relocated. In 1963, the lake that was to cover more than 25,000 acres began to fill and by 1966, the lake was at full pool.

If you hike here in the summer, the impoundment should be at full pool—795 feet in elevation. This is a good time to visit if you want to use the fishing pier or swim beach or launch your canoe or kayak. The park is also a preferable winter hiking alternative if you do not want to tackle the chill of the high mountains west of Roanoke. The North Shore Trail is a singletrack path coursing through prototypal Piedmont woods of maple, shortleaf pine, beech, and white oak. Views extend through the trees no matter the season, and a good view is a simple matter of walking a few feet to the shoreline.

At 0.3 mile, a shortcut leads back to the parking area. Continue paralleling the red-clay shoreline. At 0.8 mile, a spur trail leads to the park entrance. Stay left and cross the park entrance road, joining the South Shore Trail. It soon comes alongside the water's edge, in places forming slender tan beaches. At 1.0 mile, circle by the swim beach, arguably the most popular place here. The path reenters woods, then reaches a spur trail at 1.3 miles. Take this spur right to explore the farthest point of the park, a peninsula on a peninsula. Make a little loop on this evergreen-clad point, enjoying more watery panoramas.

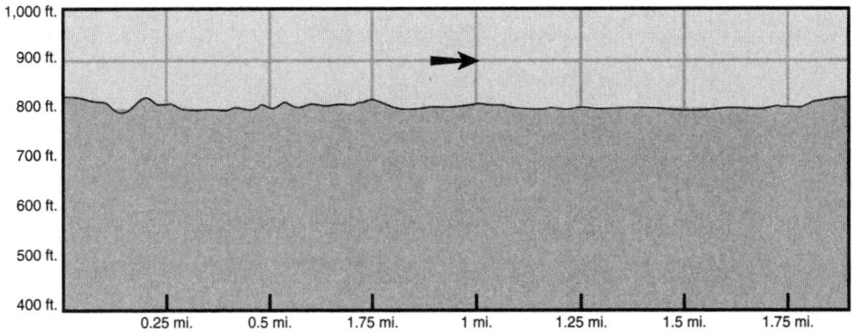

Soon return to the fishing pier area, then backtrack to the trailhead on the Picnic Point Trail.

Nearby Attractions

Smith Mountain Lake is a huge reservoir with loads of aquatic activities, from fishing to swimming to boating and more. The lake is ringed with accesses and includes land-based recreation at Smith Mountain Lake State Park, located just across the water—but a 20-minute drive—from this park.

Directions

From Exit 6 on I-581 in downtown Roanoke, turn left on Elm Avenue toward Vinton. Go 0.5 mile to a traffic light and turn right on Ninth Street. Follow Ninth Street 1.1 miles, then turn left on VA 116 South. Follow VA 116 South 14 miles to a traffic light and turn right on VA 122 South toward Rocky Mount (do not be tempted to turn left toward Smith Mountain Lake State Park). Follow VA 122 South just a short distance, then turn left on VA 670 (Burnt Chimney Road) and follow it 6.9 miles to turn left on Lovely Valley Road. Follow Lovely Valley Road 2.4 miles, then turn right on Scruggs Road. Follow Scruggs Road 1.7 miles and then turn left onto Blue Water Drive. Follow Blue Water Drive 1.1 miles, then turn right on Saunders Farm Road and follow it 0.4 mile to turn right on Winding Waters Drive (you are now in a subdivision). Continue another 0.4 mile, then turn left on Park Way Avenue and follow it to dead-end in Smith Mountain Lake Community Park at a turnaround and parking area, a little beyond the swim beach.

31 Turtle Island Hike

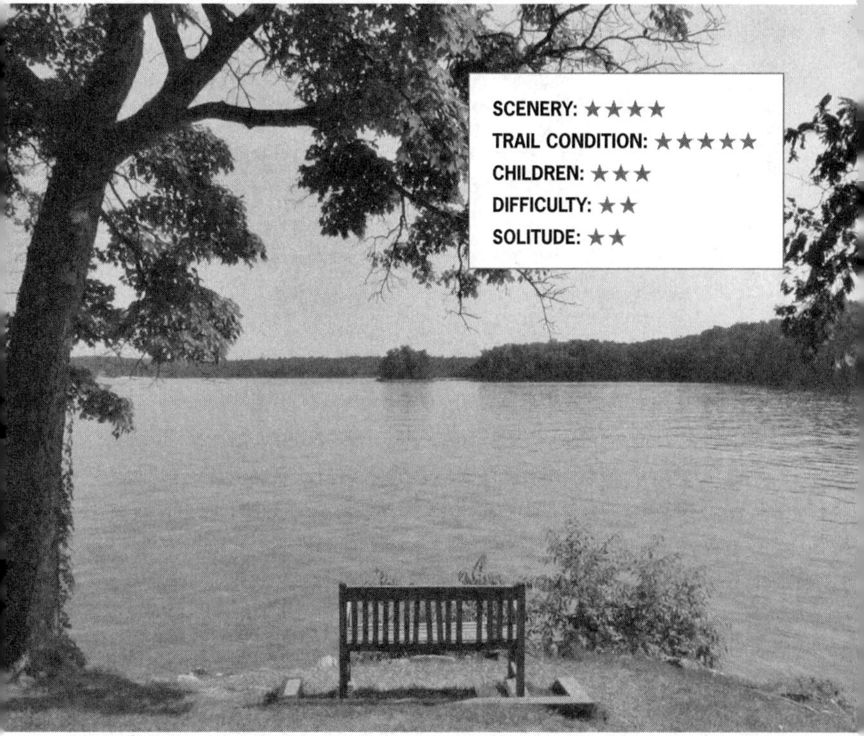

SCENERY: ★★★★
TRAIL CONDITION: ★★★★★
CHILDREN: ★★★
DIFFICULTY: ★★
SOLITUDE: ★★

LOOKING OUT ON TURTLE ISLAND FROM A POINT ENHANCED BY A CONTEMPLATION BENCH

GPS TRAILHEAD COORDINATES: N37° 4.903' W79° 36.491'

DISTANCE & CONFIGURATION: 4.4-mile loop

HIKING TIME: 2.5 hours

OUTSTANDING FEATURES: Lake views, historic structures

ELEVATION: 865 feet at trailhead, 796 feet at low point

ACCESS: Entrance fee required

MAPS: Smith Mountain Lake State Park Trails, USGS *Smith Mountain Dam*

FACILITIES: Visitor center, dock, interpretive center, campground, picnic and swim areas

WHEELCHAIR ACCESS: None

INFO: Smith Mountain Lake State Park, 1235 State Park Road, Huddleston, VA 24104; 540-297-7381, virginiastateparks.gov

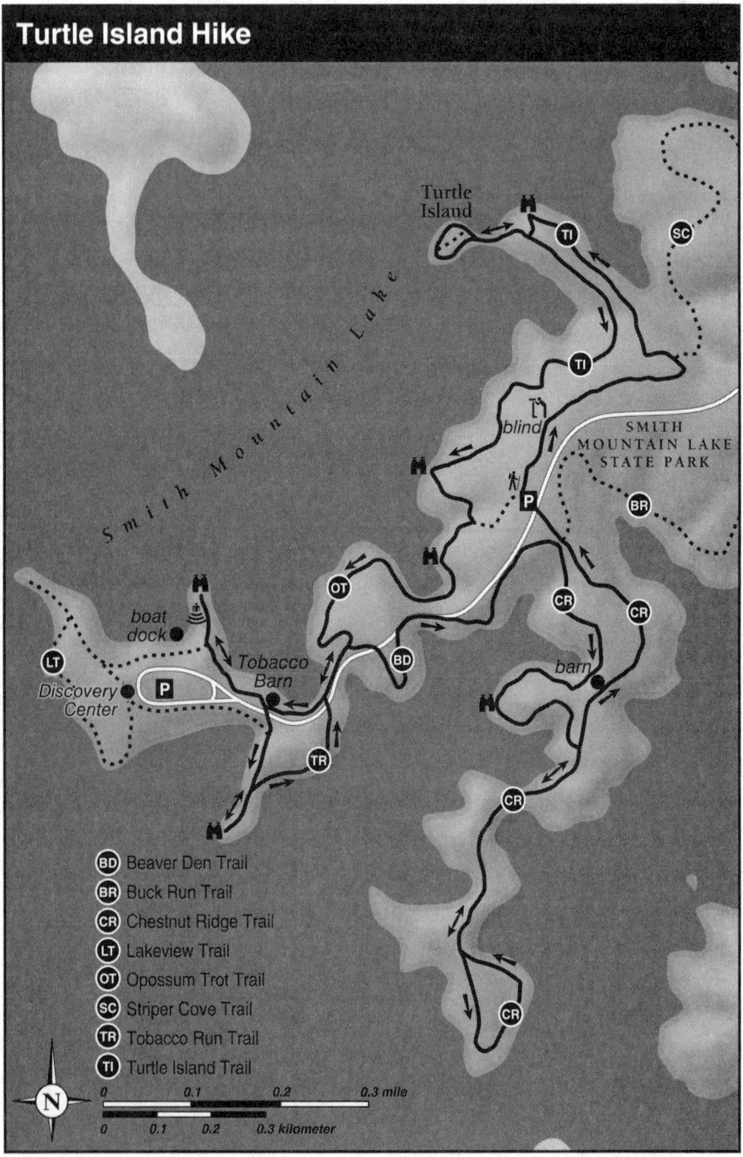
Turtle Island Hike
Turtle Island
Smith Mountain Lake
SMITH MOUNTAIN LAKE STATE PARK
blind
boat dock
Tobacco Barn
Discovery Center
barn
BD Beaver Den Trail
BR Buck Run Trail
CR Chestnut Ridge Trail
LT Lakeview Trail
OT Opossum Trot Trail
SC Striper Cove Trail
TR Tobacco Run Trail
TI Turtle Island Trail
0 0.1 0.2 0.3 mile
0 0.1 0.2 0.3 kilometer
N

In Brief

This hike explores the shoreline within the confines of Smith Mountain Lake State Park. Along the way, head out to Turtle Island, linked by a bridge to the mainland, and gain many views of the impoundment from vistas complete with benches. Finally, visit a restored tobacco barn, as well as one left to the elements and time.

Route Details

Smith Mountain Lake State Park is a significant resource for Roanoke recreational enthusiasts. The low-elevation Piedmont impoundment offers alternative scenery and landscapes from the mountain-rimmed immediate Roanoke and New River Valley area. The Roanoke River was dammed at Smith Mountain to create the huge lake. Luckily, the state of Virginia acquired nearly 1,800 acres of land to use as a state park. They created quite a trail network—well marked and maintained, too—for hikers like us, as well as numerous other facilities to accentuate the hiking opportunities. Truthfully, though, most park visitors are water-oriented. However, you will find this hike is as water oriented as a trail experience can be—nearly the entire circuit goes along the shoreline, and if the hike is not along the shoreline

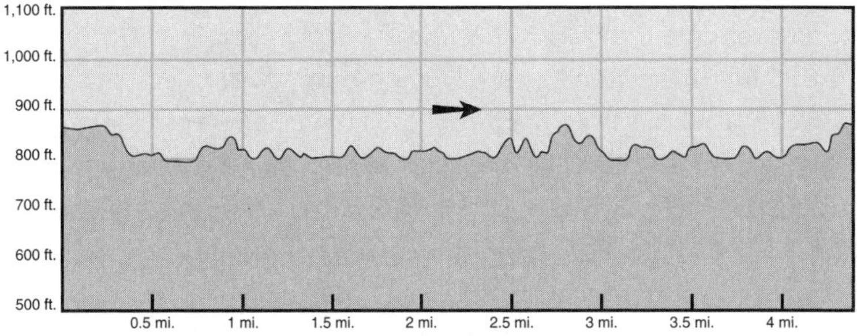

it is near the shoreline. You are never far from water while hiking at Smith Mountain Lake State Park.

Consider coming here when the blast of winter chills the mountains, or come here during the warm season when you can fully engage in the aquatic opportunities here. Or visit when you desire more level, easy trails. Start the adventure at the Turtle Island trailhead. Join the Turtle Island Trail heading right (it also goes straight), parallel to Interpretive Trail Road. Soak in the interpretive information along the path as you traipse under oaks, cedar, and pines. A short spur goes left to a wildlife observation blind overlooking a small meadow. If it is near dusk or dawn and you are patient, consider trying to view a deer or other critter. Otherwise, continue along the Turtle Island Trail in former fields now turned to forest.

At 0.2 mile, near a steep hollow, the Striper Cove Trail splits right toward the main visitor center. Stay left with the Turtle Island Trail, soon coming along the shoreline on a peninsula. Look for a clear view with a contemplation bench before meeting the spur trail leading right toward Turtle Island at 0.5 mile. Head to the former hill turned island, connected to the mainland by a short, arched wood bridge. Loop around the island. It is bisected with a short cross trail of its own. Enjoy the views. Smith Mountain Lake Community Park is just across the cove from you. Ironically, you could swim there quicker than you could drive there from Smith Mountain Lake State Park.

Resume the shoreline jaunt, passing more views to meet the Opossum Trot Trail at 1.3 miles. It is a short distance left to the Turtle Island trailhead if you forgot anything. Otherwise, continue the circuit, passing near Interpretive Trail Road. Come along the park road again at 1.6 miles. Stay along the shore, joining the Tobacco Run Trail to immediately pass a restored tobacco barn. Beyond there, continue hiking. The park's Discovery Center stands to your left. Emerge at an amphitheater and vista point with a picnic table and bench. This is my favorite view here. Turtle Island is clearly visible to the north.

Backtrack to the tobacco barn, then cross the road, treading new trail. Come to a vista point at 2.2 miles. Grab a southerly view, including a look at Smith Mountain rising in the distance. The lake dam is in that direction. Complete the Tobacco Run Trail at 2.4 miles. Keep east, now back along Interpretive Trail Road; then split right with the Beaver Den Trail. This is the steepest trail segment of this hike, as you cut through hollows.

Meet the Chestnut Ridge Trail at 2.8 miles. You are near the trailhead again. This path makes its own way along a peninsula. Head south, winding through pine/oak woods to pass an unrestored barn at 3.0 miles. This is the fate of most tobacco barns that once dotted the Piedmont countryside. The peninsula narrows and you stay right at an intersection, keeping south. Make a mini loop at the peninsula tip. Enjoy your closest views of Smith Mountain, rising in the distance, at 3.6 miles. Make your way back toward the trailhead, meeting the Buck Run Trail just before completing the hike at 4.4 miles.

Nearby Attractions

This Virginia state park has it all—miles of hiking and bicycling trails, a campground, a swim beach, picnic areas, boat ramps, cabins, a visitor center, and the Discovery Center. Consider overnighting it here and taking part in the many outdoor recreational opportunities.

Directions

From Exit 4 on I-58 in downtown Roanoke, take Orange Avenue East/US 220 East 1.5 miles to turn right on Gus Nicks Boulevard. Gus Nicks becomes Washington Avenue, then Stewartsville Road/VA 24. After 17 miles from Orange Avenue, turn right onto Stony Fork Road and follow it 3.2 miles to turn right on VA 122/Moneta Road. Follow VA 122/Moneta Road 2.8 miles, then turn left on White House Road. Follow it 5.9 miles to turn right on VA 626/Smith Mountain Lake Parkway. Follow it 2.1 miles, then turn right onto State Park Road. Follow State Park Road 0.3 mile, then turn left at the visitor center onto Interpretive Trail Road. Follow Interpretive Trail Road 1.1 miles to reach the Turtle Island trailhead, on your right.

32 Mill Mountain Park Loop

SCENERY: ★★★★
TRAIL CONDITION: ★★★★★
CHILDREN: ★★
DIFFICULTY: ★★★
SOLITUDE: ★

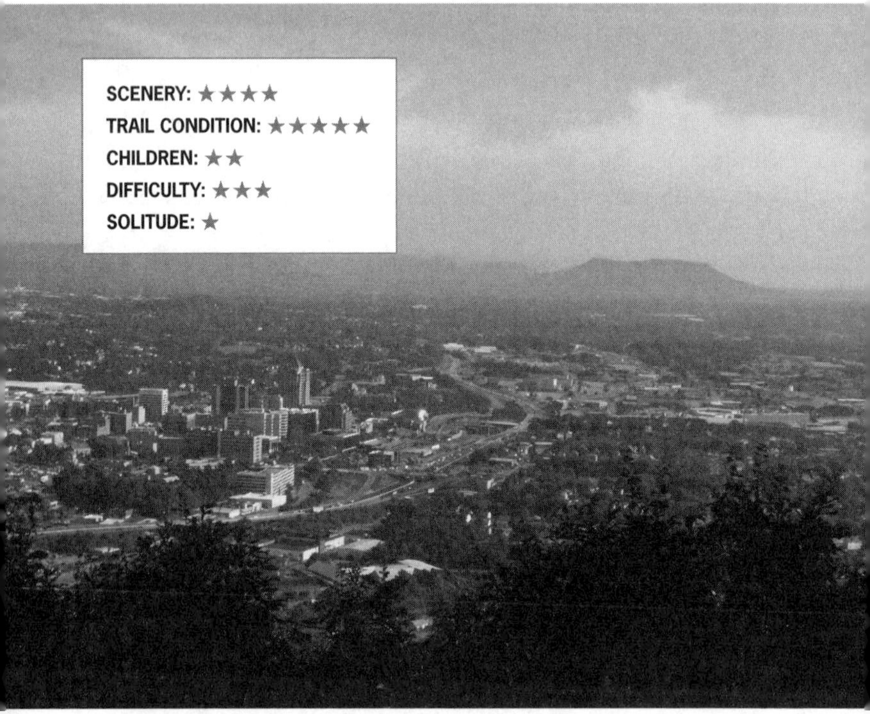

THE VIEW OF DOWNTOWN ROANOKE FROM MILL MOUNTAIN STOKES LOCAL PRIDE.

GPS TRAILHEAD COORDINATES: N37° 14.917' W79° 56.164'

DISTANCE & CONFIGURATION: 5.2-mile loop

HIKING TIME: 3 hours

OUTSTANDING FEATURES: Views of Roanoke and more, Roanoke Star, old trailside jalopy

ELEVATION: 1,700 feet at trailhead, 1,080 feet at low point, 1,847 feet at high point

ACCESS: No fees or permits required

MAPS: Mill Mountain Park; USGS *Roanoke, Garden City*

FACILITIES: Interpretive center, picnic area, water, playground, restrooms

WHEELCHAIR ACCESS: First 0.2 mile to overlook and Roanoke Star

INFO: Mill Mountain Park, J. P. Fishburn Parkway, Roanoke, VA 24014; 540-853-1236, playroanoke.com

In Brief

This hike above downtown Roanoke delivers stellar vistas of the city and adjacent mountains, then visits the famed Roanoke Star. From there, the circuit uses an amalgam of pathways to circle Mill Mountain, passing an old jalopy. Reach a low point before making a final 700-foot ascent on the Star Trail, returning for encore views before completing the circuit.

Route Details

Mill Mountain rises above downtown Roanoke and upon its peak stands the famous Roanoke Star. For more than 60 years, the star has shone onto Roanoke to become its symbol. Mill Mountain is also home to a fine city park laced with hiking trails, a nature center, and even a zoo. The following hike visits not only the Roanoke Star but also another overlook where you can see the Roanoke Valley and mountains beyond. Ultimately, switchback down the steep north side of the mountain to make a counterclockwise circuit that encircles Mill Mountain, returning you to the famed star.

The Roanoke Star came to be back in 1949, when city boosters decided to erect a massive Christmas decoration to inspire both locals and visitors and hopefully improve the Christmas shopping season. The Roanoke Merchants Association footed the bill for the 90-foot-high, 10,000-pound beacon, built by Kinsey Sign Company. Their neon tubing is still in use today. The star sits 1,045 feet above the city and 1,847 feet above sea level. The 2,000 feet of neon tubing is fashioned into three separate stars: a small star in the center, then a larger, midsize star, and finally the outermost, largest star. Purportedly the world's largest man-made star, it cost $28,000 to build—in 1949 dollars, that is. No telling what the Roanoke Star would cost today.

After that first Christmas season, the star was such a hit with the populace that it was kept up and lighted year-round. It is still lit up to this day every evening, the bright white light illuminating Mill Mountain. It is colored red, white, and blue during patriotic holidays.

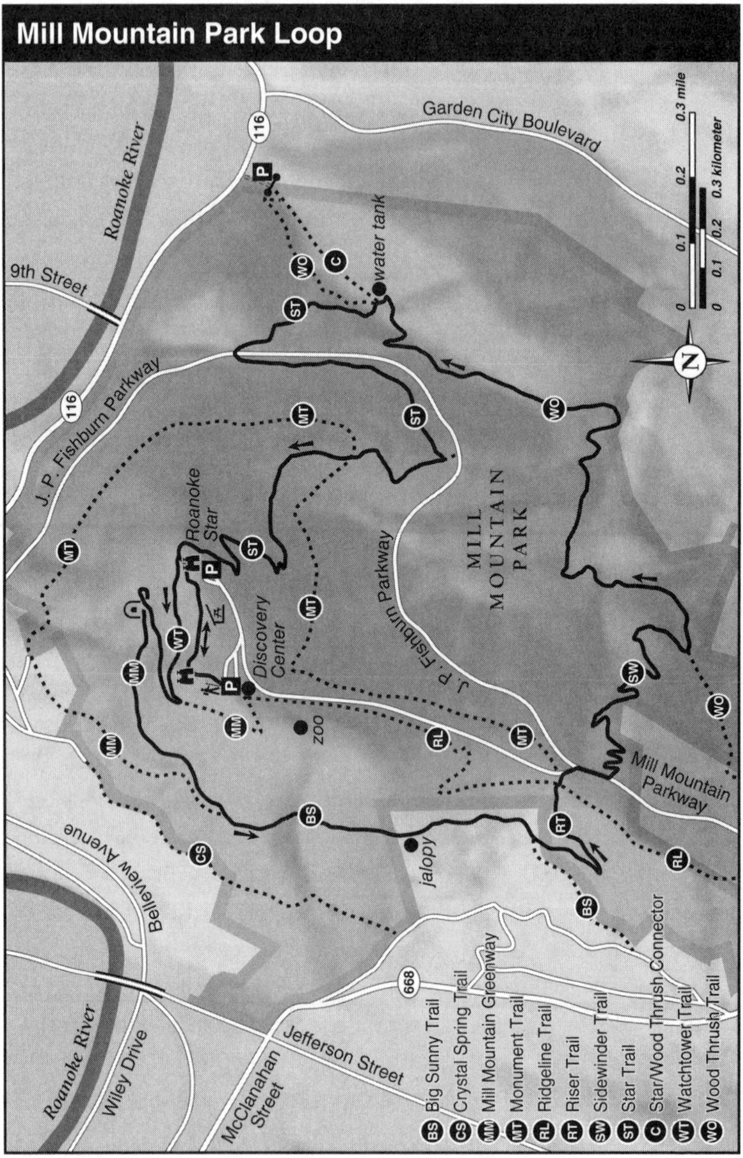
Mill Mountain Park Loop
Garden City Boulevard
Roanoke River
9th Street
116
J. P. Fishburn Parkway
water tank
Roanoke Star
Discovery Center
zoo
MILL MOUNTAIN PARK
J. P. Fishburn Parkway
Mill Mountain Parkway
jalopy
Belleview Avenue
668
Jefferson Street
McClanahan Street
Wiley Drive
Roanoke River
0 0.1 0.2 0.3 mile
0 0.1 0.2 0.3 kilometer
N
BS Big Sunny Trail
CS Crystal Spring Trail
MM Mill Mountain Greenway
MT Monument Trail
RL Ridgeline Trail
RT Riser Trail
SW Sidewinder Trail
ST Star Trail
C Star/Wood Thrush Connector
WT Watchtower Trail
WO Wood Thrush Trail

You get to visit the Roanoke Star early in this hike. First, leave the Discovery Center parking area northbound on an asphalt track. (Trail maps and interpretive information are available at the Discovery Center.) A picnic area/playground is on your right. In 200 feet, reach an overlook of downtown Roanoke and mountains beyond. Curve right beyond the overlook, passing a picnic shelter on your right to reach another overlook and the Roanoke Star at 0.2 mile. The views are stupendous, and a visual guide points out the distinct mountains near and far.

Continue beyond the star on a gravel path, descending to quickly reach the Watchtower Trail. Head left down the hiker-only, natural-surface path to meet the paved Mill Mountain Greenway, formerly Prospect Road. Leave right, descending to circle under a tunnel near a lone private residence; then meet the Big Sunny Trail at 1.1 miles. Stay straight on a natural-surface hiking trail that shortly joins a former dirt road, proof of which is a tumbled jalopy beside the path at 1.4 miles.

Come to the Riser Trail at 1.5 miles. Stay left, switchbacking uphill through gravelly woods to meet the Ridgeline Trail at 1.8 miles. Keep straight at the intersection, quickly finding Mill Mountain Parkway. Walk right along the road, then cross the road at 1.9 miles, joining the newer Sidewinder Trail at the entrance sign for Mill Mountain Park. This singletrack path curves down the mountainside like a stony snake to meet the Wood Thrush Trail at 2.5 miles.

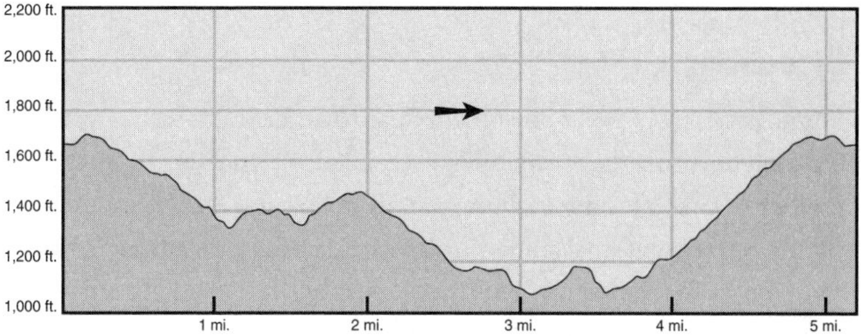

You are continuing your counterclockwise trip around Mill Mountain. The Wood Thrush Trail crosses tributaries of Garnand Branch, most likely dry, though bridges span these drainages at 2.8 miles and 3.0 miles. Reach a low point at 3.1 miles, then turn north, ascending a draw. At 3.4 miles, cut through a gap between Mill Mountain and a knob to your right. Descend past a water tank, reaching a trail intersection at 3.6 miles. Head left, joining the Star Trail. The walking is easy at first, until you cross J. P. Fishburn Parkway at 3.8 miles, then you make a nearly continuous climb, eased by a moderate gradient and switchbacks, the first of which comes at 4.2 miles, in pine woods rising from pale rocks. Bisect the Monument Trail at 4.4 miles. The climbing continues in pines and blueberry bushes on a gravel-and-stone-pocked path.

A few final switchbacks lead you to a wide gravel trail and alternative parking near the Roanoke Star. From here, head right, soon reaching the symbol of Roanoke. Grab one more view, and then backtrack the asphalt trail, reaching the Discovery Center parking lot at 5.2 miles.

Nearby Attractions

Mill Mountain Park has not only hiking and biking trails but also a zoo with more than 175 animals, from a red panda to a red wolf. It also participates in an endangered-animal breeding program. The zoo is open Thursday–Sunday and has an admission fee. For more information, visit exemplum.com.

Directions

From Exit 6 on I-581 in downtown Roanoke, take Elm Avenue west 0.2 mile to turn left on Jefferson Street. Follow Jefferson Street 0.5 mile, then veer left onto Walnut Avenue. Follow it 0.3 mile to a stop sign. Keep straight as Walnut Avenue turns into J. P. Fishburn Parkway (you'll see a sign for the Blue Ridge Parkway). Keep straight on J. P. Fishburn Parkway and follow it 2.1 miles to turn right at the signed turn for the Discovery Center. After 0.5 mile, turn left and park in the Discovery Center lot.

33 Chestnut Ridge Loop

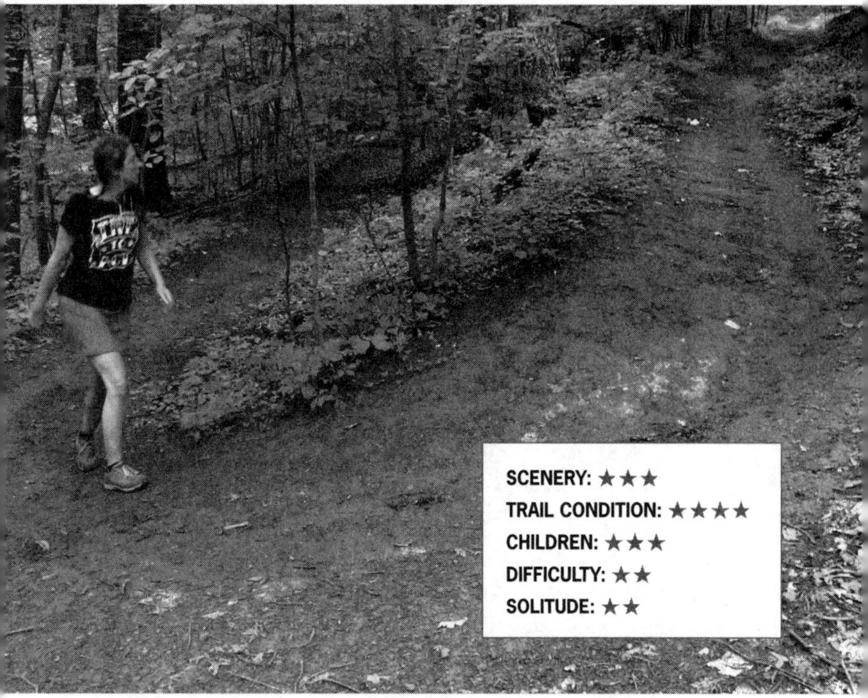

SCENERY: ★★★
TRAIL CONDITION: ★★★★
CHILDREN: ★★★
DIFFICULTY: ★★
SOLITUDE: ★★

A SWITCHBACK EASES AN ASCENT ON THE CHESTNUT RIDGE LOOP.

GPS TRAILHEAD COORDINATES: N37° 13.716' W79° 57.051'

DISTANCE & CONFIGURATION: 5.6-mile loop

HIKING TIME: 3 hours

OUTSTANDING FEATURES: Ideal loop with varied distances available, picnic areas

ELEVATION: 1,470 feet at trailhead, 1,270 feet at low point, 1,540 at high point

ACCESS: No fees or permits required

MAPS: Blue Ridge Parkway–Roanoke Valley, USGS *Garden City*

FACILITIES: Picnic area, water and restrooms near trailhead and along hike

WHEELCHAIR ACCESS: None

INFO: Blue Ridge Parkway, 199 Hemphill Knob Road, Asheville, NC 28803-8686; 828-298-0398, nps.gov/blri

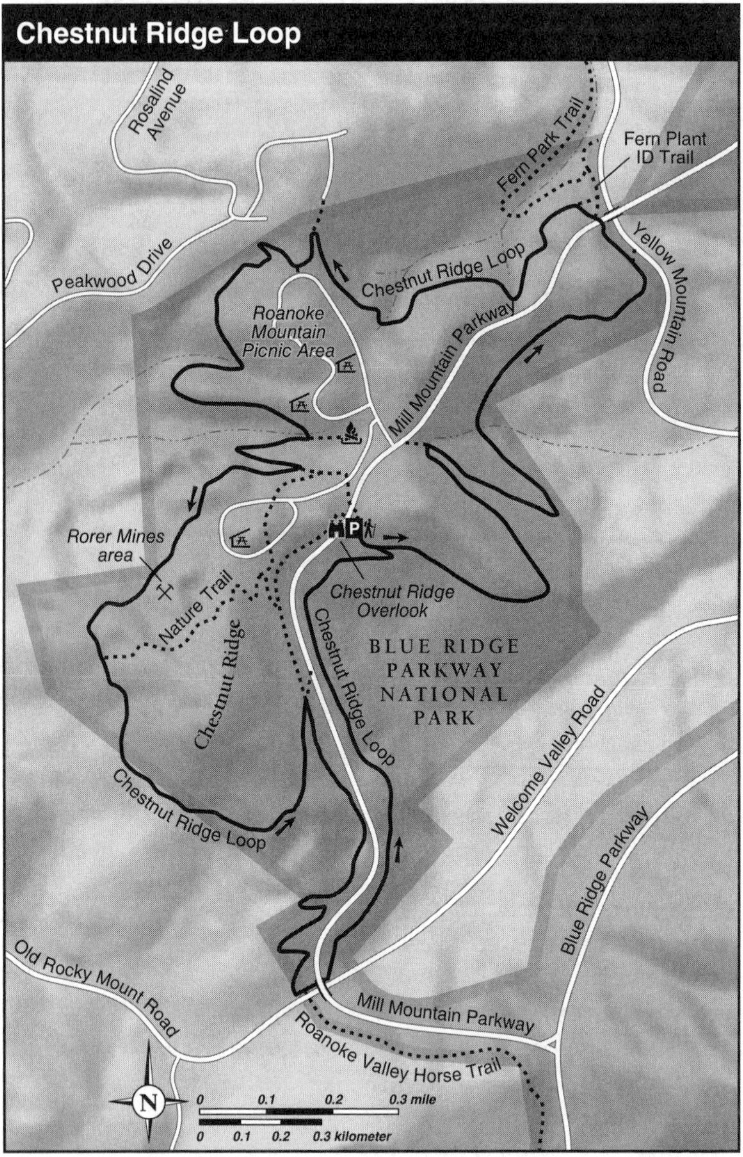
Chestnut Ridge Loop
Rosalind Avenue
Peakwood Drive
Fern Park Trail
Fern Plant ID Trail
Chestnut Ridge Loop
Yellow Mountain Road
Roanoke Mountain Picnic Area
Mill Mountain Parkway
Rorer Mines area
Nature Trail
Chestnut Ridge
Chestnut Ridge Overlook
Chestnut Ridge Loop
BLUE RIDGE PARKWAY NATIONAL PARK
Welcome Valley Road
Chestnut Ridge Loop
Blue Ridge Parkway
Old Rocky Mount Road
Mill Mountain Parkway
Roanoke Valley Horse Trail
N
0 0.1 0.2 0.3 mile
0 0.1 0.2 0.3 kilometer

In Brief

This hike, just minutes from downtown Roanoke, loops through woods of Blue Ridge Parkway National Park above the city. Start at Chestnut Ridge Overlook, then hike through rocky, oak-dominated woods. Circle near Roanoke Mountain Picnic Area, with its ample facilities. Connector trails allow hikers to vary the length of their circuit. Beyond the picnic area, the trail bisects a former iron mining area from the 1800s, now woodlands, before returning to the trailhead.

Route Details

Founded as a railroad hub, Roanoke is well situated deep in the valley of the Roanoke River, nestled by the Blue Ridge Mountains. No one knew the town was also to become a recreation hub a century later, helped along by the nearby passage of the Blue Ridge Parkway just a few miles above downtown. Fortunately for us, this part of the parkway presents the Chestnut Ridge Loop, a circuit trail with several useful connectors offering numerous hike possibilities, all within the realm of the former Roanoke Mountain campground, now a well-outfitted picnic area. This convenient hike not only offers numerous loop possibilities, but with gentle grades and a vertical variation of

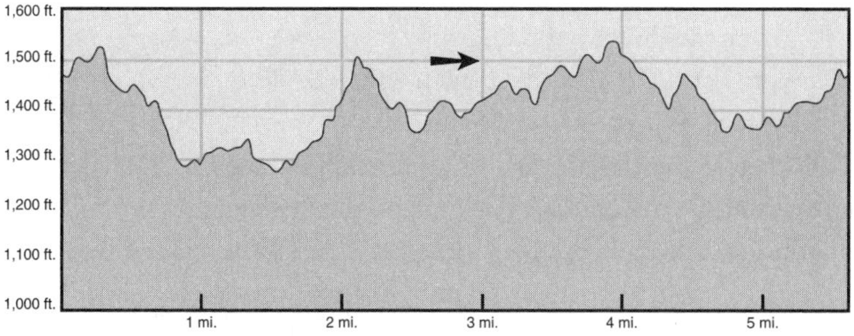

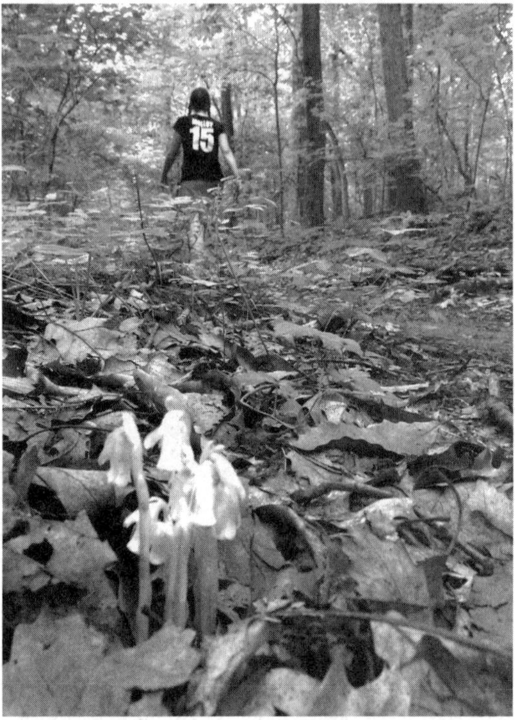

INDIAN GHOST PIPE AND A TRAIL TREKKER GIVE EACH OTHER PERSPECTIVE.

less than 300 feet, it also makes a good starter hike that is not too steep or long—and you can cut it short if necessary.

Start by leaving the Chestnut Ridge Overlook heading east. Do not take the trail heading left toward the old campground. The rocky singletrack path—open to hikers only—travels 200 feet under oaks before reaching the first of many trail intersections. Head left, beginning the counterclockwise circuit. Cruise under prototypal xeric hardwoods: chestnut oaks, pignut hickory, black gum, and sourwood. Curve around a knob above Gum Spring Branch. At 0.3 mile, turn back west. At 0.6 mile, a connector trail leads left to Mill Mountain Parkway, a spur of the Blue Ridge Parkway, and the Roanoke Mountain picnic area. Stay with the main track as it descends in long, loping switchbacks on a stone-strewn hillside. At 1.0 mile, cross an intermittent drainage. Arc left around a piney knob before reaching a spur trail dropping right to Yellow Mountain Road, which you can see below. Cross over Mill Mountain Parkway at 1.5 miles, and reenter dry-slope hardwoods of oak and sourwood. The short Fern Plant ID Trail drops right, while the Chestnut Ridge Loop heads west.

Ahead, you will begin to see picnic tables and parts of the former Roanoke Mountain Campground, now renamed a picnic area. The campground infrastructure is still intact. Make the first real climb of the hike to reach an intersection at 2.1 miles. A spur leads right to a residential area and Lockridge Road. The Chestnut Ridge Trail heads sharply left and comes to a signed spot at the north end of the old tent camper's loop. Here is a shortcut opportunity—and a maze of user-created trails that may temporarily throw you off. The blazed Chestnut Ridge Trail drops to turn into a wet-weather drainage at 2.5 miles. At 2.8 miles, come to another trail intersection in another drainage. Here, a spur leads left toward the old Campfire Circle, where campground ranger programs were held.

The trail wanders away from the former campground then returns, reaching a major trail intersection at 3.0 miles. Here, a connector trail leaves east to cross Mill Mountain Parkway and reach Chestnut Ridge Overlook, making a 3.3-mile loop. To go the full distance, stay with the Chestnut Ridge Trail, heading southwest. Join a flat, wide trail. You are now traveling the former railroad line used to transport iron ore from the Rorer Mines, owned by noted Roanoke businessman Ferdinand Rorer. The mine and rail line operated in the late 1800s. Look at the lay of the land—it just doesn't look natural, despite the tree cover. Hills are where they shouldn't be, and drainages look suspiciously carved. You may even spot crumbled iron ore. At 3.3 miles, the trail spans a drainage on an elevated berm erected to aid the railroad's passage through these hills.

At 3.5 miles, the Nature Trail leaves left and presents another shortcut opportunity. Keep straight on the Chestnut Ridge Trail. Begin circling around the actual Chestnut Ridge. Come very near some houses. This area can be brushy in summer. At 4.1 miles, a spur leaves left to Mill Mountain Parkway. Stay right (south) for the full circuit. Travel parallel to Mill Mountain Parkway. Switchback downhill, criss-crossing a power line, to emerge at Welcome Valley Road (VA 672) at 4.7 miles. Turn left and follow the road, passing under Mill Mountain Parkway; then cut left, northbound, back on foot trail at 4.8 miles.

The Chestnut Ridge Loop heads north, again paralleling Mill Mountain Parkway. Negotiate brushy woods, rife with huckleberries and blackberries in summer. After a final uptick, Chestnut Ridge Overlook comes into view. The trail turns away then makes a quick switchback. Complete the circuit and backtrack just a short distance, finishing the hike.

Nearby Attractions

Roanoke Mountain Picnic Area, a former campground, is located near this trailhead and offers numerous picnic sites, water, and restrooms. **Mill Mountain Park,** with high-quality trails and facilities of its own, is just 2 miles away.

Directions

From downtown Roanoke, from Exit 143 on I-81, take I-581 to where it morphs into US 220 South 5.4 miles to veer right and join the Blue Ridge Parkway. Head northbound on the Blue Ridge Parkway and drive 1.1 miles; then veer left onto Mill Mountain Parkway. Follow Mill Mountain Parkway 1.1 miles to reach the Chestnut Ridge Overlook on your right.

34 Poor Mountain Natural Area Preserve

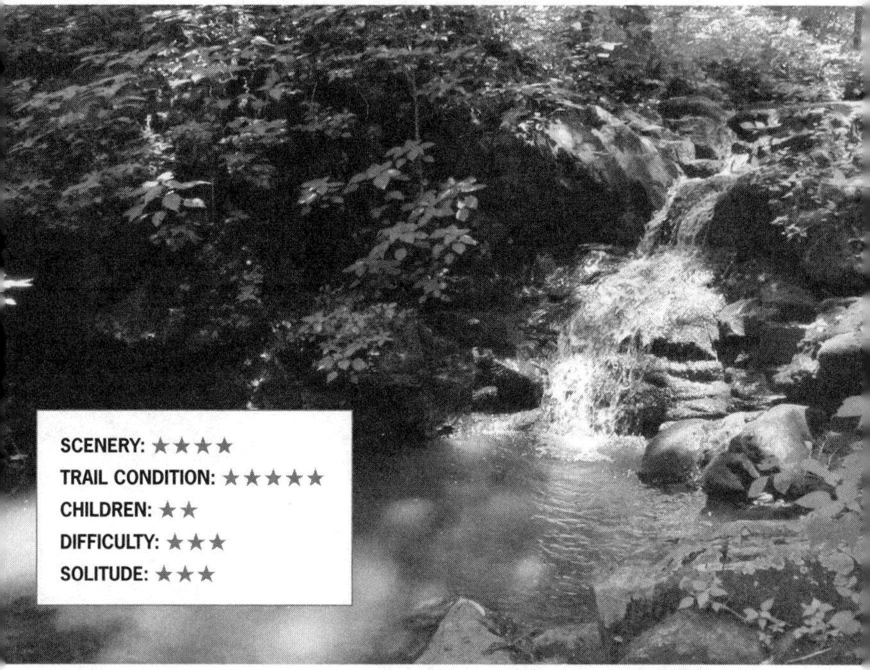

SCENERY: ★★★★
TRAIL CONDITION: ★★★★★
CHILDREN: ★★
DIFFICULTY: ★★★
SOLITUDE: ★★★

THIS WATERFALL FLOWS AT THE LOWERMOST REACHES OF THE PRESERVE.

GPS TRAILHEAD COORDINATES: N37° 13.757' W80° 5.308'

DISTANCE & CONFIGURATION: 3.7-mile loop

HIKING TIME: 2.5 hours

OUTSTANDING FEATURES: Rare plant environment, views, cascades, stellar trail construction

ELEVATION: 2,250 feet at trailhead, 1,550 feet at low point

ACCESS: No fees or permits required

MAPS: Poor Mountain Natural Area, USGS *Bent Mountain*

FACILITIES: None

WHEELCHAIR ACCESS: None

INFO: Virginia Department of Conservation and Recreation, 217 Governor St., Richmond, VA 23219; 804-786-7951, dcr.virginia.gov

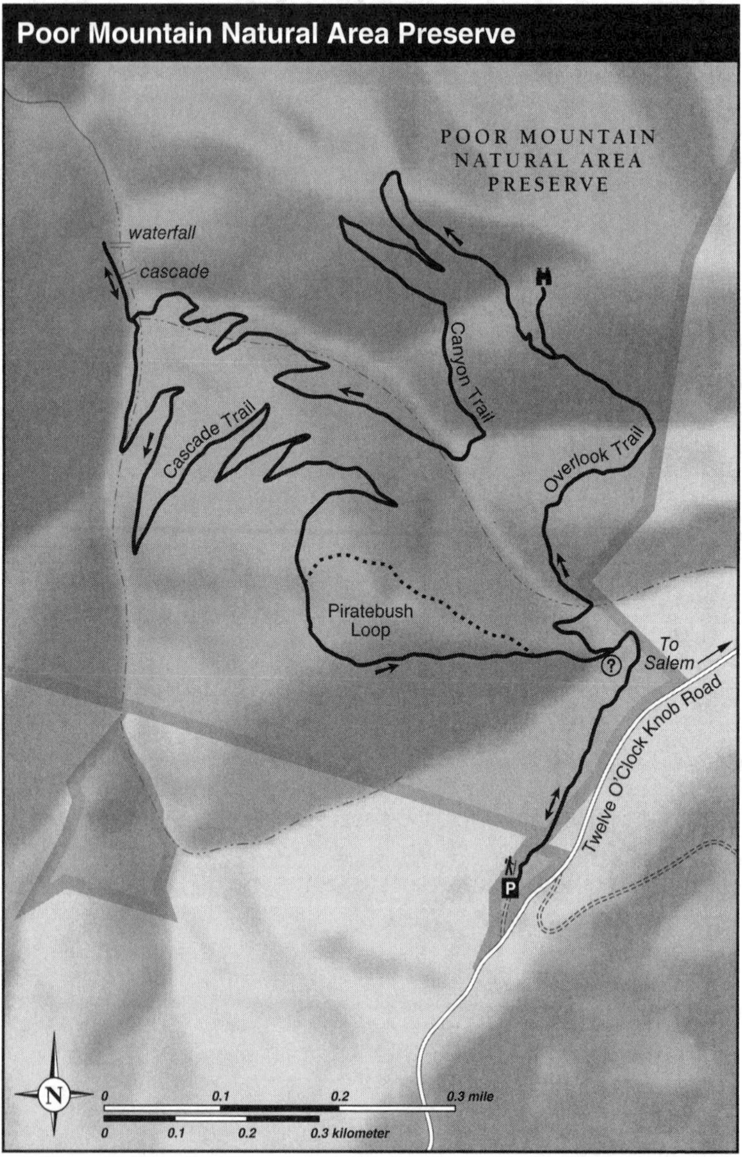
Poor Mountain Natural Area Preserve
POOR MOUNTAIN
NATURAL AREA
PRESERVE
waterfall
cascade
Canyon Trail
Cascade Trail
Overlook Trail
Piratebush
Loop
To
Salem
Twelve O'Clock Knob Road
P
N
0
0.1
0.2
0.3 mile
0
0.1
0.2
0.3 kilometer

In Brief

An abundance of the rare piratebush is the reason for the preservation of this parcel of Poor Mountain. You can not only see this plant in season but also enjoy a varied loop on well-built trail. First, visit an overlook of the valley below and mountains beyond before dropping to visit a pair of waterfalls. Climb back to the trailhead with more views between the pines.

Route Details

Poor Mountain Natural Area Preserve is rich with a rare plant known as piratebush, found in limited locations in the states of Virginia, North Carolina, and Tennessee and nowhere else in the world. Poor Mountain hosts more piratebush plants than all other known planetary locations combined. Botanists cannot explain this concentration of piratebush. For that reason, this 925-acre parcel of Poor Mountain deserves to be in the Virginia Natural Heritage Program, whose mission is to conserve "Virginia's biodiversity through inventory, protection, and stewardship."

Poor Mountain Natural Area Preserve came to be after first being acquired and held by The Nature Conservancy. It was then purchased by the state of Virginia in 1992. Today, the acreage acts as a safe

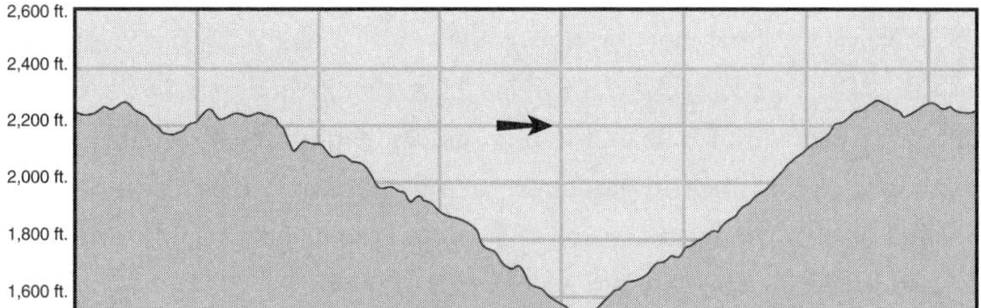

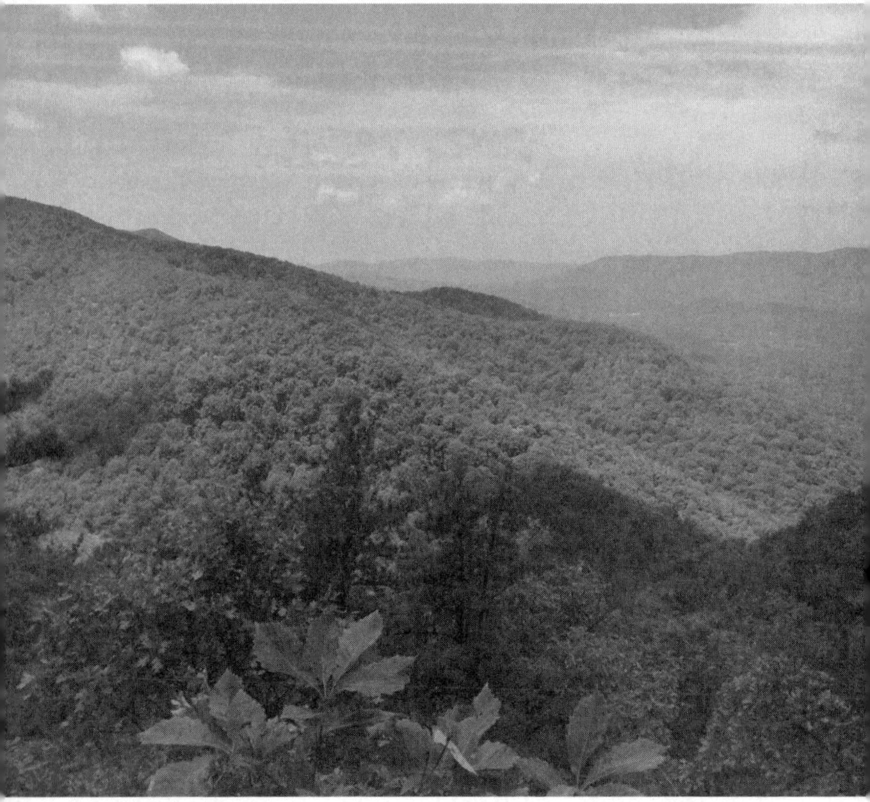

GAZING OUT FROM POOR MOUNTAIN INTO THE ROANOKE RIVER VALLEY

harbor for the piratebush and as a scenic and biologically significant destination for hikers like you and me. High-quality hiking trails on the preserve provide a venue to see the wonders within, which include not only rare plants like the piratebush but also multiple views from the slopes of Poor Mountain as well as steep mountain streams, culminating in a pair of waterfalls at the lower end of the tract.

Leave the parking area on the singletrack Piratebush Loop Trail, heading north on a steep slope. Bisect a transmission-line clearing at 0.2 mile, then curve left downhill to reach a kiosk and trail intersection at 0.3 mile. Begin the loop portion of the hike by taking the

Overlook Trail right, saving the rest of the Piratebush Loop Trail for last. A narrow, well-constructed path leads you across a small creek then into xeric, shale-rich woods of Table Mountain pine, scarlet oak, and chestnut oak, rising in gnarled forms, often with spaces open between the trees, allowing views across the Roanoke River Valley to Fort Lewis Mountain.

At 0.7 mile, take the spur trail right, toward the overlook. At 0.8 mile, reach the spur's end. Here, a bench faces west above a chasm below, a canyon created by a nameless tributary cutting through the western slope of Poor Mountain. You can see a transmission tower atop a peak of Poor Mountain to the west, the Roanoke River Valley below, and ranks of ridges extending toward West Virginia.

Thus far, the hike has been easy, and a trip to the aforementioned overlook and back would be a short, easy there-and-back walk. However, this loop goes on, rejoining the Overlook Trail to where it arbitrarily becomes the Canyon Trail at 1.0 mile. A resting bench stands at this point. Here comes a series of switchbacks painstakingly constructed using stone found on-site. A high-quality path with a steady but moderate gradient like this not only makes life easier on hikers, but the trail also conserves the landscape, cutting down on erosion, and keeps trail maintainers from having to rework the path as it snakes through stunted oaks and pines on a declivitous slope.

At 1.5 miles, circle around a wet-weather drainage in richer, viney woods contrasting with the sun-burnished pines. Beyond the stream valley, reenter xeric woods salted with talus slopes. More switchbacks drop you to a trail intersection and the confluence of two streams draining Poor Mountain at 2.0 miles. Rock-hop the clear creek and head downstream. Quickly reach the first of two modest waterfalls. The first slides over an irregular slope into a surprisingly deep plunge pool. The second cataract is just downstream. It slides over a rock slab then dives off a ledge, crashing into rocks. The official path ends just beyond the lower fall.

Join the Cascade Trail after backtracking past the falls. This path aims south, roughly paralleling the more southerly creek of the preserve. It's now time to make up the 750 or so feet you lost traversing the canyon. More switchbacks moderate the gradient, but you remain on an upward angle, rising into pines and regaining views. Reach the Piratebush Loop at 3.1 miles. Stay right and begin looking for the main reason this preserve exists. Interestingly, piratebush is a parasite; hence the name. They tap into the root systems of neighboring plants, often hemlock trees, but here on Poor Mountain their primary host is the Table Mountain pine. Walk through the densest concentration of piratebush on the planet.

At 3.3 miles, reach the other end of the Piratebush Loop. Keep straight to reach the trail kiosk and Overlook Trail. From this point it's a 0.3-mile backtrack to complete the circuit at 3.7 miles.

Nearby Attractions

The **Roanoke River Greenway** travels through the town of Salem off East Riverside Drive and provides a level hiker- and biker-friendly experience.

Directions

From Exit 137 on I-81, take VA 112 East 0.5 mile into Salem and US 460/US 11/Main Street. Turn left onto US 460/US 11/Main Street and follow it 0.8 mile to turn right onto Mill Lane. Cross the Roanoke River and railroad tracks to turn left on West Riverside Drive after 0.4 mile. Follow West Riverside Drive 0.8 mile to reach Twelve O' Clock Knob Road/VA 694. Turn right on Twelve O'Clock Knob Road/ VA 694 and follow it 4.8 winding miles to the sharp right turn into the preserve parking area, a little before reaching Farm Hill Drive.

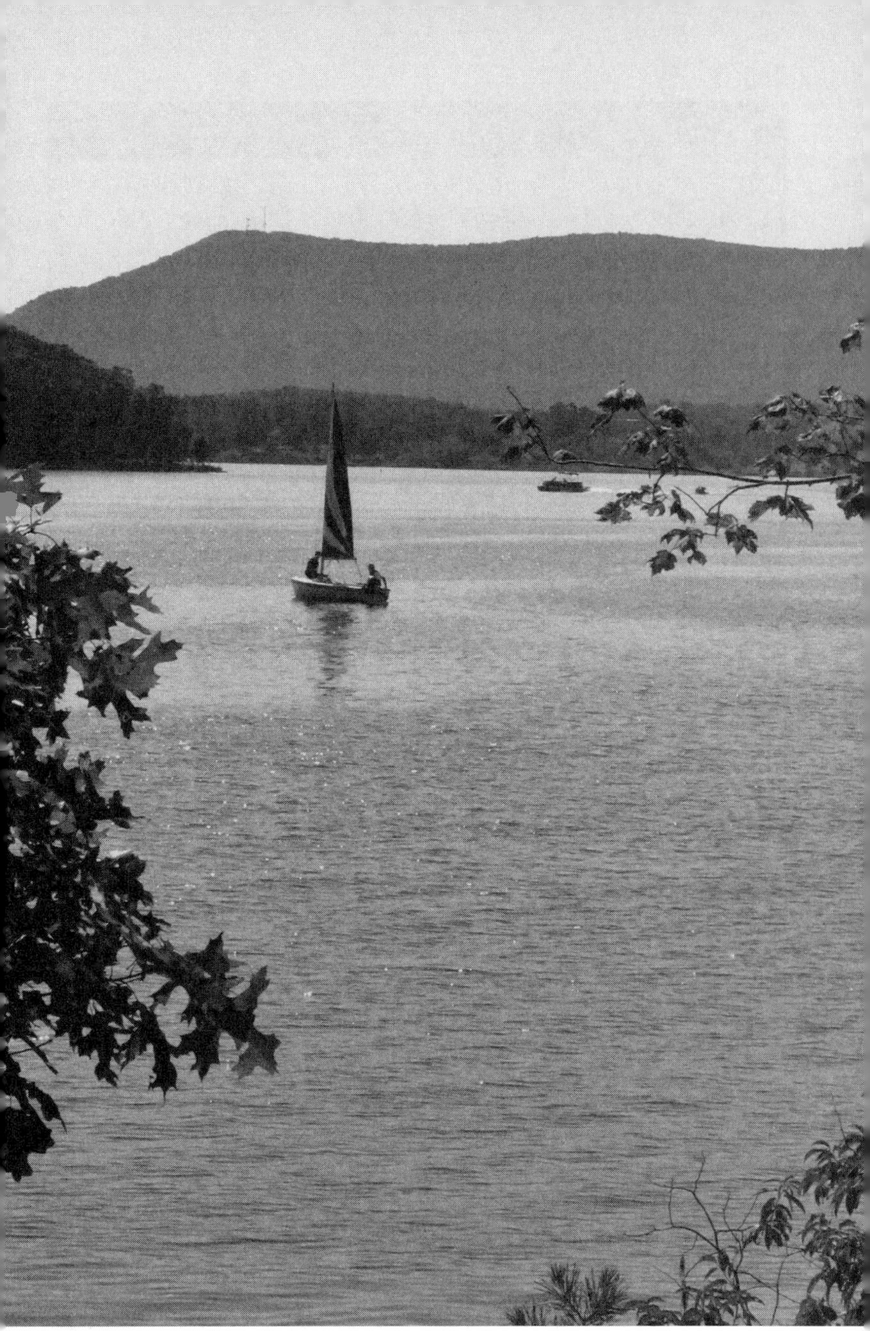

SMITH MOUNTAIN RISES ABOVE SAILING WATERS ON THE TURTLE ISLAND HIKE.
(See Hike 31, page 189.)

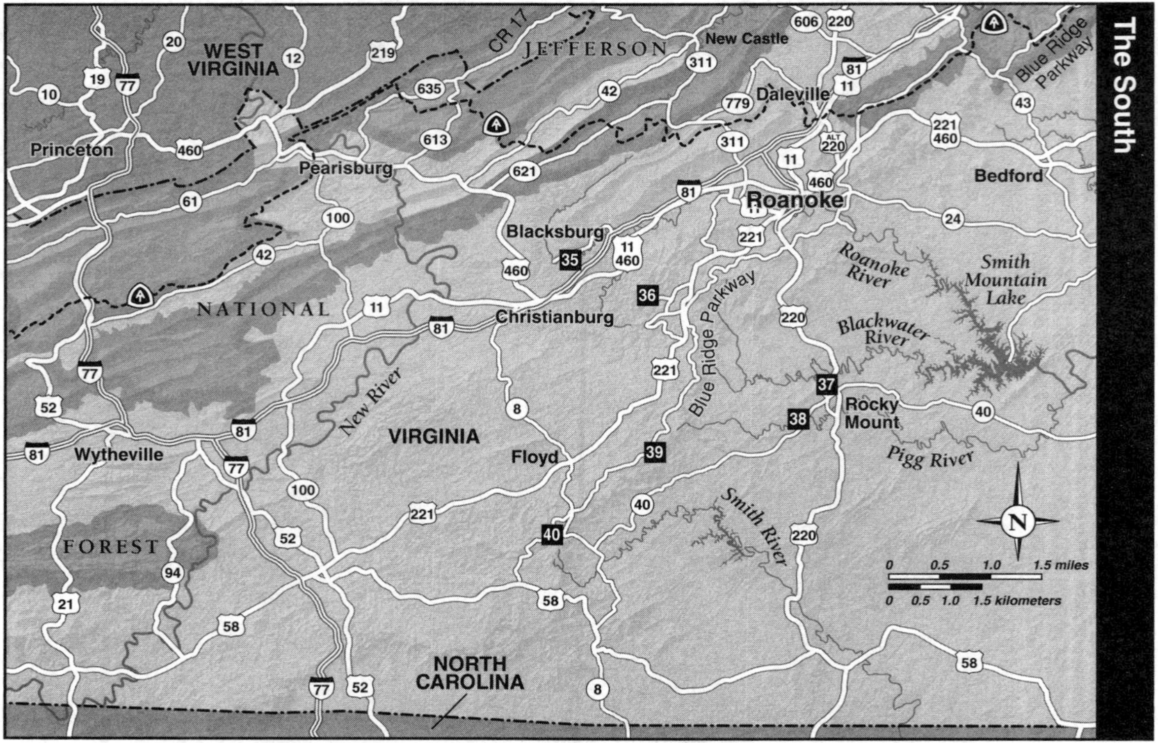
The South
WEST VIRGINIA
JEFFERSON
CR 17
NATIONAL
FOREST
VIRGINIA
NORTH CAROLINA
Princeton
Pearisburg
New Castle
Daleville
Roanoke
Bedford
Blacksburg
Christianburg
Wytheville
Floyd
Rocky Mount
Blue Ridge Parkway
Blue Ridge Parkway
New River
Roanoke River
Blackwater River
Smith Mountain Lake
Pigg River
Smith River
N
0 0.5 1.0 1.5 miles
0 0.5 1.0 1.5 kilometers

The South

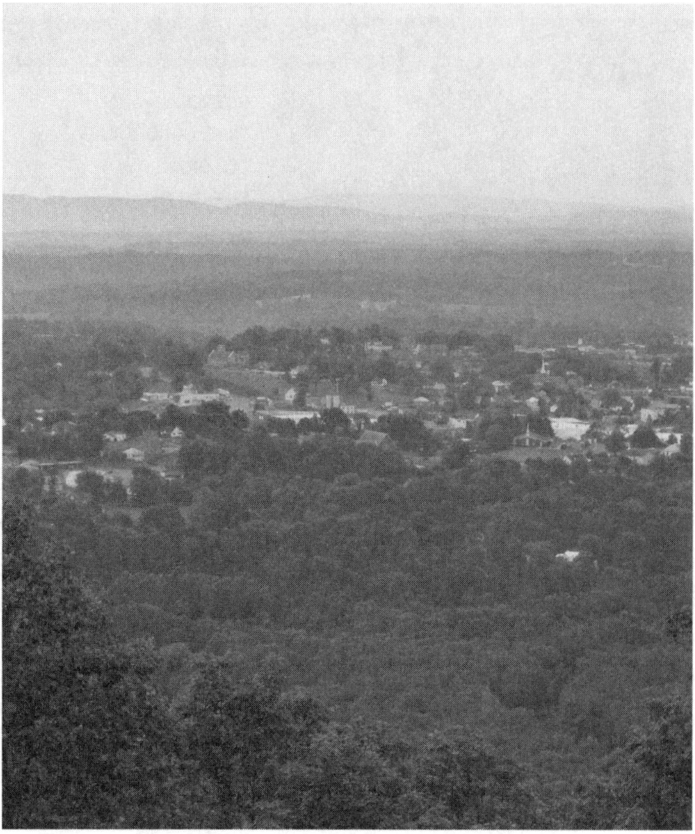

THE TOWN OF ROCKY MOUNT STANDS AT THE BASE OF GRASSY HILL.
(See Hike 37, page 224.)

35 Falls Ridge Preserve

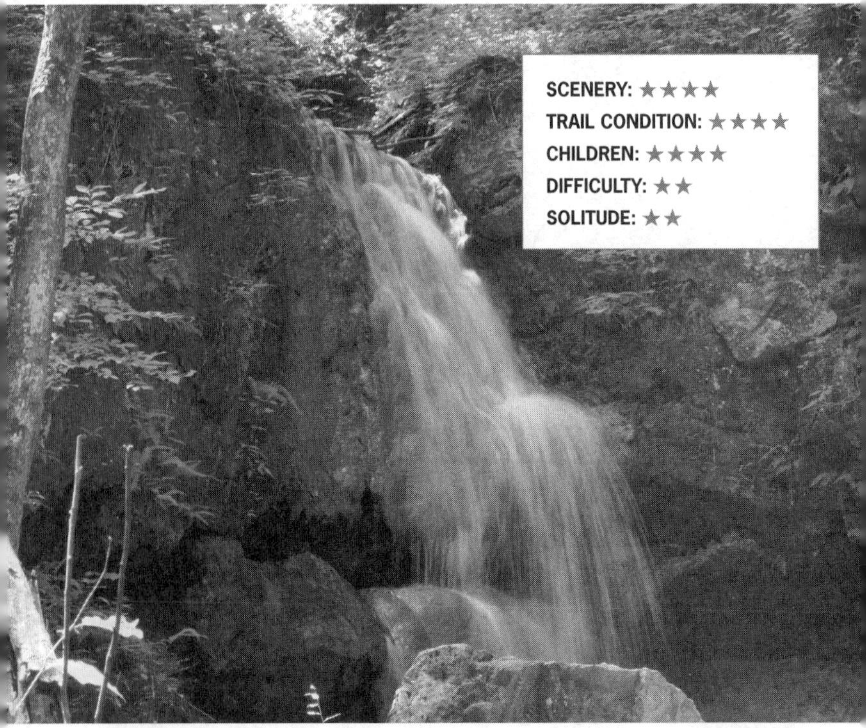

SCENERY: ★★★★
TRAIL CONDITION: ★★★★
CHILDREN: ★★★★
DIFFICULTY: ★★
SOLITUDE: ★★

THE STRANGE AND WONDERFUL CATARACTS OF FALLS RIDGE PRESERVE RESULT FROM CALCIUM CARBONATE DEPOSITS.

GPS TRAILHEAD COORDINATES: N37° 11.590' W80° 19.293'

DISTANCE & CONFIGURATION: 3.7-mile double balloon loop

HIKING TIME: 2 hours

OUTSTANDING FEATURES: Multiple waterfalls, caves, exposed calcium carbonite displays

ELEVATION: 1,460 feet at trailhead, 2,040 feet at high point

ACCESS: No fees or permits required

MAPS: Falls Ridge Preserve, USGS *Ironto*

FACILITIES: None

WHEELCHAIR ACCESS: None

INFO: The Nature Conservancy–Virginia, 490 Westfield Road, Charlottesville, VA 22901; 434-295-6106, nature.org

In Brief

View waterfalls flowing over some of the largest calcium carbonate displays in the world. The geological wonderment continues among rock bluffs entrenched with caves. The hike then takes off, passing a concrete kiln from yesteryear. Finally circle around Mill Knob, completing the visit to this Nature Conservancy preserve. *Note:* Dogs are not allowed.

Route Details

The waterfalls of Falls Ridge Preserve are undoubtedly the star attraction of this Nature Conservancy property. However, the formation of the falls is the bigger story. It is in Falls Hollow that one of the world's largest deposits of exposed calcium carbonate forms. Here, minerals and lime dissolve as the stream of Falls Hollow flows downward, creating calcium deposits. Over time these calcium carbonate deposits, commonly known as travertine, have built up, steepening the stream's gradient and creating the roughly 80-foot stair-step waterfalls that attract so many visitors. Not only is the water attractive in its own right, but the travertine deposits over which it flows seem strange and otherworldly, almost like melted rock or some queer combination of soil and stone. Elsewhere, erosion has fashioned caverns in nearby bluffs, adding yet another geological component to this preserve. Furthermore, unexplored underlying caverns add an air of mystery.

In earlier days, the land in Falls Hollow was owned by the Dudley clan. On it they farmed, cut timber, raised dairy cattle, and at one time even had a general store and post office. In the 1930s, Harry Dudley saw money to be made in the calcium carbonate deposits that he could turn into lime to sell. Dudley built a concrete kiln to convert the calcium deposits into lime. This kiln still stands today. Later, William P. Bradley realized the important natural features of Falls Hollow and bought it. The photographer lived here in retirement then deeded the property to The Nature Conservancy in 1974.

Falls Ridge Preserve

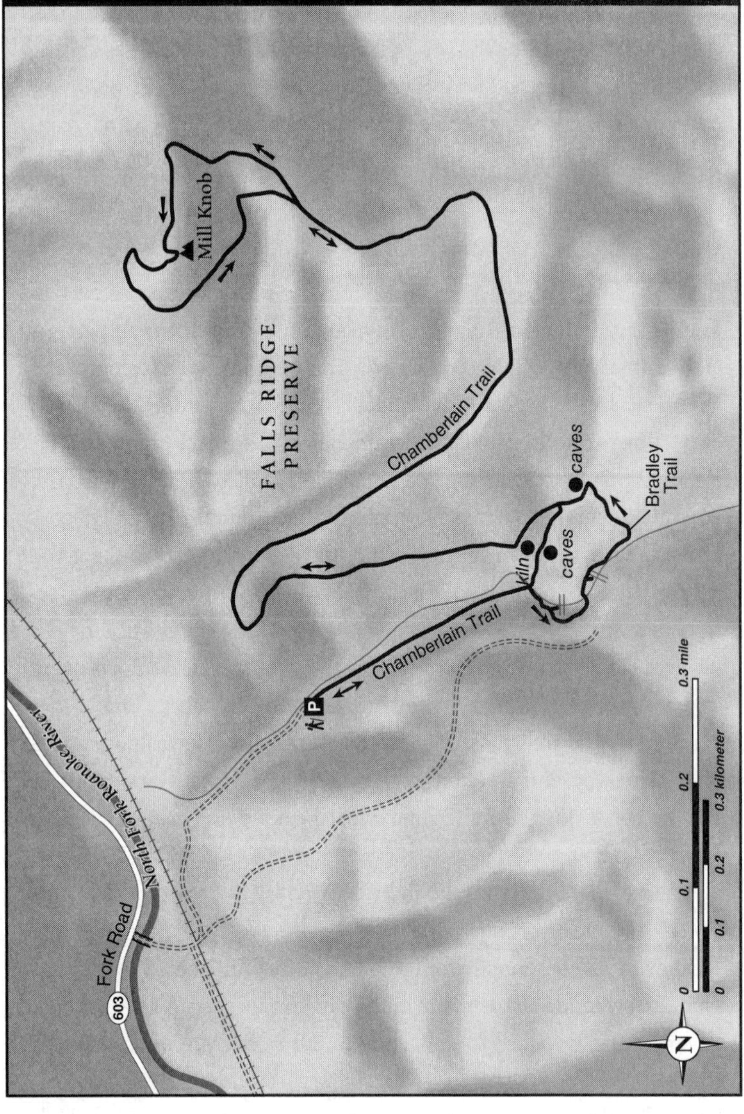

Today, The Nature Conservancy manages the tract and trails leading to the waterfalls as well as other parts of the 655-acre preserve. Although primarily created to safeguard the strange and wonderful cataracts, the preserve also harbors rare plants such as the Allegheny plum, goldenseal, and Addison's leatherflower. Elsewhere, as you will see on this hike, the hilly woods are covered in a hickory–oak–pine complex.

Depart the trailhead on a grassy track, southbound through a linear meadow. Leave the meadow at 0.2 mile and reach a trail junction. Head right on the Bradley Trail, which is also the way to the falls. Ascend a bit, then reach the main falls of the preserve on a short spur trail left. Here, the stream spills 30 feet over a tan travertine ledge into a shallow, rock-dotted pool, collects, then pushes downstream in small rapids. Depending on the flow, the water will be falling over different parts of the ledge at different rates. Upon closer inspection, you see the odd look and texture of the rock over which the falls spill.

The falls may be the most unusual cascades in the Old Dominion. Continue on the Bradley Trail, circling around the lowermost fall then bridging the stream at yet another fall. This cataract is much lower but has a much deeper pool. Pass more small but weird waterfalls. Turn away from the stream at 0.4 mile. Turn into a lesser hollow, passing smaller caves. At 0.5 mile, split right with the Chamberlain

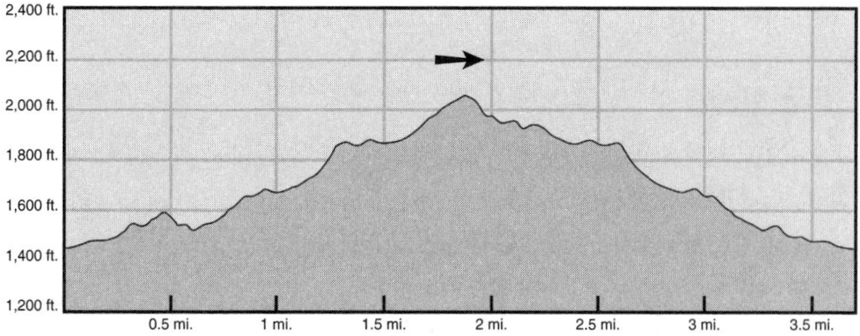

Trail. It leads above the concrete lime kiln. When this was operating, pieces of the calcium carbonate were blasted from the stream area, loaded onto carts, and then pulled by mule to the top of the kiln, where the minerals were processed.

Continue beyond the kiln, with the lower part of Falls Hollow to your left. Curve right around the point of a ridge, gently rising toward Mill Knob in woods. At 1.5 miles, just after turning north, drop to a gap. Gently ascend to reach a trail intersection at 1.7 miles. Stay right as the Chamberlain Trail circles Mill Knob. Reach a high point at 1.9 miles, then continue circling around the knob, now on the north side of the ridge in pines. Here you can look down through the trees into the North Fork Roanoke River valley. Continue circling around, and complete the loop portion of the Chamberlain Trail at 2.2 miles. From here, backtrack to the Bradley Trail, reaching it at 3.3 miles. Walk a bit of new trail, passing stone bluffs harboring intriguing caves to your left. Ahead you will pass the lower part of the concrete lime kiln on your right. Finally, bridge the stream of Falls Hollow. From there it's a 0.2-mile backtrack to the trailhead.

Nearby Attractions

Anglers can fish the North Fork Roanoke River, along which you will drive en route to Falls Hollow Preserve. Roadside pullovers allow access for anglers who can then wade the river for smallmouth bass and other species.

Directions

From Exit 128, Ironto, on I-81 southwest of Roanoke, follow North Fork Road/VA 603 for 7 miles to Falls Ridge Road and the community of Fagg. Cross a narrow bridge over North Fork Roanoke River to then cross railroad tracks just ahead. Turn left on a dirt road immediately after crossing the railroad track. Follow the dirt road 0.2 mile, then split left at the sign for Falls Ridge Preserve to end at a parking area.

36 Bottom Creek Gorge

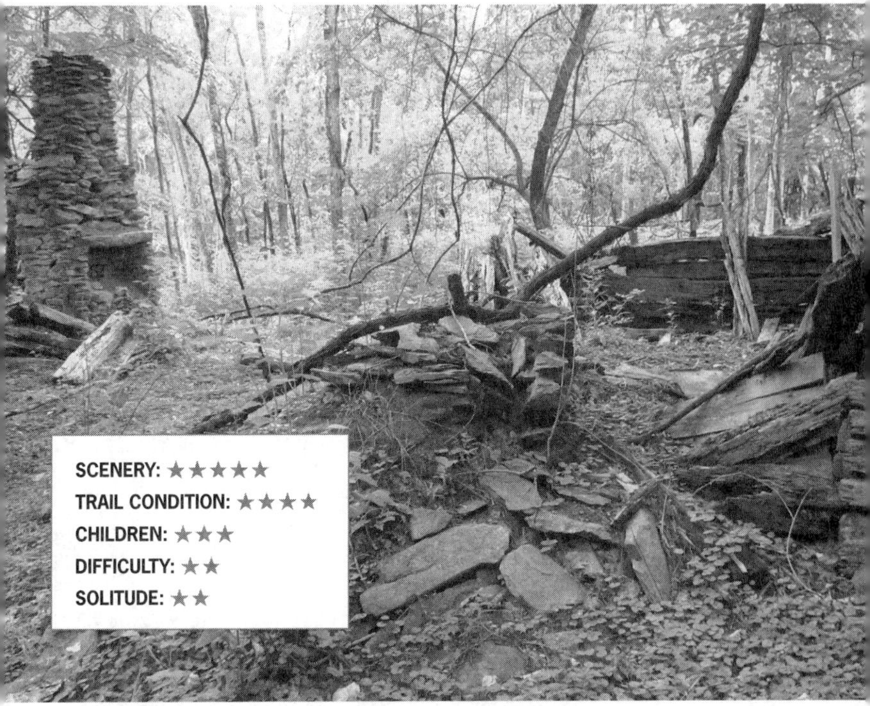

SCENERY: ★★★★★
TRAIL CONDITION: ★★★★
CHILDREN: ★★★
DIFFICULTY: ★★
SOLITUDE: ★★

PEOPLE LIVED IN WHAT IS NOW BOTTOM CREEK GORGE PRESERVE INTO THE 1950S.

GPS TRAILHEAD COORDINATES: N37° 7.984' W80° 10.969'

DISTANCE & CONFIGURATION: 4.6-mile balloon loop

HIKING TIME: 2.5 hours

OUTSTANDING FEATURES: Bent Mountain Falls, Bottom Creek Gorge, pioneer homesites

ELEVATION: 2,470 feet at trailhead, 2,670 feet at high point

ACCESS: No fees or permits required

MAPS: Bottom Creek Gorge Preserve; USGS *Elliston, Check*

FACILITIES: None

WHEELCHAIR ACCESS: None

INFO: The Nature Conservancy–Virginia, 490 Westfield Road, Charlottesville, VA 22901; 434-295-6106, nature.org

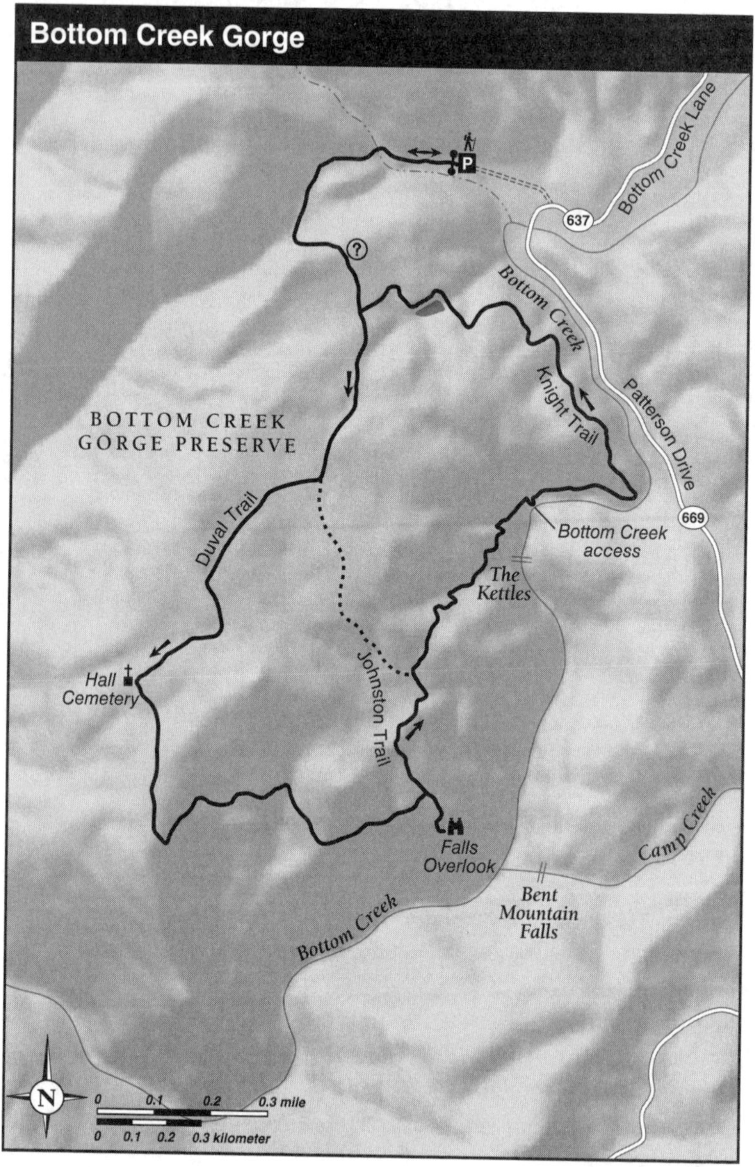
Bottom Creek Gorge
Bottom Creek Lane
637
Bottom Creek
Patterson Drive
669
Knight Trail
BOTTOM CREEK
GORGE PRESERVE
Duval Trail
Bottom Creek
access
The
Kettles
Johnston Trail
Hall
Cemetery
Falls
Overlook
Camp Creek
Bent
Mountain
Falls
Bottom Creek
N
0 0.1 0.2 0.3 mile
0 0.1 0.2 0.3 kilometer

In Brief

This balloon loop cobbles together a network of old settler roads and newer foot trails to explore the Bottom Creek valley. First, climb to a ridgetop plateau and enter a formerly settled area with evidence of the past, from chimneys to fence posts and more. Next, enjoy natural features such as 200-foot Bent Mountain Falls, then finally visit Bottom Creek, where pools and cascades form an area known as The Kettles.

Route Details

Back in the 1970s, scientists came to realize that Bottom Creek not only was home to one-tenth of all the native freshwater fishes of Virginia, but also, more important, contained three very rare species—the riverweed darter, orangefin madtom, and bigeye jumprock. The Nature Conservancy stepped in and began purchasing lands along Bottom Creek, ultimately acquiring more than 1,600 acres to protect not only these rare fish but also special plants such as old-growth Carolina hemlocks and the chestnut lipfern. In doing so, they also preserved the deep shale-and-granite gorge of Bottom Creek where The Kettles—a series of pools and shoals—forms. Furthermore, Appalachian Power Company donated additional acreage preserving Bent Mountain Falls, a 200-foot cataract that is Virginia's second-highest

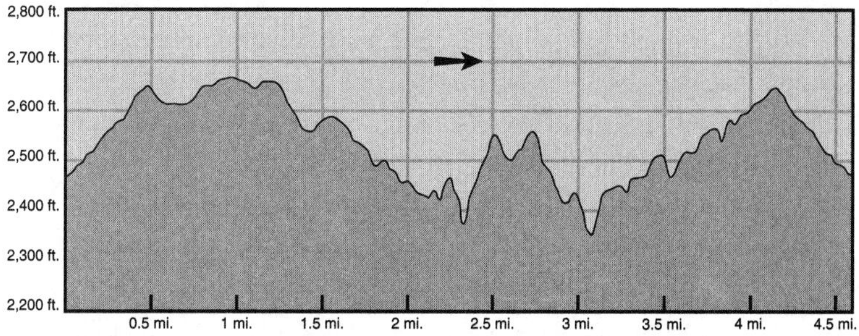

waterfall. Additionally, the lands acquired by The Nature Conservancy contained homesites, graveyards, and other evidence of the families that called the Bottom Creek valley home. Therefore, a hike here in the shadows of Poor Mountain ends up being an excursion into both human and natural history.

Leave the parking area, passing around a gate. Remember, no dogs are allowed in the preserve. Take a doubletrack path west up a hollow, passing homesites of the Craighead family. The path rises to a gap, a clearing, and a trailside kiosk at 0.5 mile. This signboard provides copious human and natural history about Bottom Creek Gorge, giving context to the preserve.

Continue straight on the doubletrack, entering the preserve proper. Descend past growing-over fields to pass the Knight Trail at 0.6 mile. This is your return route. For now, keep straight on the settler road, bordered by old fencing. Folks lived on this plateau into the 1950s but had originally settled here in the late 1700s—families like the Funks, the Halls, and the Kings. Today, the fields are reverting to woods, but the gorge was always wild. Local residents called it "The Roughs" for how difficult it was to get about along Bottom Creek.

At 0.9 mile, leave right on the Duval Trail, in transitioning forest. Most folks are going straight with the Johnston Trail, the quickest way to Bent Mountain Falls, but we will first explore some of the homesites found on the Duval Trail. At 1.4 miles, look right for a short spur leading to the small, fence-bordered Hall Cemetery. Only the grave of Emily Hall has an engraved memorial. The others are simply flat fieldstones. Walk just a bit farther, then find the Woods Hall homesite on the right, with crumbled chimney, hewn logs, and metal relics. Just ahead on the left are the remains of the Jesse Hall homestead.

The trail turns into the Bottom Creek Gorge, passing sloped terrain with pioneer rock piles. Stream sounds rise from below. At 2.2 miles, split right at a trail intersection, heading toward Bent Mountain Falls. Reach the falls overlook at 2.3 miles. Here, you can peer across the gorge as Camp Creek tumbles into the Bottom Creek chasm, dropping 200 feet over naked rock, angling on a cliff. It is hard to capture the fall in its entirety, but the sight is worthy nonetheless as Virginia's second-highest cataract.

Backtrack from the overlook spur, then take the Johnston Trail uphill on log-and-earth steps. At 2.6 miles, after crossing a small branch, turn right on the Knight Trail. This path rises to bisect a gap, then drops you into the gorge. Pass a notable seven-trunked basswood tree. Reach a water-access spur at 3 miles. Here, hikers follow a short path to reach the pools, boulders, and cascades of Bottom Creek Gorge—The Kettles—where the rare fishes live and part of why The Nature Conservancy preserved this tract.

Return to the Knight Trail, keeping up the gorge. Shoals and rapids play in your ears from below. Turn away from the gorge, then come upon a small pond at 3.8 miles, yet another relic of a time when this land was settled. The Knight Trail ends at 4.0 miles. From here, it is a 0.6-mile backtrack to the trailhead.

Nearby Attractions

On the way, you pass an access to the Blue Ridge Parkway. Not only does the parkway offer scenic driving but also the Smart View Picnic Area (see Hike 39, page 234).

Directions

From the intersection of US 221 and US 49 in Cave Spring near Roanoke, take US 221 South 14 miles to County Line Road (VA 644), 0.5 mile after passing a signed left turn toward the Blue Ridge Parkway. Turn right on County Line Road and follow it 1.1 miles to bear right onto VA 669 (Bottom Creek Road) at the Floyd–Roanoke County line. Stay with VA 669 for 0.9 mile. Here, Bottom Creek Road turns right but you stay straight on VA 669, which changes names to Patterson Drive. Follow Patterson Drive 1.8 miles to bridge Bottom Creek. Just after this bridge turn left into the signed entrance to Bottom Creek Gorge Preserve. Reach a gate at 0.1 mile. Parking is limited here, so please be considerate.

37

Grassy Hill Natural Area Preserve

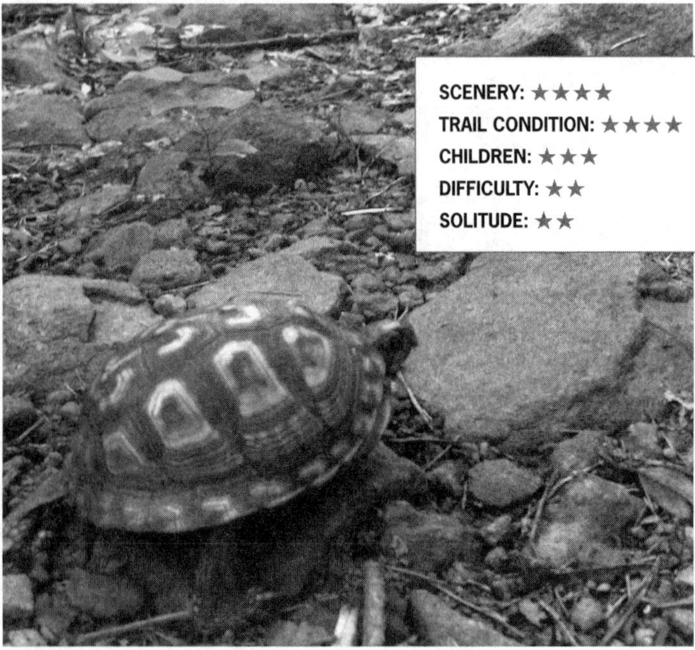

SCENERY: ★★★★
TRAIL CONDITION: ★★★★
CHILDREN: ★★★
DIFFICULTY: ★★
SOLITUDE: ★★

EVEN THE TURTLES LIKE GRASSY HILL NATURAL AREA PRESERVE.

GPS TRAILHEAD COORDINATES: N37° 0.905' W79° 53.654'

DISTANCE & CONFIGURATION: 6.4-mile balloon loop

HIKING TIME: 3.5 hours

OUTSTANDING FEATURES: Views, good trail system

ELEVATION: 1,200 feet at trailhead, 1,710 feet at high point

ACCESS: No fees or permits required

MAPS: Grassy Hill Natural Area Preserve Hiking Trail System; USGS *Boones Mill, Rocky Mount*

FACILITIES: None

WHEELCHAIR ACCESS: None

INFO: Department of Conservation and Recreation, Natural Heritage Program, 600 E. Main St., 24th Floor, Richmond, VA 23219; 804-786-7951, dcr.virginia.gov

In Brief

This is a low-elevation mountain hike near the town of Rocky Mount. Explore this preserved parcel of the Virginia Natural Heritage Program using a pair of loops that run atop Grassy Hill, wooded in rich forests of oak and hickory. Three overlooks provide views of Rocky Mount and the Piedmont below.

Route Details

It all starts with the soil. Here on Grassy Hill, the magnesium-rich soils, known as mafic soils, combined with the dry, rocky conditions on this ridge overlooking Rocky Mount, have created a habitat worth preserving. In the late 1990s, the 1,295-acre preserve was added to the Virginia Natural Heritage Program. In former times, Grassy Hill resembled more what its name implies, and grasses swayed on its slopes; however, fewer fires have allowed the forest to increase. Yet there are still vestiges of the prairielike openings harboring plants such as grass-leaf blazing star and glade wild quinine that make the preserve worth preserving. The Virginia Department of Conservation and Recreation is using fire to restore parts of Grassy Hill to its former state. The challenge has been to be able to make prescribed burns considering the proximity of Rocky Mount and other populated areas. Therefore, burning has been limited to the uppermost slopes of the preserve. The DCR is also thinning the forest in places, as well as controlling invasive species.

However, it is the views that attract many hikers. They are stretched out along the 3-mile ridge that forms Grassy Hill. In addition to these clear vistas, winter hikers will be rewarded with near-continuous leaf-off panoramas. In fact, Grassy Hill Preserve makes for an ideal winter hike, since it is low elevation and stream crossings are not an issue. Conversely, the low elevation and south-facing slope will be hot in summer. Additionally, hikers can easily alter their Grassy Hill adventure, doing the full 6.5-mile circuit, cutting the loop in half, or executing a there-and-back hike to the East Loop overlook—the preserve's finest.

Grassy Hill Natural Area Preserve

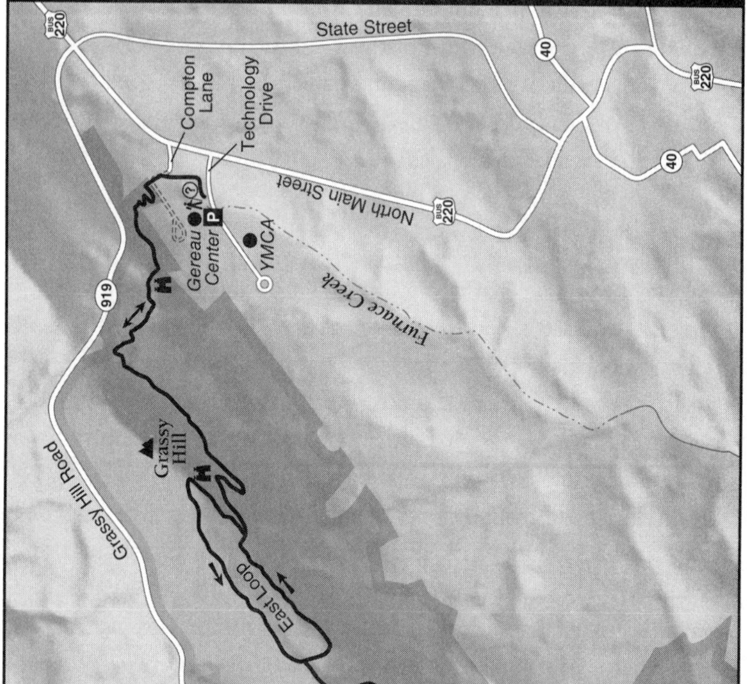

After parking at either The Gereau Center or the YMCA, walk back toward US 220 Business, then look for the kiosk on the woods' edge. Join a gravel doubletrack heading through woods to soon reach Compton Street. Head left here and walk the road for a moment, then pick up actual hiking trail entering woods and the preserve proper at 0.2 mile. The reason for this unusual beginning is to accommodate adequate trail parking.

Once in the preserve, the path switchbacks uphill in oak woods along the dry, rocky south slope of the mountain. Curve around a rib ridge, then come to a stone overlook at 0.4 mile. Here, you can look down into the Pigg River Valley and beyond. Ahead, hop over a little spring branch, the only perennial water along the hike. At 0.7 mile, head west, joining an old access road. The proper trail is marked as you cruise a nearly level track in oaks, pocked with reddish ore.

At 1.4 miles, after a pair of switchbacks, reach a trail intersection. Turn right onto the East Loop Trail and crest Grassy Hill. Easy walking lies ahead. Take the short spur right to another overlook at 1.6 miles. This is the premier vista on Grassy Hill. Here, you can gaze southeast down to the town of Rocky Mount, viewing the individual buildings with clarity, and onward to the declining hills of the Virginia Piedmont.

The East Loop continues northeast just a short distance beyond the view, then curves southwest, along the other side of Grassy Hill. Gain

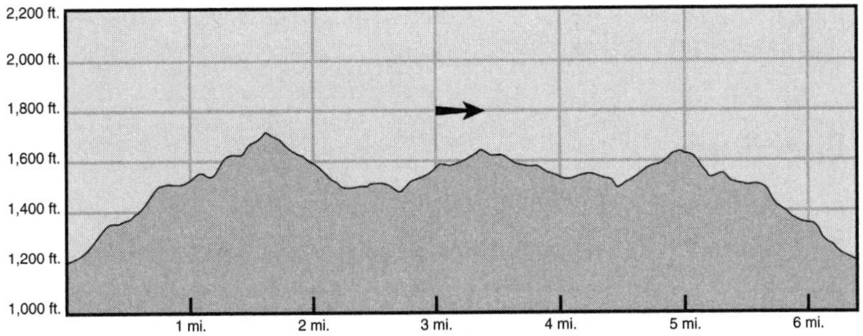

winter views through the trees of the Blackwater River Valley below. At 2.2 miles, come to the Connector Trail. Keep southwest, dropping to a doubletrack access road; then meet the West Loop Trail. Keep straight on the access road, then quickly veer right, back on singletrack path. The West Loop Trail continues southwest on a nearly level grade, rolling among hardwoods. Pass under a power line at 2.6 miles. Cross wet-weather drainages flowing off the hill.

Rise to the ridgecrest at 3.3 miles. Here, the West Loop Trail turns east and joins a doubletrack path. Ramble atop Grassy Hill, traversing areas managed by fire. See if you can tell the difference in the woods here versus elsewhere in the preserve. Pass larger oaks with widespread limbs, indicating a once grassier forest floor. At 3.8 miles, a spur leads right to the West Loop overlook. This one is more limited but still presents views down to Rocky Mount.

At 4 miles, pass back under the power line. After returning to woods, the West Loop splits from the doubletrack then rejoins it before returning to the Connector Trail at 4.5 miles. Backtrack on the Connector Trail, then split right on the East Loop, enjoying new pathway. Curve around to the southeast slope of Grassy Hill, making a stony but easy forest walk to complete the East Loop at 5.1 miles. Backtrack from here, reaching the trailhead at 6.5 miles.

Nearby Attractions

Waid Park (see next hike), a Franklin County preserve on the Pigg River, has several trails worth exploring.

Directions

From Roanoke, take US 220 South to Rocky Mount. Leave US 220 at US 220 Business upon reaching Rocky Mount. Drive south on US 220 Business 0.5 mile, then turn right on Technology Drive. The trail starts on the right shortly before reaching The Gereau Center on the right. Parking is available at The Gereau Center outside school hours or at the Franklin County YMCA, beyond The Gereau Center on the left.

38 Waid Park

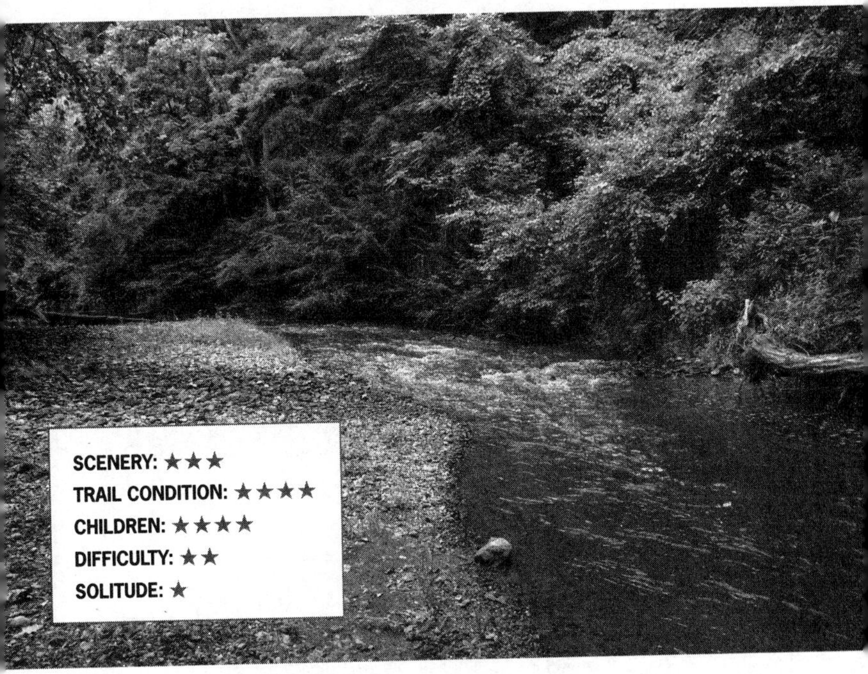

VIEW OF THE PIGG RIVER FROM A TRAILSIDE GRAVEL BAR

GPS TRAILHEAD COORDINATES: N36° 58.290' W79° 56.359'

DISTANCE & CONFIGURATION: 4.7-mile loop

HIKING TIME: 2.5 hours

OUTSTANDING FEATURES: Pigg River, Falling Run waterfall, multiple environments and route possibilities

ELEVATION: 1,140 feet at trailhead, 1,260 feet at high point, 1,050 feet at low point

ACCESS: No fees or permits required

MAPS: Waid Park Recreation Area Trail Map, USGS *Rocky Mount*

FACILITIES: Restrooms, picnic shelter, water, baseball fields

WHEELCHAIR ACCESS: First 0.5 mile of trail

INFO: Waid Park, 701 Waid Park Road, Rocky Mount, VA 24151; 540-483-3030, franklincounty.gov

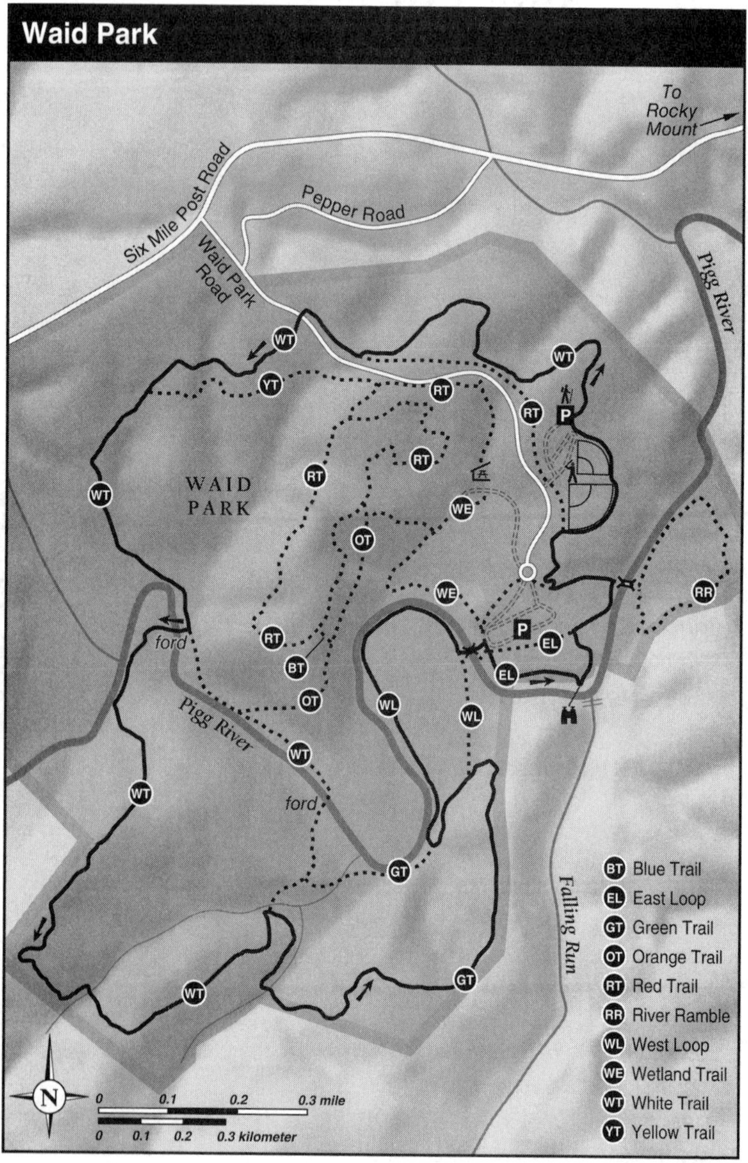
Waid Park
To Rocky Mount
Six Mile Post Road
Pepper Road
Waid Park Road
Pigg River
WAID PARK
ford
Pigg River
ford
Falling Run
WT
YT
RT
OT
BT
WE
EL
RR
WL
GT
P
0
0.1
0.2
0.3 mile
0
0.1
0.2
0.3 kilometer
N
BT Blue Trail
EL East Loop
GT Green Trail
OT Orange Trail
RT Red Trail
RR River Ramble
WL West Loop
WE Wetland Trail
WT White Trail
YT Yellow Trail

In Brief

Make a 4-plus-mile loop at this Franklin County Park near Rocky Mount. A network of trails leads throughout the preserve. Leave the primary trailhead, going on and off historic roads to ford the Pigg River. Circle through hills and hollows, returning to the Pigg a second time, where you hike along the waterway, stopping to watch Falling Run create a waterfall as it meets the Pigg.

Route Details

Waid Park is combination recreation and nature destination. Situated on a part of the Pigg River Valley, the park is named for a family that had settled here by 1750, at the ford on the Pigg where the Old Carolina Road crossed. The Waidses' stagecoach stop formed the basis of a family home and business. The family hung on until the coming railroad rendered stagecoach travel obsolete. Some Waid lands were sold to satisfy debts, but Waid descendants hung on to the heart of the tract until 1993, when the final heir sold what became Waid Park to Franklin County.

Over time, the park was developed into what we see today. Facilities such as picnic areas, trails, parking lots, baseball fields, and bridges were integrated into the natural lay of the land. Historical elements,

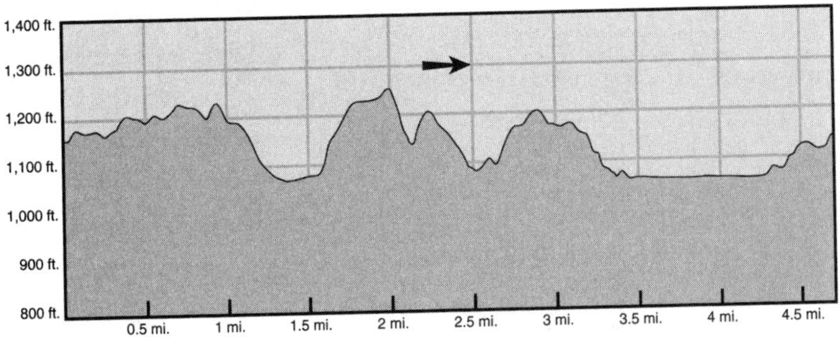

including long-cultivated fields, the Old Carolina Road, Old Floyd Pike, and even a relic barn, remain from the Waid family era.

Start at the signed official trailhead parking area, just above the baseball fields. Take the pea gravel, all-access White Trail. This wide path immediately enters woods of pine, sourwood, and oaks aplenty. Cruise gentle hills on a path level enough for a wheelchair hiker. By the way, elevation changes throughout the hike amount to just over 200 feet. At 0.6 mile, the White Trail meets the Red Trail, and this ends the White Trail's all-access status. Follow a grass-and-dirt track, part of the Old Carolina Road formerly linking the Carolinas to Philadelphia, to cross alive-and-well Waid Park Road at 0.7 mile. Wander through pine–oak woods to join Old Floyd Turnpike at 0.9 mile. This is a wider track, a "newer" historic road gone to seed. Soon meet the Yellow Trail. Keep straight on the White Trail.

At 1.1 miles, at a cornfield, Old Floyd Turnpike goes straight, but the White Trail heads left and descends a doubletrack to reach the Pigg River and a trail intersection at 1.3 miles. Here, the White Trail splits right to ford the Pigg River at a shallow shoal, and goes straight. Take off your shoes and go right with the ford. Walk a wet-weather stream braid, then rise to rejoin trail astride a field. The White Trail soon leaves the field, then climbs a hill in black gum/pine woods. Circle the "back 40" of the park, dropping to step over a fern-bordered tributary of the Pigg at 2.1 miles. Climb from the tributary among straight-trunked tulip trees, and open to an active agricultural field. Interestingly, parts of Waid Park are being leased for farming, offsetting park expenses. The signed path leaves left, traveling the margin between field and woods. Look for a huge old barn to the right of the path. Drop to find the Green Trail at 2.5 miles. Head right on the Green Trail, circling back around the barn. Cross yet another tributary of the Pigg at 2.6 miles. Climb again to pick up another portion of the Old Carolina Road.

Continue circling the perimeter of the park. Meet the pea gravel, all-access West Loop Trail at 3.3 miles. Follow the loop left as it circles past an arm of the Green Trail, then comes alongside the Pigg River.

Hike along the walnut-bordered Pigg with grassy fields to your right. Watch for accesses to the seasonal trout stream used by anglers and other water lovers. Follow a sharp bend, then reach the pedestrian bridge over the Pigg at 3.6 miles. Bridge the Pigg, then quickly head right on the East Loop, passing the Pigg River paddler access.

Keep along the river, reaching the Falling Run waterfall overlook at 4.1 miles. Here, you can observe Falling Run falling 15 feet in stony stages into a big pool of the Pigg River. At 4.2 miles, stay right, crossing a small bridge over a drainage; then come to another bridge over the Pigg River and the Wetland Trail at 4.3 miles. The Wetland Trail, a loop, offers an additional 0.3 mile of path. Otherwise, bypass the Wetland Trail, then find a winding uphill path at 4.4 miles. It leads right, up to the baseball fields, which you circle around before returning to the trailhead, completing the hike at 4.7 miles.

Nearby Attractions

Grassy Hill Natural Area Preserve offers more than 6 miles of hiking trails through hickory–oak habitat and features three vistas. A 6.5-mile circuit hike at Grassy Hill is detailed in this guide (see Hike 37, page 224).

Directions

From Roanoke, take US 220 South to Rocky Mount. Leave US 220 at US 220 Business upon reaching Rocky Mount. Drive south on US 220 Business/Main Street for 1.6 miles to turn right at a traffic light onto Franklin Street/VA 40 West. Follow Franklin Street/VA 40 West through downtown Rocky Mount and continue 2.4 miles to a traffic light. Turn right on Six Mile Post Road/VA 640. Follow Six Mile Post Road 1.8 miles, then turn left onto Waid Park Road. Follow the road through the park 0.6 mile, then turn left into the trailhead parking area.

39 Smart View

SCENERY: ★★★★
TRAIL CONDITION: ★★★★★
CHILDREN: ★★★★
DIFFICULTY: ★★
SOLITUDE: ★★★

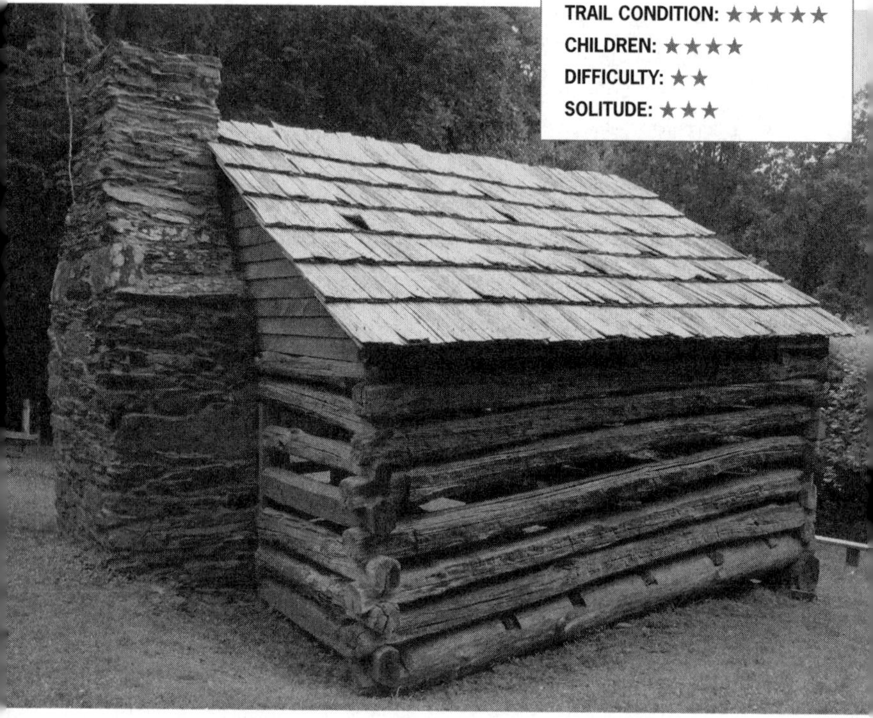

THE TRAIL CABIN HELPS INTERPRET BYGONE LIFEWAYS ALONG THE BLUE RIDGE PARKWAY.

GPS TRAILHEAD COORDINATES: N36° 55.688' W80° 11.227'

DISTANCE & CONFIGURATION: 3.0-mile loop

HIKING TIME: 1.5 hours

OUTSTANDING FEATURES: Views, historic cabin, meadows, trailside picnic area

ELEVATION: 2,500 feet at trailhead, 2,410 feet at low point, 2,630 feet at high point

ACCESS: No fees or permits required

MAPS: Blue Ridge Parkway–Smart View, USGS *Endicott*

FACILITIES: Picnic shelter, picnic area, restrooms near trailhead

WHEELCHAIR ACCESS: None

INFO: Blue Ridge Parkway, 199 Hemphill Knob Road, Asheville, NC 28803; 828-298-0398, nps.gov/blri

In Brief

This is a moderate hike with ample rewards. Situated on the Blue Ridge Parkway, the Smart View Picnic Area features a loop that starts at a historic cabin, then visits a creek. After that, you wander through woods and fields, culminating in a far-reaching view of the Piedmont before returning to the trailhead.

Route Details

This is the type of hike on which you take your willing but out-of-shape and woods-wary cousin. It isn't too difficult, with elevation changes of just over a couple of hundred feet. It offers human history at the Trail Cabin. And hikers can enjoy a "Smart View" of the Piedmont in the distance along the way. Furthermore, the well-marked and -maintained trail network starts at a picnic area with a shelter, water, and restrooms, so your citified cousin won't feel too disconnected from civilization. Hikers can cut the loop short if need be, in case your cousin decides there are just too many icky spiders in the woods. And a ride on the Blue Ridge Parkway will warm your cousin up to the idea of reconnecting with the nature of Western Virginia.

After parking, walk down to examine the hand-hewn log cabin built by W. J. Trail in the 1880s. The cabin has almost no windows. The chinking in between the logs is now missing. Note the sizable stone chimney, built to render a roaring fire to ward off the chill of mountaintop winter nights in the Appalachians. The original floor has been removed, and the wood shingle roof has been replaced numerous times, as the cabin was one of the first structures targeted for preservation along the fledgling Blue Ridge Parkway.

Leave left from the Trail Cabin on the Smart View Loop Trail, making a counterclockwise loop. You are circling around the Smart View Picnic Area in oak woods. It isn't long before you reach the first of several short paths connecting the Smart View Loop Trail to the picnic area. Keep northbound. The slope of the Blue Ridge drops sharply to your right, yet the trail remains mostly level. At 0.3 mile,

Smart View

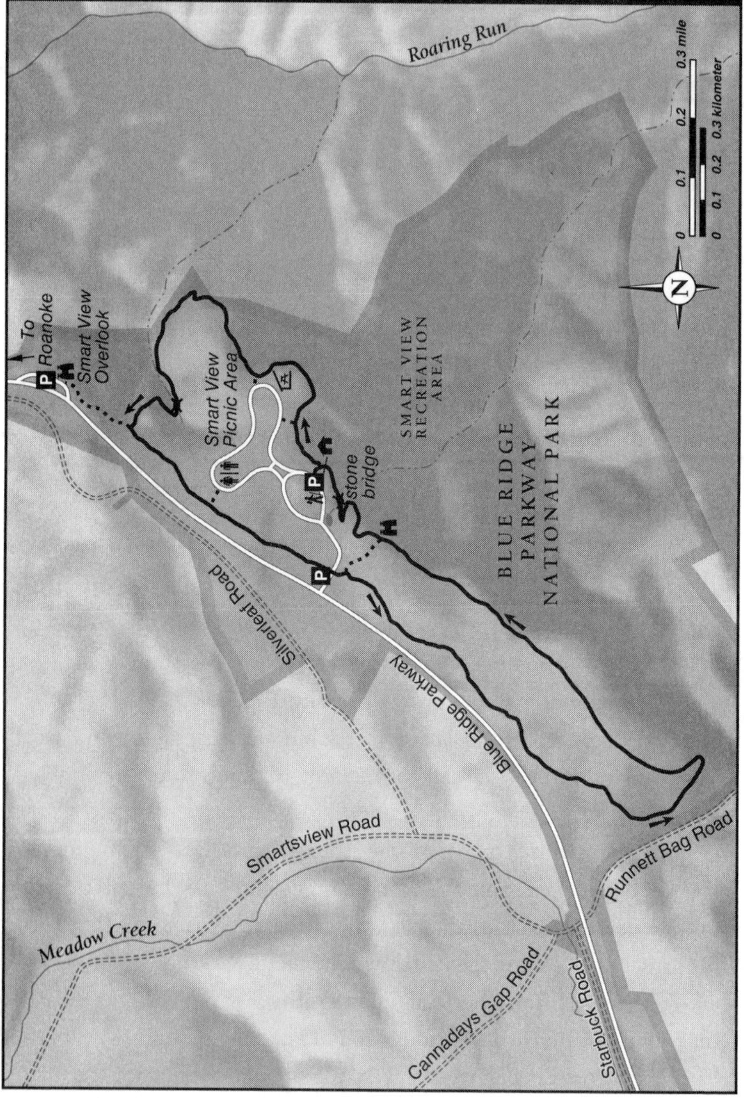
Roaring Run
To Roanoke
Smart View Overlook
Smart View Picnic Area
stone bridge
SMART VIEW RECREATION AREA
BLUE RIDGE PARKWAY NATIONAL PARK
Silverleaf Road
Blue Ridge Parkway
Smartsview Road
Meadow Creek
Runnett Bag Road
Cannadays Gap Road
Starbuck Road
0 0.1 0.2 0.3 mile
0 0.1 0.2 0.3 kilometer
N

meet an asphalt segment of pathway linking to the picnic area very near the picnic shelter. The asphalt trail segment is short and you are soon back on natural-surface track. Pass by yet another connector to the picnic area at 0.4 mile.

Turn away from the picnic area, descending in switchbacks. Straight-trunked tulip trees are prevalent down in the hollow you are entering. Wildflowers such as dwarf crested iris rise colorful here in spring. Come alongside a trickling branch. Smaller springs flow across the path, adding water to the main branch. Rhododendron and ferns reflect the increased moisture content of this valley. Span the clear, gurgling stream, a nameless tributary of Roaring Run, at 0.7 mile.

You are on the right bank of the creek, heading upstream. At 0.8 mile, come to a trail intersection. Here, a path leads right a short piece to the Smart View Overlook and the parkway. Our hike heads left, southbound, and parallels the parkway in broken woods, running alongside an old fence line. Imagine the picnic area being a pasture, or a field of row crops where corn was grown by W. J. Trail. At 1.0 mile, another connector leads left to the picnic area, not far from the restrooms.

At 1.1 miles, open onto a relic field. This grassland would have been reclaimed by encroaching forest, but the park service keeps it mowed to increase habitat for songbirds and other wildlife. Leave

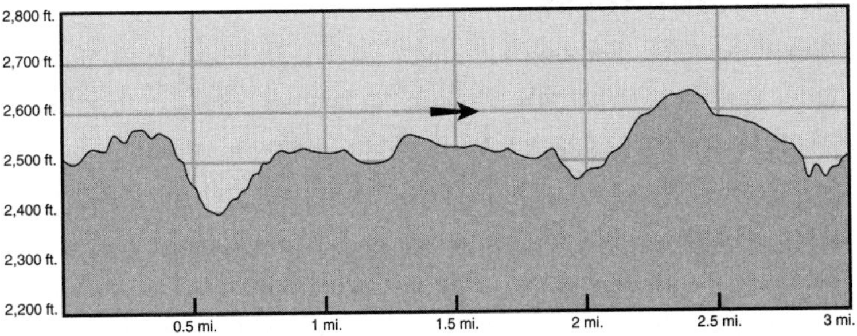

the field, crossing the picnic area entrance road at 1.2 miles. Walk through a stile to quickly meet the loop shortcut. We're going the longer route, so keep right, still heading south under rolling woods of oak and pine. The hiking is very easy as it meanders along gentle slopes parallel to the Blue Ridge Parkway. The large oaks you see were likely here before the parkway, shading adjacent pastures. Now, occasional benches overlook the risen forest.

The path is heading toward Cannaday Gap on the Blue Ridge, but limited publicly held parkland forces the trail to slowly turn back north before reaching the gap. At 2.1 miles, climb a bit to a knob, reaching the high point of the hike at 2.5 miles. Now, the land drops off precipitously to your right, easterly, setting up the view ahead. At 2.8 miles, come to the loop shortcut and, more important, a cleared view to the east, a panorama stretching to the Piedmont and the Smith River Valley below—a "right smart view," as goes the saying that gave the area its name.

From here, the loop nears the picnic area, passing a spur trail leading left to a pond, then drops to cross a trickling branch emanating from the pond using an interestingly constructed rock slab bridge. From here, it is a short distance before you emerge at the historic Trail Cabin, completing the moderate yet rewarding adventure, which your cousin will likely like.

Nearby Attractions

Rocky Knob Recreation Area is located a dozen miles south on the Blue Ridge Parkway. It has trails of varying difficulties, a visitor center, a picnic area, and a campground that's open in season.

Directions

From Roanoke, take the Blue Ridge Parkway south 34 miles to milepost 154.5. Enter the Smart View Picnic Area and follow the loop road a short distance to start your hike at the Trail Cabin on the right. There is alternative parking at the picnic area entrance.

40 Rock Castle Gorge

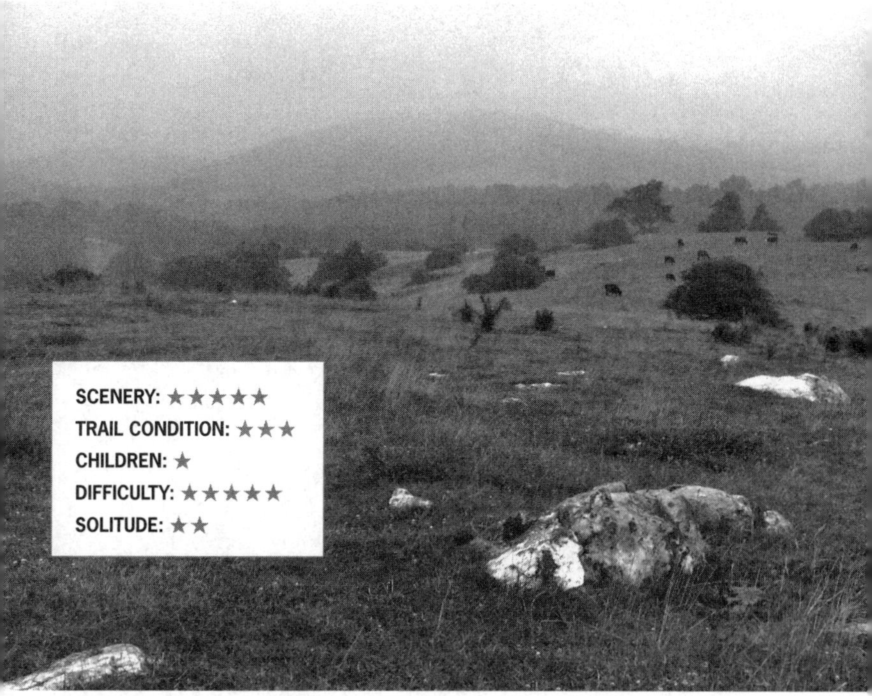

SCENERY: ★★★★★
TRAIL CONDITION: ★★★
CHILDREN: ★
DIFFICULTY: ★★★★★
SOLITUDE: ★★

THE HIGHLANDS ABOVE ROCK CASTLE GORGE

GPS TRAILHEAD COORDINATES: N36° 48.597' W80° 21.005'

DISTANCE & CONFIGURATION: 10.7-mile loop

HIKING TIME: 6.5 hours

OUTSTANDING FEATURES: Views, rugged gorge, human history, falls, geology

ELEVATION: 3,210 feet at trailhead, 1,720 feet at low point, 3,560 feet at high point

ACCESS: Permit required for overnight backpacking

MAPS: Blue Ridge Parkway–Rocky Knob Trail, USGS *Woolwine*

FACILITIES: Backcountry campsite on trail, picnic area, campground near trailhead

WHEELCHAIR ACCESS: None

INFO: Blue Ridge Parkway, 199 Hemphill Knob Road, Asheville, NC 28803; 828-298-0398, nps.gov/blri

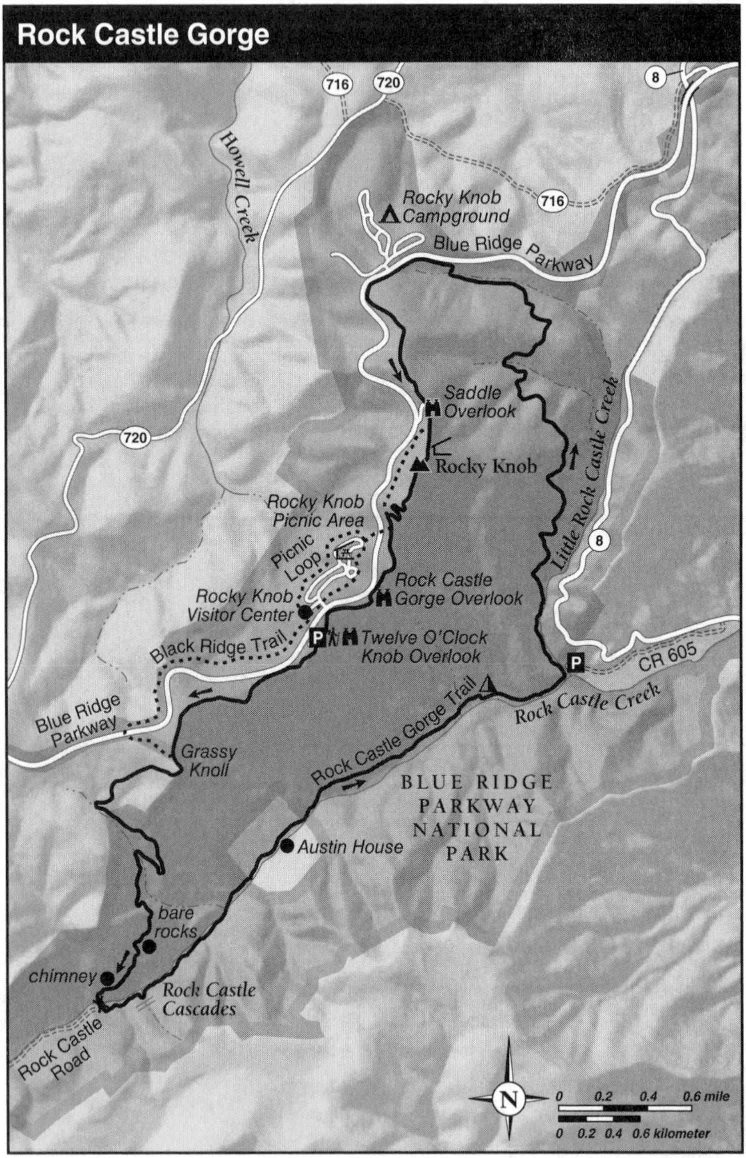
Rock Castle Gorge
716
720
8
Howell Creek
Rocky Knob Campground
716
Blue Ridge Parkway
Saddle Overlook
Rocky Knob
Little Rock Castle Creek
720
Rocky Knob Picnic Area
Picnic Loop
8
Rock Castle Gorge Overlook
Rocky Knob Visitor Center
Twelve O'Clock Knob Overlook
Black Ridge Trail
CR 605
Rock Castle Gorge Trail
Rock Castle Creek
Blue Ridge Parkway
Grassy Knoll
BLUE RIDGE PARKWAY NATIONAL PARK
Austin House
bare rocks
chimney
Rock Castle Cascades
Rock Castle Road
N
0 0.2 0.4 0.6 mile
0 0.2 0.4 0.6 kilometer

In Brief

This long loop has it all—widespread panoramas, human history, waterfalls, wildflowers, geological wonders, and trail challenges galore. Make a circuit over highland meadows, down the gorge of Rock Castle Creek, then up a steep track, past pioneer homesites, to the crest of the Blue Ridge and Rocky Knob, where more highland vistas put an exclamation point on this both rewarding and demanding federally designated National Recreation Trail.

Route Details

This trek is a classic that should be on every Old Dominion hiker's checklist. It can be done as a long day hike. However, a primitive campsite is situated about halfway along the trek; a permit is required.

The Twelve O'Clock Knob Overlook on the Blue Ridge Parkway features a map of the Rock Castle Gorge Trail and is your starting point. Leave the asphalt parking area, walking south down the grassy clearing to join the Rock Castle Gorge Trail. Turn right, southbound, doing the loop counterclockwise.

Quickly enter woods, passing a spur going right back to the parking area. Stay with the well-maintained singletrack path. The Rock Castle Gorge drops sharply to your left. Cruise locust, maple, hickory, and

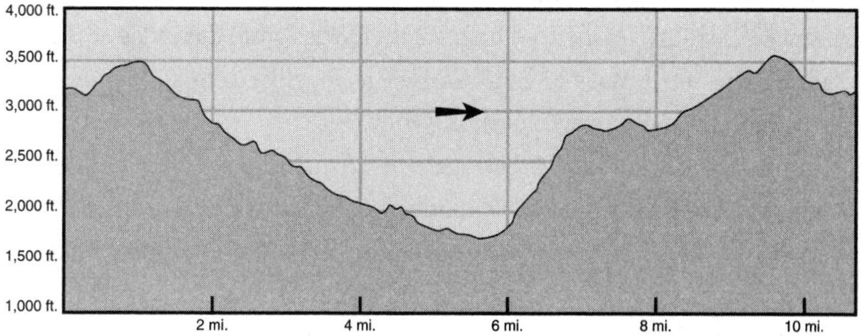

oak woods. At 0.5 mile, cross a stile, entering grazing land, with big-time views north, where ranks of mountains meld into the distance. Wander over truly grassy Grassy Knoll, where more Virginia country-side rolls away to infinity. At 0.9 mile, the Black Ridge Trail leaves right. Keep straight, and the Rock Castle Gorge Trail reenters woods after passing through a stile, then curves near a communication tower to surmount another stile. Descend to open onto a meadow at 1.2 miles and begin a near-constant, 4-plus-mile downgrade. Reenter woods and find a tributary of Rock Castle Creek at 1.4 miles. The rhododendron-choked feeder crashes down a cleft of its own making. Trace the stream, then temporarily split away, switchbacking to rock-hop the stream just above a 40-foot-high, 100-foot-long sloped cascade at 2.1 miles.

Leave this tributary, then continue angling toward Rock Castle Creek, crossing smaller streams divided by rocky slopes. Navigate a boulder jumble known as the Bare Rocks at 2.5 miles. The going is slow. Out of nowhere, come to an old chimney at 2.8 miles. At one time, more than 30 families lived in the Rock Castle Creek valley, doing subsistence farming. It is hard to believe there were ever clearings and homes considering how finely the native trees, ferns, and wildflowers have reclaimed the hillsides.

Bridge Rock Castle Creek at 2.9 miles as it crashes in rapids and pools as you might expect. Just ahead, intersect the Rock Castle Fire Road, open only to official personnel. Head left, and trace the primitive doubletrack down the Rock Castle Gorge, where everywhere-you-look beauty is evidenced by reaching Rock Castle Cascades at 3.1 miles. Here, a tributary of Rock Castle Creek spills 70 or so feet over an irregular rock spillway, splashing your feet.

Bridge Rock Castle Creek again at 3.7 miles and 3.8 miles. The gorge widens. Wooded flats, old roadbeds, and rock piles indicate past habitation. At 4.0 miles, pass the privately held Austin House. Built in 1916, the white, two-story clapboard structure was considered the finest in the valley. Walnut trees abound here. Bridge Rock Castle at 4.3 miles. Hardwoods abound in the wider bottomland. Look for evidence of homesites, such as nonnative planted yuccas.

At 5.2 miles reach the primitive camping area where a Civilian Conservation Corps camp once stood. You can still see the stone slab foundations of the buildings. It is now a campsite with multiple fire rings and bear-proof food-storage boxes. Rock Castle Creek gurgles nearby. At 5.6 miles, the Rock Castle Gorge Trail splits left as a singletrack path, heading up the Little Rock Castle Creek valley. The fire road keeps straight a short distance farther to reach alternative parking off VA 605.

Head up the valley. At 5.9 miles, the trail steepens and you wind up rocky terrain. Gain 1,000 feet in the next 1.2 miles, much of it on irregular, steep slope on a singletrack path. The going is slow and tough. Resume a moderate, rising path that joins a settler road. Bridge a stream at 7.3 miles, then curve right past the remains of a settler's home, including a crumbled fireplace, stone piles, and ancient cedars. As you surmount a minor gap, look for large trees astride the former road.

At 7.6 miles, curve sharply left, west, and turn up yet another valley rife with the cool-climate specialist yellow birch. Cross what is left of this stream at 8.2 miles. Pass over a stile, then enter grazed lands, mostly grassy but pocked with old gnarled oaks—and blackberries in season. At 8.5 miles, a spur leads right a short distance to Rocky Knob Campground. The Rock Castle Gorge Trail then meanders through view-rich meadows near the Blue Ridge Parkway. In Florida, they swim with the dolphins; here in Virginia we hike with the cattle. Watch your feet. Look for wooden posts marking the trail as you ascend a knob then enter woods at 9.0 miles, after passing through a small corral and stile.

Quickly reach Saddle Overlook on the parkway at 9.1 miles. Walk along the parking area to enter woods yet again. Reach a trail split at 9.2 miles. Head left, uphill, toward Rocky Knob. The other way curves through wooded hillside, bypassing the knob. Instead, climb through forest to reach a former Appalachian Trail shelter at 9.4 miles. This part of the path was once the AT. The shelter stands on the precipice of Rocky Knob, overlooking the gorge below. The easterly panoramas extend beyond the gorge onward through the Piedmont. Keep south on the knife edge of Rocky Knob, eventually descending to meet the bypass at 9.8 miles.

At 9.9 miles, a spur leads right to Rocky Knob Picnic Area. Stay straight on the Rock Castle Gorge Trail, straddling the gorge edge. The drop-off below is a doozy. Emerge at the Rock Castle Gorge Overlook and the parkway at 10.2 miles. Auto tourists looking out have little idea of the depth and ruggedness of the gorge.

Resume the trail in woods. At 10.5 miles, a spur goes right to the Rocky Knob visitor center. Keep straight and shortly emerge at the Twelve O'Clock Knob Overlook, completing the challenging hike at 10.7 miles.

Nearby Attractions

Rocky Knob Recreation Area on the Blue Ridge Parkway has not only this hike but also other trails of varying difficulty, a visitor center, a picnic area, and a campground open in season.

Directions

From Roanoke, take US 221 South to Floyd, then take VA 8 South 6 miles to the Blue Ridge Parkway and milepost 165.3. From there, take the parkway southbound to milepost 169.1 and the Twelve O'Clock Knob Overlook, on the left, just past the Rocky Knob Picnic Area and Visitor Center.

Appendix A: Area Outdoor Retailers

BACKCOUNTRY SKI & SPORT
bcski.com
3710 S. Main St.
Blacksburg, VA 24060
540-552-6400

1931 Apperson Drive
Salem, VA 24153
540-389-8602

BLUE RIDGE MOUNTAIN SPORTS
brms.com
1560 S. Main St., Suite 100
Blacksburg, VA 24060
540-953-7060

DICK'S SPORTING GOODS
dickssportinggoods.com
100 New River Road
Christiansburg, VA 24073
540-381-0102

GANDER MOUNTAIN
gandermountain.com
8195 Gander Way
Roanoke, VA 24019
540-362-3658

OUTDOOR TRAILS
outdoortrails.com
28 Kingston Drive
Daleville, VA 24083
540-992-5850

SPORTSMAN'S WAREHOUSE
sportsmanswarehouse.com
3550 Ferncliff Ave. NW
Roanoke, VA 24017
540-366-9700

WALKABOUT OUTFITTER
walkaboutoutfitter.com
301 Market St.
Roanoke, VA 24011
540-777-2727

4822-J Valley View Blvd. NW
Roanoke, VA 24012
540-777-0990

Appendix B: Hiking Clubs

ROANOKE APPALACHIAN TRAIL CLUB

ratc.org
PO Box 12282
Roanoke, VA 24024

ROANOKE OUTDOOR & SOCIAL CLUB

meetup.com/roanoke-outdoor-club

OUTDOOR CLUB AT VIRGINIA TECH

www.outdoor.org.vt.edu

YMCA AT VIRGINIA TECH

vtymca.org
1000 N. Main St.
Blacksburg, VA 24060
540-961-9622

Index

G

H

V *(continued)*

W

Y

Z

About the Author

Photo: Keri Anne Molloy

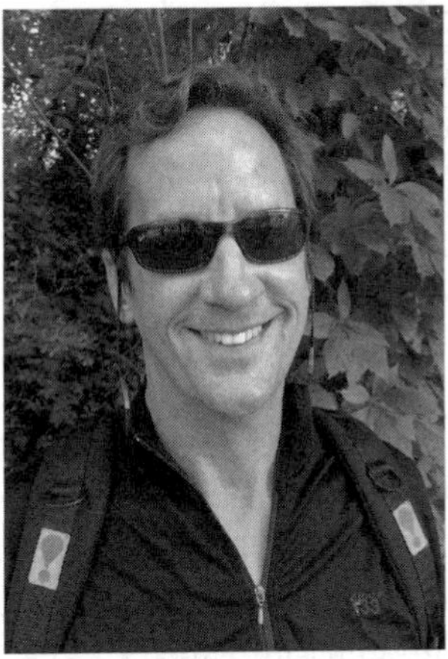

JOHNNY MOLLOY is a writer and adventurer based in Johnson City, Tennessee. His passion for the outdoors was ignited on a backpacking trip in Great Smoky Mountains National Park while he was a student at the University of Tennessee. That first foray unleashed a love of the outdoors that led this native Tennessean to spend more than 3,500 nights backpacking, canoe camping, and tent camping over the past three decades.

Friends enjoyed his outdoor-adventure stories; one even suggested that he write a book. Johnny pursued his friend's idea and soon parlayed his love of the outdoors into an occupation. His efforts have resulted in more than 60 books and guides, including hiking guidebooks, camping guidebooks, paddling guidebooks, comprehensive guidebooks about specific areas, and books about true outdoor adventure throughout the eastern United States—including several guides about Virginia's outdoors.

Though he's primarily involved with books, Johnny writes for various magazines and websites and is a columnist and feature writer for his local paper, the *Johnson City Press*. He continues writing and traveling extensively throughout the United States, endeavoring in a variety of outdoor pursuits.

A Christian, Johnny is an active member of First Presbyterian Church in Johnson City, Tennessee. His wife, Keri Anne, accompanies him on the trail. Johnny's nonoutdoor interests include reading, American history, and University of Tennessee sports. For the latest on Johnny, please visit johnnymolloy.com.

DEAR CUSTOMERS AND FRIENDS,

SUPPORTING YOUR INTEREST IN OUTDOOR ADVENTURE, travel, and an active lifestyle is central to our operations, from the authors we choose to the locations we detail to the way we design our books. Menasha Ridge Press was incorporated in 1982 by a group of veteran outdoorsmen and professional outfitters. For many years now, we've specialized in creating books that benefit the outdoors enthusiast.

Almost immediately, Menasha Ridge Press earned a reputation for revolutionizing outdoors- and travel-guidebook publishing. For such activities as canoeing, kayaking, hiking, backpacking, and mountain biking, we established new standards of quality that transformed the whole genre, resulting in outdoor-recreation guides of great sophistication and solid content. Menasha Ridge Press continues to be outdoor publishing's greatest innovator.

The folks at Menasha Ridge Press are as at home on a whitewater river or mountain trail as they are editing a manuscript. The books we build for you are the best they can be, because we're responding to your needs. Plus, we use and depend on them ourselves.

We look forward to seeing you on the river or the trail. If you'd like to contact us directly, visit us at menasharidge.com. We thank you for your interest in our books and the natural world around us all.

SAFE TRAVELS,

BOB SEHLINGER
PUBLISHER